Memory: Interdisciplinary Approaches

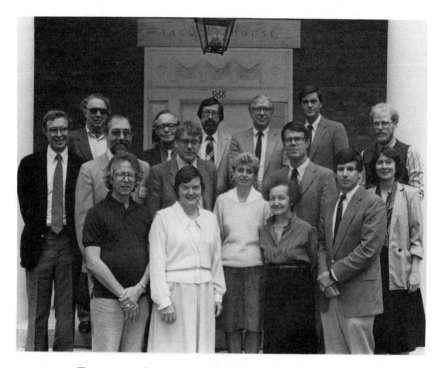

Front row (l–r): Robert Wyer, Katherine Nelson,
Carolyn Rovee–Collier, Brenda Milner, Paul Solomon
Middle row: George Goethals, Thomas Ostrom, Alan Baddeley,
Robert Kail, Colleen Kelley
Back Row: George Mandler, Ulric Neisser, Richard Thompson,
James McGaugh, David Hamilton, Benjamin Stephens

Paul R. Soloman   George R. Goethals
Colleen M. Kelley   Benjamin R. Stephens
Editors

Memory:
Interdisciplinary
Approaches

With 31 Illustrations

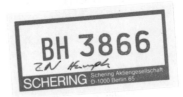

Springer-Verlag
New York Berlin Heidelberg
London Paris Tokyo

Paul R. Solomon
George R. Goethals
Colleen M. Kelley
Department of Psychology
Williams College
Williamstown, MA 02167, USA

Benjamin R. Stephens
Department of Psychology
Clemson University
Clemson, SC 29631, USA

Library of Congress Cataloging-in-Publication Data
Memory: interdisciplinary approaches.
  Bibliography: p.
  Includes indexes.
  1. Memory—Physiological aspects.   2. Memory.
I. Solomon, Paul R.
QP406.M455 1988   153.1'2   88-4923

Printed on acid-free paper

Typeset by TCSystems, Inc., Shippensburg, Pennsylvania.
Printed and bound by R.R. Donnelley & Sons, Harrisonburg, Virginia.
Printed in the United States of America.

9 8 7 6 5 4 3 2 1

ISBN 0-387-96724-9 Springer-Verlag New York Berlin Heidelberg
ISBN 3-540-96724-9 Springer-Verlag Berlin Heidelberg New York

G. Stanley Hall

received his bachelor's degree from Williams College in 1867. To commemorate his contribution to the discipline, the Psychology Department at Williams has instituted a series of symposia. In the tradition of Hall, these symposia will focus on the potential integration of varying approaches to enduring psychological issues. The goal is to demonstrate how psychologists approach similar problems from varying perspectives.

Preface

G. Stanley Hall received his bachelor's degree from Williams College in 1867. Prepared at the Williston Seminary in Easthampton, Hall entered Williams College in 1863, having walked most of the distance from Ashfield to Williamstown. The student–teacher relationship at the college was intimate and personal. Of his 12 instructors, Professor Bascom influenced him the most. Bascom held the college's chair in rhetoric, but was far more interested in philosophy and political economics, and passed along these interests to his student. In Hall's time, board at the college ranged from $1.75 to $3.00 per week, and tuition was $45.00 for the year.

Hall had little interest in athletics, except for baseball, but he failed to make the team. His other extracurricular interests were wide. He sang bass in the Williams Amateur Serenaders. He took part in the Mills Theological Society, the Lyceum of Natural History, the Williams Art Association, and the Kieseritzky Chess Club, and was editor of the Williams Quarterly. He was elected to Phi Beta Kappa in his senior year.

During his years at Williams, Hall was described as a good conversationalist with a warm regard for his friends, but a morbid bashfulness with regard to women—an attitude that changed little in later years (Straker, 1934).

To commemorate Hall' contribution to the discipline, the Psychology Department at Williams College decided to institute a series of symposia. The first conference was held at Williams College on October 2–5, 1986. In the tradition of Hall, this meeting focused on the potential integration of varying approaches to enduring psychological issues. The goal was to demonstrate how psychologists approach similar problems from differing perspectives.

The topic of the first symposium was memory. To discuss this issue, we invited behavioral neuroscientists, developmental psychologists, cognitive psychologists, and social psychologists, each with an interest in memory. Our goals for the conference include asking the participants to indicate (1) how research in their subspecialty approaches the problem of memory, (2) what they consider to be the critical questions in the study of memory, and (3) what information provided by people working in other subspecialties would be most helpful to their work.

During the course of the conference we attempted to keep a balance between formal presentations and informal discussions. As such, each participant gave a presentation of his work, which was followed by a period for questions and discussion. At the end of each day, we scheduled a "Round Table Discussion" featuring the presenters of that day and moderated by two of the conference organizers. Abstracts of many of the presentations and the full texts of some were circulated in advance of the meeting. The chapters in this volume are based on the presentations, revised to reflect the discussion as well as subsequent editorial review.

Although participants in this conference came with widely divergent views on the nature of memory and how and why it should be studied, the 3 days of meetings provided the opportunity to understand and appreciate better both the points of contention and agreement among the various approaches. We hope G. Stanley Hall would have approved.

Even though the conference lasted only 3 days, we depended on many people to help plan and conduct the meeting. We are pleased to offer our thanks to them. We are most grateful to President John Chandler of Williams College for providing the funds to conduct the conference. It was this generous grant that allowed the participants to gather and work. The meetings were held at the Clark Art Institute on the edge of the Williams campus. These surroundings made our work more pleasant and from time to time provided a necessary distraction. We are grateful to John H. Brooks for cheerfully availing this facility. Steven Chick and his staff at the Williams College food service took care of our day-to-day needs. It was their efforts that allowed us to devote our full attention to the business at hand. Several Williams College students served as aides at the conference. Bernadette Gaffney and Julie James often took care of within 10 minutes what had eluded us for 10 months. We are also grateful to Sharon Band for providing some fascinating background material on G. Stanley Hall. Finally, we wish to acknowledge Angie Giusti for handling what seemed like endless correspondence in her usual cheerful manner.

Springer-Verlag agreed early on to publish the proceedings. We are grateful for their encouragement and help.

PAUL R. SOLOMON

Contents

Contributors

BADDELEY, A., MRC Applied Psychology Unit, Cambridge CB2 2EF, England

GOETHALS, G.R., Department of Psychology, Williams College, Williamstown, MA 01267

HAMILTON, D.L., Department of Psychology, University of California, Santa Barbara, CA 93106

KAIL, R.V., Department of Psychological Sciences, Purdue University, West Lafayette, IN 47907

KELLEY, C.M., Department of Psychology, Williams College, Williamstown, MA 01267

McGAUGH, J.L., Center for the Neurobiology of Learning and Memory and Department of Psychobiology, University of California, Irvine, CA 92717

MANDLER, G. Center for Human Information Processing, University of California, La Jolla, CA 92093

NEISSER, U., Department of Psychology, Emory University, Atlanta, GA 30322

NELSON, K., CUNY Graduate School, New York, NY 10036

OSTROM, T.M., Department of Psychology, Ohio State University, Columbus, OH 43210

ROVEE-COLLIER, C., Department of Psychology, Rutgers University, New Brunswick, NJ 08903

SOLOMON, P.R., Department of Psychology, Williams College, Williamstown, MA 01267

STEPHENS, B.R., Department of Psychology, Clemson University, Clemson, SC 29631

THOMPSON, R.F., Department of Psychology, Stanford University, Stanford, CA 94305

WYER, R.S., JR., Department of Psychology, University of Illinois, Champaign, IL 61820

CHAPTER 1

Interdisciplinary Perspectives on the Study of Memory

George R. Goethals and Paul R. Solomon

Why choose memory as the subject of the first G. Stanley Hall Symposium? It strikes us as the obvious choice for several reasons. First, no other phenomenon is as central to human existence and human experience. Not surprisingly, memory occupies a central place in both basic and applied studies of human functioning. Second, it is a topic that figures prominently in each of the subfields of psychology represented at this conference: neuroscience, cognitive psychology, developmental psychology, and social psychology. As such, it is a phenomenon that is highly amenable to interdisciplinary study within the broad field of psychology. In addition, attempting to synthesize the various strands of memory research at the end of the 1980s is timely. The 1880s have been called the "golden decade of memory research" (Squire, 1987). We might argue that the 1980s have also been a golden decade for work on memory. A tremendous amount has been done in a variety of areas. This volume gives us the special opportunity to consider the relationships between some of these lines of research.

What justifies the claim that memory is of first importance in human functioning? Memory is clearly the enabling capacity of human existence. Without memory's capacity to store information in the remarkable quantities we generally take for granted, human behavior, human consciousness, and human identity would bear no relation to their present form. Without memory we couldn't engage in even the simplest and most familiar behaviors—tying our shoes, writing our names, or giving our telephone numbers—not to mention much more complex behaviors, such as preparing our meals, driving our cars, or filing our taxes. Consciousness without reminiscing or ruminating, awareness without last week's knowledge, and thinking without the information of a life history are hard to imagine. Identity without a sense of "enduring sameness and continuity" (Erikson, 1968) is empty. We might argue that none of these human achievements would actually be possible without memory. In short, memory allows us to be fully human. Its centrality in human experience, and the interest it holds for a range of different psychologists, have made it seem natural as the focus of our first G. Stanley Hall symposium.

Investigations Into Memory: A Brief History

Like psychological functioning as a whole, memory is a subject that has been explored for centuries. The Greek philosophers considered the problem of "representation in absence" (Posner & Shulman, 1979). How do people keep in mind or consciousness representations of people, objects, and experiences that are no longer directly present in the person's environment? That is, how is information recalled? The Greek's answer to this question was that some trace of specific experiences with the object or person was in some way stored in the mind. Both Plato and Aristotle recognized that there were difficulties with this "trace theory," but it was debated and pursued until the experimental psychology of the past century enabled scholars to move beyond it. Still, it has not been forgotten, and informs work in several areas of memory research, particularly the neurosciences.

Basic Perspectives on Memory

One of the pioneers of the early experimental studies of memory was Hermann Ebbinghaus. Ebbinghaus conducted studies of his own capacity to remember nonsense syllables during the early 1880s and published his classic *On Memory* in 1885. In this volume, Ebbinghaus charted the decay of memories and postulated two basic and enduring principles: (1) that a great deal of learned material is forgotten very soon after it is originally acquired, and (2) that if the information is remembered for as long as a day or two, it is likely to be retained for a much longer period. Ebbinghaus was influenced by the associationism propounded by English philosophers, including John Locke, who discussed memory and its laws. The basic idea of associationism—that very complex ideas can be built up from extremely simple ones—is still highly influential today, as is evident in several chapters in this volume.

Although Ebbinghaus' work and the basic point of view that it represented continues to occupy a central place in memory research, there have been other quite different approaches to understanding our capacity to store information. Some, like Ebbinghaus', began before the turn of the century. One important departure emphasizing what we think of today as the cognitive approach to memory was articulated by Alfred Binet, who is more well known for his pioneering work on intelligence testing. Binet's early research on children's memory for verbal material (Binet & Henri, 1894) suggested that children remember the basic idea or the underlying message of long passages (Cairns & Ornstein, 1979). In other words, people do not simply passively register experience and recall it by relying on traces of those registrations, but actively construct a representation of experience that attempts to abstract its basic significance in light of what the person's other experience is.

While Binet's work is remarkably compatible with cognitive approaches that emerged in the 1950s, it was largely forgotten due to the strong influence of Ebbinghaus and the dominance of the behavioral viewpoint that marked the first half of the present century. However, Bartlett's classic 1932 book, *Remembering: A Study in Experimental and Social Psychology*, also emphasized the ideas of active organization and the impact of what a person already knows. Bartlett suggested that memory was based on the general impression that results from combining recalled details with the overall schema an individual forms of what has occurred. That schema in turn is affected by a person's general knowledge and the expectations that result from it.

Another approach emerging around the turn of the century has had relatively little impact on experimental psychology, though its importance has been acknowledged by Neisser (1982), one of the contributors to this volume. That is the work of Sigmund Freud. Freud considered the functions of memory and argued that recalled experiences and ideas were related to other symbolically and emotionally important thoughts and feelings. We remember something because it is personally meaningful and significant, though that significance may be hidden. Freud also shared the perspective of Binet and Bartlett in emphasizing the active construction of memory, and, more than they, how such active construction can lead to emotionally significant errors and distortions.

While Binet and Freud were working on the active construction of significant memories, the associationistic approach represented by Ebbinghaus was strengthened in the very early years of the 20th century by Pavlov's work on conditioning and Watson's writings on behaviorism. One of those strongly influenced by Watson was one of his students at Johns Hopkins University, Karl Lashley. Lashley believed that if learning involved the construction of specific connections between behavior and events, and memory the impact of that connection on behavior (the behaviorist perspective), then that connection ought to be stored in a specific location in the cerebral cortex. This idea goes back to the trace theory of the Greeks. Lashley devoted most of his career, which spanned the greater part of the first half of this century, to finding those locations in the brain where memory traces, or engrams, were stored. In 1950 he wrote an important paper signaling the major direction of his life's work, "In search of the engram."

Since Lashley, other physiological psychologists and neuroscientists have explored the physiological basis of learning and memory. In the 1930s and 40s scientists such as Gantt (a student of Pavlov's) and Loucks and Brogden studied the use of electrical brain stimulation as conditioned or unconditioned stimuli (Thompson & Robinson, 1979). Later, researchers explored the electrophysiological, anatomical, and chemical changes involved in long-term and short-term memory.

In short, the history of memory research shows the impact of the same perspectives that have dominated psychology in general, notably the behavioral, cognitive, biological, and psychoanalytic approaches (Crider, Goethals, Kavanaugh, & Solomon, 1986). Although in recent years memory research reflecting these and other perspectives has flourished, the question of integration remains. In the remainder of this chapter we will discuss both areas of divergence and possible areas of convergence as represented in the chapters in this book, and in the field as a whole.

Areas of Divergence

As the chapters in this volume attest, the study of memory spans many of the major areas of psychology. Equally apparent is that memory is treated both conceptually and empirically in different ways by the various subspecialties. What one group considers to be a central problem in the study of memory may be seen as secondary by another. There is even debate about what aspects of behavior and mental processes can be considered memory. Although fundamental areas of divergence such as these may at first glance appear to preclude a volume on interdisciplinary approaches to memory, upon more careful consideration they can provide a useful starting point for considering this important topic.

During the course of this conference, two primary points of divergence concerning fundamental issues in memory emerged. These points are instructive in terms of elucidating issues in the cross-disciplinary study of memory.

What Changes in Behavior and Mental Processes Constitute Memory?

Contemporary research now makes it clear that memory is not a unitary phenomena. This is clearly exemplified by the research demonstrating spared memory abilities in amnestics (e.g., Milner, 1962; Squire, 1987; Weiskrantz, 1985) as well as work demonstrating similar dissociations in normal subjects (e.g., Jacoby & Witherspoon, 1982). As Thompson (Chap. 2) aptly points out, "Memory is a deceptively simple word." But even allowing for different memory systems, both at the cognitive and neurobiological levels, there is still disagreement. To paraphrase Neil Miller (1967) in his discussion of learning, there is considerable debate as to what constitutes "grade A certified memory."

The broad definition of memory argues that any experience that later affects thought and behavior constitutes memory (see Oakley, 1983, Rozin, 1976; Nelson, Chap. 7, this volume). Whether these memories are conscious or unconscious, formed by invertebrates or humans or mediated by language is not crucial. (This is not to imply that important distinctions need not be made as to subtypes of memory.) Psychologists working with animal models (see Chaps. 2 and 3) and those attempting to study memory in young infants (Rovee-Collier, Chap. 8) or in brain-damaged patients necessarily subscribe to this model. This is because these preparations both require and exploit paradigms of relative simplicity.

A second and more narrow conceptualization of memory significantly limits the behaviors and mental processes that constitute memory. Tulving (1983) began his book on episodic memory by stating that, "Remembering past events is a universally familiar experience. It is also a uniquely human one." Although this was a provocative statement that has since been softened (see Tulving, 1984), there is still a tendency to ascribe memory, or at least the more important aspects of it, to humans (see Mandler, Chap. 5; Nelson, Chap. 7). Others (see Thompson, Chap. 2) take exception to this limitation, indicating that memory must evolve in small steps and it seems unlikely that any aspect of memory is uniquely human (see Squire & Zola-Morgan, 1985).

Can the issue of what constitutes memory represent an irreconcilable difference? We think that a resolution is suggested by the work indicating that there are various types of memory, and that these may be represented differently and take on varying degrees of importance in species of varying complexity. Table 1.1 suggests possible divisions of long-term memory (Squire, 1987). Whether any of these ultimately account for the data may not be as important as recognizing that systems such as these can coexist and interact. For example, Mishkin (see Mishkin & Petri, 1984) has made the distinction between memories and habits. This

TABLE 1.1. Divisions of long-term memory

Fact memory	Skill memory
Declarative	Procedural
Memory	Habit
Explicit	Impicit
Knowing that	Knowing how
Cognitive mediation	Semantic
Conscious recollection	Skills
Elaboration	Integration
Memory with record	Memory without record
Autobiographical memory	Perceptual memory
Representational memory	Dispositional memory
Vertical association	Horizontal association
Locale	Taxon
Episodic	Semantic
Working	Reference

(Squire, L. R. *Memory and Brain.* New York: Oxford University Press. (p. 169))

distinction is in many ways similar to the now classic debate between S-R and cognitive explanations of learning. Recent work in monkeys (Mishkin & Appenzeller, 1987) and amnestic humans (Squire, 1987) suggests that these types of memory can be separated neurobiologically (in patients with different types of brain damage) and developmentally (in monkeys of varying ages). These dichotomies of memory provide a way out of the apparent dilemma of broad versus limited views of memory by suggesting that behavior dependent upon memory could be a combination of automatic responses to stimuli and action guided by cognition. This does not in any way relegate the automatic forms of memory to second-class citizenship. The information stored in these systems is as essential and as worthy of study as the more cognitive forms. Rather, dichotomies such as this pose the challenge of understanding different types of memory systems and how they interact to guide behavior and mental processes.

What are the Fundamental Issues in the Study of Memory?

Specifying the fundamental issues in memory would seem to be a straightforward task. Indeed, some contributors to this volume attempt to do so. McGaugh (Chap. 3), for example, suggests that selection, organization, modulation, and identification of the nature and loci of neural changes constitute fundamental issues in memory storage. Thompson (Chap. 2), in advocating a model systems approach (see Kandel, 1976; Thompson, 1976), presents a similar view, but a different strategy for approaching the problem. Rovee-Collier (Chap. 8) takes a somewhat different approach by presenting paradigms that characterize what she identifies as the fundamental processes—encoding, storage, and retrieval over the long term. Whereas these issues have historically been central to the study of memory, as other contributors to this volume point out, they are not the final word.

Perhaps the greatest dissent stems from the social psychological point of view. Ostrom (Chap. 10) presents three "catechisms" for social memory: (1) how social stimuli (e.g., things that form schema) are represented cognitively, (2) the role of social behavior (such as language) in memory formation, and (3) collective memory—that is, that an understanding of memory is necessarily linked to the social milieu in which the person resides. This last point raises a serious challenge to how memory has traditionally been conceptualized and studied. Hamilton (Chap. 11) suggests that memory for the social psychologist may be most useful as a tool for understanding more complex aspects of social cognition. That is, memory in individuals is only likely to provide a partial account of what social psychologists need to know about complex tasks. Wyer (Chap. 12) makes similar arguments in the context of social judgment and points out the differences in how social and cognitive psychologists study memory and what they hope to learn from this enterprise. Nevertheless, despite the differences between the social and cognitive approaches, we are struck by the similarities between the types of experiments conducted by the two groups. This is perhaps best exemplified by the work on scripts and schemas, and social perception (e.g., Spiro, 1977).

There are many other points of divergence regarding the fundamental issues. Neisser (Chap. 4) argues again (see Neisser, 1982) that the first consideration in the study of memory is what areas of memory should be studied. He points out that memory can be studied profitably in natural contexts, and goes on to introduce the term *memoria* to encompass those situations.

It seems, then, that there is little agreement on the fundamental issues in memory. On the one hand, there are specific questions generated by those working in specific paradigms. Here the definition of memory has been specified, albeit in a single context, and specific questions concerning memory can be addressed. For other approaches, the specific questions are not as clear. Here, there are broader issues that must be grappled with. For these psychologists, the issues of what types or domains of memory should be studied is paramount. This might be analogous to a comparative approach to memory; a comparison not between species, but between memoria with the goal of determining to what extent the rules generalize. Using this inductive approach, specific questions about memory in general will have to await formulation.

The divergent views of the fundamental issues and goals of memory research tempt us to paraphrase Baddeley's (Chap. 6) question about working memory and ask, "What is Memory Research For?"

Possible Areas of Convergence

It seems that only a few years ago the notion of a cross-disciplinary conference on the nature of memory would not have been thinkable. Psychologists studying memory from different perspectives had little in common, little to offer one another, and spoke in very different languages. Although the previous section highlights some fundamental differences, the boundaries between the subdisciplines are blurring and there is an ever-growing list of topics in the study of memory that can profitably be approached by joint efforts of psychologists with different perspectives.

Table 1.2 presents some possible areas of convergence. This list is by no means exhaustive, and we intend it only to illustrate areas in which an interdisciplinary approach has been used and can be used. In the remainder of this section we would like to elaborate on several of these areas that we feel are most promising.

TABLE 1.2. Potential areas for interdisciplinary memory research.

	Behavior Neuroscience	Cognitive	Developmental	Social Personality
Age-related memory disorders	X	X	X	
Dissociation of memory systems	X	X	X	
Assessment of memory and memory disorders	X	X		X
Depression and memory	X	X		X
Infantile amnesia		X	X	
Context and memory	X	X		X
Development of memory	X	X	X	
Scripts and schemas		X		X
Memory in natural contexts		X		X
Parallel distributed models of memory	X	X	X	
Social psychophysiology and memory	X			X

Dissociable Memory Systems

Perhaps the most concentrated interdisciplinary effort in the study of memory has come as the product of collaborative efforts between cognitive psychologists and behavioral neuroscientists studying dissociable memory systems in brain-damaged patients (see also Schachter, 1984). Although the two subspecialties often approach memory from different perspectives, both have profited greatly from research on amnestic patients. Cognitive psychologists have used data from these patients to help understand distinctions and relationships between the various memory systems. As Baddeley (Chap. 6) points out, the study by Shallice and Warrington (1970) of a patient with severe short-term memory (STM) deficits but intact long-term memory (LTM) makes a strong statement regarding the flow of information through these two memory stores.

Behavioral neuroscientists have used similar cases to draw different types of conclusions. They have used data from amnestics to form hypotheses about which structures are critical for memory (Zola-Morgan, Squire, & Amaral, 1986), how different structures may mediate different aspects of memory (Squire, 1987), and how these deficits may be modeled in animals (Kesner & DiMattia, 1984; Mishkin, 1982; Winocur, 1984; Zola-Morgan & Squire, 1986). Similar strategies have been used in the study of infantile amnesia (Schachter & Moskovitch, 1984). Here, the strategy is to dissociate memory systems over the course of development. This strategy may also prove useful in the study of memory decline over the life span. This will be especially true if, within the same preparation, tasks can be used which are sensitive to damage to discrete brain areas, and if correlations between pathology and behavior can be made (Solomon, Beal, & Pendlebury, 1988). Moreover, there may be similarities between memory deficits in infants, certain amnestics, and aged subjects, suggesting an ideal area for collaboration.

Modulation of Memory

McGaugh (Chap. 3) persuasively argues for the importance of understanding factors that affect or modulate memory. In McGaugh's hands, these manipulations consist of drugs, neuromodulators, and hormones. We would like to broaden the notion of memory modulators to include other factors such as affective state, and particularly depression and context.

The role of affective state in memory has been studied from a variety of perspectives beginning with psychoanalytic and progresssing more recently to depression, especially in the elderly (Kelley, 1986).

Context is a factor that both affects memory and is studied by psychologists in a variety of subdisciplines. Context is a broad term, but it roughly corresponds to factors in the internal or external environment that may influence the memory process. Those studying animal learning have found that certain effects in classical conditioning are highly context-dependent (Wagner, 1979). Indeed, context forms a cornerstone of one influential theory of learning (Rescorla & Wagner, 1972). Context may also play an important role in animal memory (e.g., Siegal, 1976), disorders of memory (Huppert & Piercy, 1976), and development of memory (Kail, 1979). Context may also be implicated in processing of spatial (Kubie & Ranck, 1984) or temporal (Rawlins, 1985; Solomon, 1980) information. Context also forms an important aspect of neurobiological theories of memory (see Hirsch, 1974; O'Keefe & Nadel, 1978).

Disorders of Memory:
Etiology, Intervention, and Assessment

Memory disorders play a central role in a variety of neuropsychological sequalae including stroke, closed head injury, herpes encephalitus, and most predominantly in dementia (Lezak, 1984). Dementia alone now affects 7% of adults over age 65 and 25% of those over age 85 (Cross &

Gurland, 1986), and because the population is rapidly aging, without any change in the incidence of dementia, the prevalence will quintuple by the year 2040 (Office of Technology Assessment, 1987). Clearly, disorders of memory will be a problem of potentially catastrophic proportion, and it is in this area that a collaborative effort by psychologists can have a major impact.

It seems that disorders of memory can be best approached by a joint effort. For example, behavioral neuroscientists will strive to help develop drugs that can facilitate memory (see McGaugh Chap. 3, this volume, Hollister, 1984). In a related endeavor, psychologists will play a central role in testing drugs that are typically prescribed for elderly populations, but may have deleterious effects on memory.

Interventions designed to help those with mild to moderate memory disorders will be a rich area for research. Already, psychologists have applied mnemonic techniques to those suffering from dementia (e.g., Harris, 1984; Wilson, 1987). Similarly, techniques such as Reality Orientation attempt to create a social atmosphere that encourages orientation and memory.

A third area ripe for multidisciplinary approach is assessment of memory. This will be especially important in the elderly. Indeed, the American Psychological Association, recognizing the important area, recently published *The Handbook for Clinical Memory Assessment for Older Adults* (Poon, 1986). Developing sensitive tests capable of differential diagnosis will require a synthesis of knowledge from many disciplines, including neuropsychology (see Kail, Chap. 9), developmental psychology of aging, psychometric testing, and clinical and cognitive psychology.

Models of Memory—Parallel Distributed Processing

Modeling of memory presents a fruitful area for the interaction of psychologists. One recent approach that may be particularly useful is that of Parallel Distributed Processing (PDP). PDP models offer new ways of thinking about many aspects of cognition, including memory. Indeed McClelland (1984) has suggested that PDP models can account for certain aspects of distributed memory and amnesia.

There is substantial debate as to whether these models can account for complex cognitive processes; nevertheless, they provide a language in which psychologists from a variety of different areas can communicate. In the context of memory, PDP models have already been applied to such diverse areas as language development, classical conditioning, and cortical models of memory (McClelland & Rummelhart, 1986).

Diverging views of memory are often the product of differing experimental preparations and paradigms. Models such as PDP provide a common meeting ground when psychologists can devise testable hypotheses concerning memory. Areas of convergence such as the study of memory disorders provide the opportunity for a multidisciplinary approach that is driven by a common problem and not by paradigm and preparation. Efforts such as this have potential to lead a discipline guided by broad perspectives of both theoretical interest and practical application.

References

Bartlett, F.C. (1932). *Remembering: A study in experimental and social psychology*. Cambridge: Cambridge University Press.

Binet, A., & Henri, V. (1984). La mémoire des phrases (mémoire des idées). *L'année Psychologique, 1*, 24–59.

Cairns, R.B., & Ornstein, P.A. (1979). Developmental psychology. In E. Hearst (Ed.), *The first century of experimental psychology*. Hillsdale, NJ: Lawrence Erlbaum Associates.

Crider, A.B., Goethals, G.R., Kavanaugh, R.D., & Solomon, P.R. (1986). *Psychology*. Glenview, IL: Scott, Foresman.

Cross, P.S., & Gurland, G.J. (1986). *The epidemiology of dementing disorders*. Contract Report prepared for the Office of Technology Assessment, U. S. Congress.

Ebbinghaus, H. (1964/1885). *On memory*. (H.A. Ruger & C.E. Bussenius, trans.). New York: Dover.

Erikson, E. (1968). *Identity: Youth and crisis*. New York: Norton.

Harris, J. (1984). Methods of improving memory. In B.A. Wilson & N. Moffat (Eds.), *Clinical management of memory problems*. London: Aspen.

Hirsch, R. (1974). The hippocampus and contextual retrieval of information from memory: A theory. *Behavioral Biology, 12*, 421–444.

Hollister, L.E. (1984). Survey of treatment attempts in senile dementia of the Alzheimer type. In C. G. Gottfries (Ed.), *Normal aging, Alzheimer's disease and senile dementia*. Bruxelles: Editions de l'Université de Bruxelles.

Huppert, F.A., & Piercy, M. (1976). Recognition memory in amnesia patients: Effects of temporal context and familiarity of material. *Cortex, 12*, 3–20.

Jacoby, L.L., & Witherspoon, D. (1982). Remembering without awareness. *Canadian Journal of Psychology, 32*, 300–324.

Kail, R. (1979). *The development of memory in children*. San Francisco: W.H. Freeman.

Kandel, E.R. (1976). *The cellular basis of behavior*. San Francisco: Freeman Press.

Kelley, C.M. (1986). Depressive mood effects on memory and attention. In L.W. Poon (Ed.), *Handbook for clinical memory assessment for older adults*. Washington, DC: American Psychological Association.

Kesner, R.P., & DiMattia (1984). Posterior parietal association cortex and hippocampus: Equivalency of mnemonic functions in animals and humans. In L.R. Squire & N. Butters (Eds.), *Neuropsychology of memory*. New York: Guilford Press.

Kubie, J.L., & Ranck, J.B. (1984). Hippocampal neuronal firing, context, and learning. In L.R. Squire & N. Butters (Eds.), *Neuropsychology of memory*. New York: Guilford Press.

Lashley, K. (1950). In search of the engram. *Symposia of the society for experimental biology, 4,* 454–482. New York: Cambridge University Press.

Lezak, M. (1984). *Neuropsychological assessment* (2nd ed.). New York: Oxford University Press.

McClelland, J.L. (1984). Distributed models of cognitive processes: Applications to learning and memory. In D.S. Olton, E. Gamzu, & S. Corkin (Eds.), *Memory dysfunction.* New York: *Annals of The New York Academy of Sciences,* vol. 444.

McClelland, J.L., & Rummelhart, D.E. (Eds.). (1986). *Parallel distributed processing: Explorations in the microstructure of cognition.* Cambridge: Bradford Books.

Miller, N.E. (1967). Certain facts relevant to the search for its physical basis. In G.C. Quarton, T. Melnechuk, & F.O. Schmitt (Eds.), *The neurosciences.* New York: Rockefeller University Press.

Milner, B. (1962). Les troubles de la mémoire accompagnant des lésions de l'hippocampe. Paris: Center National de la Recherche Scientifique, 257–272.

Mishkin, M. (1982). A memory system in monkeys. *Philosophical Proceedings of the Royal Society of London* (Biology), *298,* 85–95.

Mishkin, M., & Appenzeller, T. (1987). The anatomy of memory. *Scientific American, 256,* 62–71.

Mishkin, M., & Petri, H.L. (1984). Memories and habits: Some implications for the analysis of learning and retention. In L.R. Squire & N. Butters (Eds.), *Neuropsychology of memory.* New York: Guilford Press.

Neisser, U. (1982). *Memory observed: Remembering in natural contexts.* San Francisco: Freeman.

Oakley, D.A. (1983). The varieties of memory: A phylogenetic approach. In A. Mayes (Ed.), *Memory in animals and humans.* Workingham, England: Van Nostrand Reinhold.

Office of Technology Assessment. (1987). *Losing a million minds: Confronting the tragedy of Alzheimer's Disease and other dementias.* Washington, DC: U.S. Government Printing Office.

O'Keefe, J., & Nadel, L. (1978). *The hippocampus as a cognitive map.* London: Oxford University Press.

Poon, L.W. (Ed.). (1986). *Handbook for clinical memory assessment for older adults.* Washington, DC: American Psychological Association.

Posner, M.I., & Shulman, G.L. (1979). Cognitive science. In E. Hearst (Ed.), *The first century of experimental psychology.* Hillsdale, NJ: Lawrence Erlbaum Associates.

Rawlins, J.N.P. (1985). Associations across time: The hippocampus as a temporary memory store. *Behavioral and Brain Sciences, 8,* 479–496.

Rescorla, R.A., & Wagner, A.R. (1972). A theory of Pavlovian conditioning: Variations in the effectiveness of reinforcement and nonreinforcement. In A.H. Black & W.F. Prokasy (Eds.), *Classical conditioning II: Current research and theory.* New York: Appleton-Century-Crofts.

Rozin, P. (1976). The evolution of intelligence and access to the collective unconscious. *Progress in Psychobiology and Physiological Psychology, 6,* 245–280.

Schachter, D.L. (1984). Toward the multidisciplinary study of memory: Ontogeny, phylogeny, and pathology of memory systems. In L.R. Squire & W. Butters (Eds), *Neuropsychology of memory.* New York: Guilford Press.

Schachter, D.L., & Moscovitch, M. (1984). Infants, amnesics and dissociable memory systems. In M. Moscovitch (Ed.), *Infant memory*. New York: Plenum.

Shallice, T., & Warrington, E.K. (1970). Independent functioning of verbal memory stores: A neuropsychological study. *Quarterly Journal of Experimental Psychology, 22*, 261–273.

Siegal, S. (1976). Morphine analgesic tolerance: Its situation specificity supports a Pavlovian conditioning model. *Science, 193*, 323–325.

Solomon, P.R. (1980). A time and a place for everything: Temporal processing views of hippocampal function with special reference to attention. *Physiological Psychology, 8*, 254–261.

Solomon, P.R., Beal, M.F., & Pendlebury, W.W. (1988). Age-related disruption of classical conditioning: A model systems approach to memory disorders. *Neurobiology of Aging*.

Spiro, R.J. (1977). Remembering information from text: "The state of schema approach." In R.C. Anderson, R.J. Spiro, & W.E. Montague (Eds.), *Schooling and the acquisition of knowledge*. Hillsdale, NJ: Lawrence Erlbaum Associates.

Squire, L.R. (1987). *Memory and the brain*. New York: Oxford University Press.

Squire, L.R., & Zola-Morgan, S. (1985). The neurology of memory: The case for correspondence between the findings for human and nonhuman primates. In J.A. Deutsch (Ed.), *The physiological basis of memory* (2nd ed.). New York: Academic Press.

Thompson, R.F. (1976). In search of the engram. *American Psychologist, 31*, 209–227.

Thompson, R.F., & Robinson, D.N. (1979). Physiological psychology. In E. Hearst (Ed.), *The first century of experimental psychology*. Hillsdale, NJ: Lawrence Earlbaum Associates.

Tulving, E. (1983). *Elements of episodic memory*. New York: Clarendon Press/Oxford University Press.

Tulving, E. (1984). Precis of elements of episodic memory. *Behavioral and Brain Sciences, 7*, 257–268.

Wagner, A.R. (1979). Habituation and memory. In A. Dickinson & R.A. Boakes (Eds.), *Mechanisms of learning and motivation*. Hillsdale, NJ: Erlbaum.

Weiskrantz, L. (1985). On issues and theories of the human amnestic syndrome. In N.M. Weinberger, J.L. McGough, & G.L. Lynch (Eds.), *Memory systems of the brain: Animal and human cognitive processes* (pp. 380–415). New York: Guilford Press.

Wilson, B.A. (1987). *Rehabilitation of memory*. London: Guilford Press.

Winocur, G. (1984). Memory localization in the brain. In L.R. Squire & N. Butters (Eds.), *Neuropsychology of memory*. New York: Guilford Press.

Zola-Morgan, S., & Squire, L.R. (1986). Memory impairment in monkeys following lesions of the hippocampus. *Behavioral Neuroscience, 100*, 155–160.

Zola-Morgan, S., Squire, L.R., & Amaral, D. (1986). Human amnesia and the medial temporal region: Enduring memory impairment following a bilateral lesion limited to the CA1 field of the hippocampus. *Journal of Neuroscience, 6*, 2950–2967.

Part I   Perspectives
from Behavioral Neuroscience

CHAPTER 2

A Model System Approach to Memory

Richard F. Thompson

Memory is a deceptively simple word. There was considerable discussion at this symposium regarding what memory is or is not. Several participants seemed to focus on what they felt to be the uniquely human aspects of memory. From a biological perspective it seems unlikely that any aspect of memory is uniquely human. Evolution proceeds by small steps—the chromosomal DNA of humans and chimpanzees is 99% identical.

I do not agree with George Mandler's "popular" definition of memory in terms of consciousness (see Chapter 5 in this volume), but this definition presents no problems from a biological point of view. Whatever consciousness is, it must have evolved in small steps like all other attributes of living organisms. If we have consciousness, so at least do other mammals. A small problem with Mandler's definition is that consciousness is much more difficult to define than memory.

Language is perhaps the most obvious species-typical behavior of humans. But there are interesting examples of natural language in other primates. Thus, vervet monkeys have developed a three word alarm call "language," one "word" for eagle, one for python, and one for leopard (Seyfarth, Cheney, & Marler, 1980). The young monkeys have to learn to utter the calls correctly. Recent evidence suggests that pigmy chimps may even be capable of learning to understand spoken English (Rumbaugh, Rumbaugh, & McDonald, 1985).

There appears to be a growing consensus in the field that memory has several forms or aspects: distinctions like declarative (learning what) verus procedural (learning how), semantic versus episodic, biographical, and so on. Evidence is very strong for the existence of several different memory systems and circuits in the brain. Thus, the amygdala seems particularly involved in fear learning, conditioning of autonomic responses (e.g., heart rate), and memory consolidation (see Chapter 2, this volume). The hippocampus and temporal lobe structures seem particularly involved in "experiential" memory, as indicated by Milner's dramatic studies of H. M. (Milner, 1966) and Mishkin's work on the

monkey (Mishkin, 1978). At least in the monkey, a very localized region
of prefrontal cortex plays a critical role in a form of short-term memory
(delayed response) (Goldman-Rakic & Schwartz, 1982). Evidence to be
reviewed here indicates that the cerebellum is critically involved in the
learning and memory of discrete behavioral responses learned to deal
with aversive events (e.g., classical conditioning of eyelid closure, leg
flexion, etc.). Indeed, the cerebellum has been suggested as the locus of
storage of memory traces for motor skills (Eccles, 1977). It seems likely
that the brain has its own categories of learning and memory, and these
may not fit the categories currently defined by psychologists.

"Procedural" Memory and the Cerebellum

Some years ago we selected classical conditioning of the eyelid closure
response as a model system in which to analyze the neuronal substrates of
basic associative learning and memory. We adopted this paradigm, and
the rabbit as the experimental animal of choice, for two key reasons:
(a) There is an extensive literature on the properties and parameters of
this basic form of associative learning in both humans and animals
(particularly the rabbit) (Black & Prokasy, 1972; Gormezano, 1972), and
(b) it obeys the basic "laws" and exhibits the basic phenomena of
associative learning in a similar manner in humans and other mammals.
When we began this work about 18 years ago, we had no idea that we
would be led to the cerebellum as the key structure that appears to store
the essential memory trace. With the advantage of hindsight, this result is
perhaps not so surprising. The conditioned eyelid closure response is a
very precisely timed movement: Over the entire effective conditioned
stimulus-unconditioned stimulus (CS-US) onset interval during which
learning occurs, from about 100 ms to over 1 s, the learned response
develops such that the eyelid closure is maximal at the time of onset of the
US. In this sense it is a maximally adaptive response. It is also a very
precisely timed "skilled" movement, perhaps the most elementary form
of learned skilled movement. Our results strongly support the general
spirit of earlier theories of the role of the cerebellum in motor learning
(Albus, 1971; Eccles, 1977; Ito, 1972; Marr, 1969) (see Fig. 2.1).

    As noted below, this conclusion is not limited to eyelid conditioning in
the rabbit but appears to hold for any discrete behavioral response
learned by mammals to deal with an aversive event. It is thus a category
of associative learning and might be described as "procedural" learning,
that is, "learning how." Some years ago we adopted the general strategy
of recording neuronal unit activity in the trained animal (rabbit eyelid
conditioning) as an initial survey and sampling method to identify putative
sites of memory storage. A pattern of neuronal activity that correlates
with the behavioral learned response, specifically one that precedes the

behavioral response in time within trials, predicts the form of the learned response within trials, and predicts the development of learning over trials, is a necessary (but not sufficient) requirement for identification of a storage locus.

We mapped a number of brain regions and systems thought to be involved in learning and memory. Neuronal activity of pyramidal cells in the hippocampus exhibited all the requirements just described (Berger, Rinaldi, Weisz, & Thompson, 1983). But the hippocampus itself is not necessary for learning and memory of such discrete behavioral responses (Thompson, Berger, & Madden, 1983). Recent evidence argues strongly that long-lasting neuronal plasticity is established in the hippocampus in these learning paradigms (Mamounas, Thompson, Lynch, & Baudry, 1984; Weisz, Clark, & Thompson, 1984). Thus, "memory traces" are formed in the hippocampus during learning, but these "higher order" traces are not necessary for learning of the basic association between a neutral tone or light CS and the precisely timed, adaptive behavioral response. However, the hippocampus can become essential when appropriate task demands are placed on the animal, even in eyelid conditioning (Thompson et al., 1983). But the hippocampus is not a part of the memory trace circuit that is essential, that is, necessary and sufficient, for basic associative learning and memory of discrete responses. Indeed, decorticate and even decerebrate mammals can learn the conditioned eyelid response (Norman, Buchwald, & Villablanca, 1977; Oakley & Russell, 1972, and animals that are first trained and then acutely decerebrated retain the learned response (Mauk & Thompson, 1987). The essential memory trace circuit is below the level of the thalamus.

In the course of mapping the brainstem and cerebellum, we discovered localized regions of cerebellar cortex and a region in the lateral interpositus nucleus where neuronal activity exhibited the requisite memory trace properties—patterned changes in neuronal discharge frequency that preceded the behavioral learned response by as much as 60 ms (minimum behavioral conditioned reflex [CR] onset latency approximately 100 ms), that predicted the form of the learned behavioral response (but not the reflex response), and that grew over the course of training (i.e., predicted the development of behavioral learning) (McCormick et al., 1981; McCormick, Clark, Lavond, & Thompson, 1982; McCormick & Thompson, 1984a; Thompson, 1986) (Fig. 2.2).

In our series of lesion studies, large lesions of the lateral cerebellar cortex and nuclei, electrolytic lesions of the lateral interpositus-medial dentate nuclear region, and lesions of the superior cerebellar peduncle ipsilateral to the learned response all abolished the learned response completely and permanently, had no effect on the reflex UR, and did not prevent or impair learning on the contralateral side of the body (Clark et al., 1984; Lavond, McCormick, Clark, Holmes, & Thompson, 1981; Lincoln McCormick, & Thomson, 1982; McCormick, et al., 1981; Mc-

Cormick, Clark, Lavond, & Thompson, 1982; McCormick, Guyer, & Thompson, 1982; Thompson et al., 1984). After our initial papers were published, Yeo, Glickstein, and associates replicated our basic lesion result for the interpositus nucleus, using light as well as tone CSs and a periorbital shock US (we had used corneal airpuff US), thus extending the generality of the result (Yeo, Hardiman, & Glickstein, 1985a).

Electrolytic or aspiration lesions of the cerebellum cause degeneration in the inferior olive. The lesion abolition of the learned response could be due to olivary degeneration rather than cerebellar damage, per se. We made kainic acid lesions of the interpositus; a lesion as small as a cubic millimeter in the lateral anterior interpositus permanently and selectively abolished the learned response with no attendant degeneration in the inferior olive (Lavond, Hembree, & Thompson, 1985). Additional work suggests that the lesion result holds across CS modalities, skeletal response systems, species, and perhaps with instrumental contingencies as well (Donegan et al., 1983; Polenchar, Patterson, Lavond, & Thompson, 1985; Yeo et al., 1984). Electrical microstimulation of the interpositus nucleus in untrained animals elicits behavioral responses by way of the superior cerebellar peduncle, for example, eye blink and leg flexion, the nature of the response being determined by the locus of the electrode (McCormick & Thompson, 1984). Collectively, these data build a case that the memory traces are afferent to the efferent fibers of the superior cerebellar peduncle, that is, in the interpositus, cerebellar cortex, or systems for which the cerebellum is a mandatory efferent.

The essential efferent CR pathway appears to consist of fibers exiting from the interpositus nucleus ipsilateral to the trained side of the body in the superior cerebellar peduncle, crossing first to relay in the contralateral magnocellular division of the red nucleus and crossing back to descend in the rubral pathway to act ultimately on motor neurons (Chapman, Steinmetz, & Thompson, 1985; Hayley, Lavond, & Thompson, 1983; Lavond, et al., 1981; Madden, Haley, Barchas, & Thompson, 1983; McCormick, Guyer, & Thompson, 1982; Rosenfield, Devydaitis, & Moore, 1985) (see Fig. 2.1). Possible involvement of other efferent systems in control of the CR has not yet been determined, but descending systems taking origin rostral to the midbrain are not necessary for learning or retention of the CR, as noted above.

Recent lesion and microstimulation evidence suggests that the essential US reinforcing pathway, the necessary and sufficient pathway conveying information about the US to the cerebellar memory trace circuit, is climbing fibers from the dorsal accessory olive (DAO) projecting via the inferior cerebellar peduncle (see Fig. 2.1). Thus, lesions of the appropriate region of the DAO prevent acquisition and produce normal extinction of the behavioral CR with continued paired training in already trained animals (McCormick, Steinmetz, & Thompson, 1985). Electrical microstimulation of this same region elicits behavioral responses and serves as an effective US for normal learning of behavioral CRs; the exact behavioral response elicited by DAO stimulation is learned as a normal CR to a CS (Mauk, Steinmetz, & Thompson, 1986).

Lesion and microstimulation data suggest that the essential CS pathway includes mossy fiber projections to the cerebellum via the pontine nuclei (see Fig. 2.1). Thus, sufficiently large lesions of the middle cerebellar peduncle prevent acquisition and immediately abolish retention of the eyelid CR to all modalities of CS (Solomon, Lewis, Loturco, Steinmetz, & Thompson, 1986), whereas lesions in the pontine nuclear region can selectively abolish the eyelid CR to an acoustic CS (Steinmetz, Rosen, Chapman, Lavond, & Thompson, 1986). Consistent with this result is current anatomical evidence from our laboratory for a direct contralateral projection from the ventral cochlear nucleus to this same region of the pons (Thompson, Lavond, & Thompson, 1986) and electrophysiological evidence of a "primary-like" auditory relay nucleus in this pontine region (Logan, Steinmetz, & Thompson, 1986).

Electrical microstimulation of the mossy fiber system serves as a very effective CS, producing rapid learning, on average more rapid than with peripheral CSs, when paired with, for example, a corneal airpuff US (Steinmetz, Lavond & Thompson, 1985a). If animals are trained with a left pontine nuclear stimulation CS and then tested for transfer to right pontine stimulation, transfer is immediate (i.e., one trial) if the two electrodes have similar locations in the two sides. This suggests that, at least under these conditions, the traces are not formed in the pontine nuclei but rather in the cerebellum, probably beyond the mossy fiber terminals (Steinmetz, Rosen, Woodruff-Pale, Lavond, & Thompson, 1986). Finally, appropriate forward pairing of mossy fiber stimulation as a CS and climbing fiber stimulation as a US yields *normal behavioral learning* of the response elicited by climbing fiber stimulation (Steinmetz, Lavond & Thompson, 1985b). Lesion of the interpositus abolishes both the CR and the UR in this paradigm. All of these results taken together would seem to build an increasingly strong case for localization of the essential memory traces to the cerebellum, particularly in the "reduced" preparation with stimulation of mossy fibers as the CS and climbing fibers as the US. In the normal animal trained with peripheral stimuli, the possibility of trace formation in brainstem structures has not yet been definitively ruled out.

We initially suggested that the memory traces might be formed in cerebellar cortex (McCormick et al., 1981); as Eccles and others have stressed, there is a vastly greater neuronal machinery there than in the interpositus nucleus. However, we have not yet found any cerebellar cortical lesion that permanently abolishes the CR. Yeo, Hardiman, and Glickstein (1985b), using more complex stimulus and training conditions (that yield less robust learning), reported that complete removal of the cortex of Larsell's lobule H VI permanently abolished the eyelid CR.

Complete removal of lobule H VI did not abolish the CR in three separate studies in our laboratory (McCormick and Thompson, 1984; Woodruff-Pak, Lavond, Logan, Steinmetz, & Thompson, 1985; Woodruff-Pak, Lavond, & Thompson, 1985). Recently, we repeated exactly the stimulus and training conditions of Yeo and colleagues and found that complete removal of lobule H VI causes only transient loss of the CR; all animals eventually relearned (Lavond, Steinmetz, Yokaitis, Lee, & Thompson, 1986). But these results do not rule out multiple parallel cortical sites (and interpositus as well?). Cortical lesions to date may not have removed all such sites; thus the flocculus has not been lesioned and it has recently been found that electrical microstimulation of the flocculus can elicit eye blinks in the rabbit (Nagao, Ito, & Karachot, 1984). In general, the larger the cerebellar cortical lesion, the more pronounced and prolonged is the transient loss of the CR. Further, cerebellar cortical lesions prior to training can prevent learning in some animals (McCormick, & Thompson, 1984a). The possibility of multiple cortical sites is consistent with the organization of somatosensory projections to cerebellum (Kassel, Shambes, & Welken, 1984; Shambes, Gibson, & Welker, 1978).

In current work we have compared electrical stimulation of the dorsolateral pontine nucleus and lateral reticular nucleus as CSs. When such stimulation is paired with a peripheral US (corneal airpuff), both yield normal and rapid learning (Knowlton, Beekman, Lavond, Steinmetz, & Thompson, 1986; Steinmetz et al., 1986). The dorsolateral pontine nucleus projects almost exclusively to an intermediate region of cerebellar cortex, whereas the lateral reticular nucleus projects in significant part to the interpositus nucleus (Bloedel & Courville, 1981; Brodal, 1975; Chan-Palay, 1977). Under these conditions, a lesion limited to the general region of cerebellar cortex receiving projections from the dorsolateral pontine nucleus completely and permanently abolishes the CR to the dorsolateral pontine nucleus stimulation CS but not to the lateral reticular nucleus stimulation CS (Knowlton et al., 1986). We have thus created a situation where a relatively restricted region of cerebellar cortex is necessary for the CR. This will be most helpful for further analysis of mechanisms of memory trace formation. More generally, these results suggest that the particular region(s) of cerebellar cortex necessary for associative memory formation depends upon the patterns of mossy fiber projections to the cerebellum activated by the CS. We hypothesize that the memory traces are formed in regions of cerebellar cortex (and interpositus nucleus?) where CS-activated mossy fiber projections and US-activated climbing fiber projections converge.

Recordings from Purkinje cells in the eyelid conditioning paradigm are consistent with the formation of memory traces in cerebellar cortex. Prior to training, a tone CS causes a variable evoked increase in frequency of discharge of simple spikes in many Purkinje cells (Donegan, Foy, & Thompson, 1985; Foy & Thompson, 1986). Following training, the majority of Purkinje cells that develop a change in frequency of simple spike discharge that correlates with the behavioral response (as opposed to being stimulus evoked) show decreases in frequency of discharge of simple spikes that precede and "predict" the form of the behavioral learned response, although increases in "predictive" discharge frequency also occur fairly frequently.

Conjoint electrical stimulation of mossy fibers and climbing fibers can yield normal learning of behavioral responses, as noted above (Steinmetz et al., 1986). The properties of these learned responses appear identical to those of the same conditioned responses learned with peripheral stimuli (e.g., eyelid closure, leg flexion). The temporal requirements for such conjoint stimulation that yields behavioral learning are essentially identical to those required with peripheral stimuli: no learning at all if CS onset does not precede US onset by more than 50 ms, best learning if CS precedes US by 200 to 400 ms, and progressively poorer learning with increasing CS precedence (Gormezano, 1972). Further, normal learning occurs if the mossy fiber CS consists of only two pulses, 5 ms apart, at the beginning of a 250-ms CS-US onset interval (Logan, Steinmetz, Woodruff-Pak, & Thompson, 1985).

Collectively, the evidence reviewed above demonstrates that the cerebellum is essential for the category of procedural memory we have studied. It also builds a very strong case that the essential memory traces are stored in very localized regions of the cerebellum.

Cognition and the Cerebellum

We hasten to add we do not argue that all types of memories are stored in the cerebellum. However, the evidence for storage of any kind of memory trace in the cerebellum is very recent, dating from our initial report in 1981 (McCormick et al.). It is at least possible that the cerebellum is much more generally involved in memory and complex information processing than was earlier believed. Indeed, there are tantalizing hints that the cerebellum may play a key role in the sequential aspects of complex cognitive processes (Leiner, Leiner, & Dow, 1986).

There is suggestive evidence from our own current work that the essential cerebellar circuit we have defined (Fig. 2.1) may in fact be capable of mediating *blocking,* a complex aspect of classical conditioning that is viewed by many as cognitive. The phenomenon of blocking (Kamin, 1969) has become a key issue of modern animal learning theory. In brief, if an animal is first trained on CS_1-US, then given additional training on CS_1 paired simultaneously with CS_2, followed by US, and then tested for response to CS_2, little conditioned responding is seen compared with animals not given the prior CS_1-US training (and other appropriate control conditions). The important message of blocking is that the informational context in which a CS appears determines the degree to which it becomes associated with the US (as opposed to simply the number of times the CS is paired with the US)—contiguity is necessary to produce conditioning, but not sufficient.

Blocking has become the cornerstone of all models of associative learning that address the Pavlovian conditioning literature (e.g., Mackintosh, 1975; Pearce & Hall, 1980; Rescorla & Wagner, 1972; Schull, 1979; Sutton, Barto, & Thompson, 1981; Wagner, 1981). In fact, it seems almost obligatory for a model to predict blocking in order to be taken seriously (see also Gluck & Thompson, 1987). One way blocking could occur is that as the CR becomes established to CS_1, the associative strength added by additional pairings of CS_1 and the US becomes increasingly less, so that after learning to CS_1 is asymptotic, no additional associative strength is added by additional CS_1-US pairings. Hence, if further training is given with CS_1 and the US while a new CS_2 is presented simultaneously, no associative strength will accrue to CS_2-US. This is the essence of the Rescorla–Wagner mathematical formulation of basic associative learning and memory (Rescorla & Wagner, 1972).

The essential learning and memory circuit involving the cerebellum (Fig. 2.1) contains within it the hypothetical potential for actualizing the Rescorla–Wagner formulation of associative learning, including blocking. The basic requirement is that as the CR develops to a US, the less effective the US becomes—the less "reinforcing" it is. We make the following assumption: The degree to which the US is reinforcing, that is, the degree to which it adds associative strength on CS-US trials, is a direct function of the occurrence of a climbing fiber volley to the cerebellum evoked by the US onset.

Since the hypothetical memory trace in the cerebellum must involve a population of Purkinje cells and a population of climbing fibers projecting from the dorsal accessory olive portion of the inferior olive, a simple way to conceptualize reinforcement strength is as the proportion of effective climbing fibers activated by the US (by "effective" is meant all those activated by the particular US prior to training).

Before learning, the tone CS does not result in any increase in the activity of interpositus neurons, that is, the efferent CR pathway from interpositus to red nucleus to motor neurons is not activated (see Fig. 2.2). As training proceeds, neurons in the interpositus increase their patterns of discharge in the CS period such that they precede and predict the occurrence of the behavioral CR, as noted above (see Fig. 2.2). In a well-trained animal, activation of neurons in the efferent CR pathway is massive in the CS period (Fig. 2.2).

Suppose that in addition to driving the behavioral CR, the efferent CR pathway also exerts an inhibitory influence on the essential US pathway. Then as the CR is increasingly well learned, activation of the US pathway by the US is increasingly attenuated. In a well-trained animal, the US

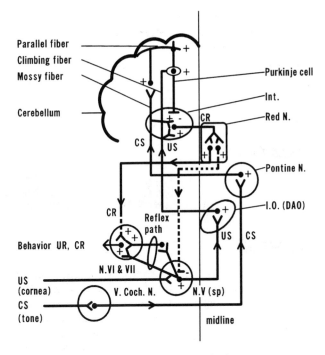

FIGURE 2.1. Simplified schematic of hypothetical memory trace circuit for discrete behavioral responses learned as adaptations to aversive events. The unconditioned stimulus (US) (corneal airpuff) pathway seems to consist of somatosensory projections to the dorsal accessory portion of the inferior olive (DAO) and its climbing fiber projections to the cerebellum. The conditioned stimulus (CS) (tone) pathway seems to consist of auditory projections to pontine nuclei (pontine N) and their mossy fiber projections to the cerebellum. The efferent (eyelid closure) conditioned reflex (CR) pathway projects from the interpositus nucleus (Int) of the cerebellum to the red nucleus (Red N) and via the descending rubral pathway to act ultimately on motor neurons. The red nucleus may also exert inhibitory control over the transmission of somatic sensory information about the US to the inferior olive (IO), so that when a CR occurs (eyelid closes), the red nucleus dampens US activation of climbing fibers. Evidence to date is most consistent with storage of the memory traces in localized regions of cerebellar cortex and possibly interpositus nucleus as well. Pluses indicate excitatory and minuses indicate inhibitory synaptic action. Additional abbreviations: N V (sp), spinal fifth cranial nucleus; N VI, sixth cranial nucleus; N VII, seventh cranial nucleus; V Coch N, ventral cochlear nucleus. From Thompson, 1986; reprinted by permission of *Science*, 1986.

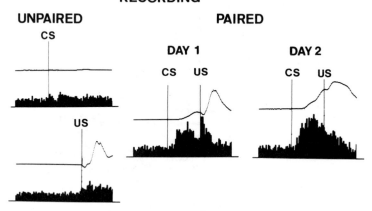

FIGURE 2.2. Neuronal unit activity recorded from the lateral interpositus nucleus during impaired and paired presentations of the training stimuli. The animal was first given pseudorandomly unpaired presentations of stimuli tone and corneal airpuff, in which the neurons responded very little to either stimulus. However, when the stimuli were paired in time, the cells began responding within the conditioned stimulus (CS) period as the animal learned the eyeblink response. The onset of this unit activity preceded the behavioral eyelid (NM = nectitating membrane) response within a trial by 36 to 58 ms. Stimulation through this recording site yielded ipsilateral eyelid closure and NM extension. Each histogram bar is 9 ms in duration. The upper trace of each histogram represents the movement of the NM, with up being extension across the eyeball. From McCormick & Thompson, 1984b).

pathway might be completely shut down. If so, additional training with the original CS_1, paired with a new CS_2, and the US will result in no association between CS_2 and the US, because the US has functionally ceased to occur at the critical regions of memory trace formation in the cerebellum (see Fig. 2.1).

Recent evidence suggests that activation of the red nucleus can inhibit somatosensory activation of the inferior olive (Weiss, McCurdy, Houk, & Gibson, 1985). Electrical stimulation of the red nucleus can produce inhibition of activation of inferior olive neurons by tactile stimulation (of the forepaw). Weiss and colleagues (1985) suggested that this inhibition acts at the somatosensory relay in the cuneate nucleus (relaying somatosensory information to the inferior olive and to higher brain structures from the forelimbs).

Assume that a comparable descending inhibitory system exists from red nucleus to the spinal trigeminal nucleus, regulating projection of somatosensory information from the face to the critical region of the inferior olive, the dorsal accessory olive (dashed line in Fig. 2.1). Similar descending inhibitory influences may exist from the interpositus to the trigeminal nucleus and perhaps to the dorsal accessory olive as well.

If this descending system inhibiting somatosensory activation of the inferior olive does in fact exist, then our cerebellar circuit provides the basic architecture for the Rescorla–Wagner formulation and can account fully for blocking. The strong prediction is that as a CR develops to a CS, activation of the essential US pathway in dorsal accessory olive–climbing fibers–cerebellum by the US no longer activates the essential US pathway at all. In current work two lines of evidence support this hypothesis. The first involves the activity of single Purkinje neurons. As noted above, there are clear and marked changes in the patterns of simple spike discharges of Purkinje neurons. (Simple spikes are evoked by the mossy fiber–granule cell–parallel fiber system, the essential CS pathway.) But there are also clear and dramatic changes in the patterns of complex spike discharges. (Complex spikes in Purkinje cells are evoked by activation of climbing fibers from the inferior olive—the essential US pathway). Prior to training, the onset of the US (corneal airpuff) consistently evokes complex spikes in those Purkinje cells receiving climbing fiber projections from the region of the inferior olive that is activated by stimulation of the eye region of the face. In well-trained animals, the US onset typically does not evoke complex spikes in the appropriate Purkinje cells (Foy & Thompson, 1986). It appears that as the CR develops, activation of the Purkinje cells by the US becomes markedly attenuated, as predicted by our blocking hypothesis.

In current and preliminary studies we are obtaining more direct evidence for our blocking hypothesis by recording activity of neurons in the dorsal accessory olive activated by the corneal airpuff US onset (Steinmetz, Donegan, & Thompson, unpublished data). US presentation alone consistently evokes a phasic increase in responses of these neurons (US onset evoked). As the behavioral CR (eyelid response) begins to develop, this US-onset-evoked response in dorsal accessory olive neurons becomes markedly attenuated. Indeed, in a well-trained animal, US-onset-evoked activity may be completely absent in the dorsal accessory olive.

Perhaps the most striking aspect of our blocking hypothesis is that the phenomenon of blocking is a mandatory emergent property of the essential memory trace circuit itself. If the circuit indeed functions as we hypothesize, the explanation of blocking is purely mechanistic. Terms like "expectation" and "surprise" favored by some cognitive psychologists to "explain" blocking become so much excess baggage. From a different perspective, an identified neuronal memory trace circuit in the mammalian brain can indeed account for the cognitive phenomenon of blocking.

In more general terms, our cerebellar circuit would seem to provide the

neuronal substrate for the Rescorla–Wagner formulation of basic associative learning. This emerges from the architecture of the circuit itself
rather than from any special synaptic processes. In our circuit, the reason
that CS-US pairings add progressively less associative strength as
learning develops is because the essential reinforcement provided by the
US becomes progressively weaker over the course of training. In a
well-trained animal the US provides no reinforcement at all.

References

Albus, J.S. (1971). A theory of cerebellar function. *Mathematics and Bioscience,*
    10, 25–61.
Berger, T.W., Rinaldi, P., Weisz, D.J., & Thompson, R.F. (1983). Single unit
    analysis of different hippocampal cell types during classical conditioning of the
    rabbit nictitating membrane response. *Journal of Neurophysiology, 50,* 1197–
    1219.
Black, A.H., & Prokasy, W.F. (Eds.) (1972). *Classical conditioning. II: Current*
    research and theory. New York: Appleton-Century-Crofts.
Bloedel, J.R., & Courville, J. (1981). Cerebellar afferent systems. In J.M.
    Brookhart, V.B. Mountcastle, V.B. Brooks & S.R. Geiger (Eds.), *Handbook of*
    physiology (Vol. 2, pp. 735–829). Baltimore: American Physiological Society.
Brodal, P. (1975). Demonstration of a somatotopically organized projection onto
    the paramedian lobule and the anterior lobe from the lateral reticular nucleus:
    An experimental study with the horseradish peroxidase method. *Brain Re-*
    search, 95, 221–239.
Chan-Palay, V. (1977). *Cerebellar Dentate Nucleus.* New York: Springer-Verlag.
Chapman, P.F., Steinmetz, J.E., & Thompson, R.F. (1985). Classical condi-
    tioning of the rabbit eyeblink does not occur with stimulation of the cerebellar
    nuclei as the unconditioned stimulus. *Society of Neuroscience Abstracts, 11*
    835.
Clark, G.A., McCormick, D.A., Lavond, D.G., & Thompson, R.F. (1984).
    Effects of lesions of cerebellar nuclei on conditioned behavioral and hippocam-
    pal neuronal responses. *Brain Research 291:* 125–136.
Donegan, N.H., Foy, M.R., & Thompson, R.F. (1985). Neuronal responses of the
    rabbit cerebellar cortex during performance of the classically conditioned eyelid
    response. *Society of Neuroscience Abstracts, 11,* 835.
Donegan, N.H., Lowry, R.W., & Thompson, R.F. (1983). Effects of lesioning
    cerebellar nuclei on conditioned leg-flexion responses. *Society of Neuroscience*
    Abstracts, 9, 331 (No. 100.7).
Eccles, J.C. (1977). An instruction-selection theory of learning in the cerebellar
    cortex. *Brain Research, 127:*327–352.
Foy, M.R., & Thompson, R.F. (1986). Single unit analysis of Purkinje cell
    discharge in classically conditioned and untrained rabbits. *Society of Neuro-*
    science Abstracts, 12, 518.
Gluck, M.A., & Thompson, R.F. (1987). Modelling the neural substrates of
    associative learning and memory: A computational approach. *Psychological*
    Review, 94, 176–191.
Goldman-Rakic, P.S., & Schwartz, M.L. (1982). Interdigitation of contralateral

and ipsilateral columnar projections to frontal association cortex in primates. *Science, 216*, 755–757.

Gormezano, I. (1972). Investigations of defense and reward conditioning in the rabbit. In Black, A.H., & Prokasy, W.F. (Eds.), *Classical conditioning. II: Current research and theory* (pp. 151–181). New York: Appleton-Century-Crofts.

Haley, D.A., Lavond, D.G., & Thompson, R.F. (1983). Effects of contralateral red nuclear lesions on retention of the classically conditioned nictitating membrane/eyelid response. *Society of Neuroscience Abstracts, 9*, 643.

Ito, M. (1972). Neural design of the cerebellar motor control system. *Brain Research, 40*, 81–84.

Kamin, L.J. (1969). Predictability, surprise, attention and conditioning. In Campbell, B.A. & Church, R.M. (Eds.), *Punishment and aversive behavior* (pp. 279–296). New York: Appleton-Century-Crafts.

Kassel, J., Shambes, G.M., & Welker, W. (1984). Fractured cutaneous projections to the granule cell layer of the posterior cerebellar hemisphere of the domestic cat. *Journal of Comparative Neurology, 225*, 458–468.

Knowlton, B., Beekman, G., Lavond, D.G., Steinmetz, J.E., & Thompson, R.F. (1986). Effects of aspiration of cerebellar cortex on retention of eyeblink conditioning using stimulation of different mossy fiber sources as conditioned stimuli. *Society of Neuroscience Abstracts, 12*, 754.

Lavond, D.G., Hembree, T.L., & Thompson, R.F. (1985). Effect of kainic acid lesions of the cerebrellar interpositus nucleus on eyelid conditioning in the rabbit. *Brain Research, 326*, 179–182.

Lavond, D.G., McCormick, D.A., Clark, G.A., Holmes, D.T., & Thompson, R.F. (1981). Effects of ipsilateral rostral pontine reticular lesions on retention of classically conditioned nictitating membrane and eyelid response. *Physiological Psychology 9*(4), 335–339.

Lavond, D.G., Steinmetz, J.E., Yokaitis, M.H., Lee, J., & Thompson, R.F. (1986). Retention of classical conditioning after removal of cerebellar cortex. *Society of Neuroscience Abstracts, 12*, 753.

Leiner, H.C., Leiner, A.L., & Dow, R.S. (1986). *Behavioral Neuroscience 100*, 443–454.

Lincoln, J.S., McCormick, D.A., & Thompson, R.F. (1982). Ipsilateral cerebellar lesions prevent learning of the classically conditioned nictitating membrane/eyelid response of the rabbit. *Brain Research 242*, 190–193.

Logan, C.G., Steinmetz, J.E., & Thompson, R.F. (1986). Acoustic related responses recorded from the region of the pontine nuclei. *Society of Neuroscience Abstracts, 12*, 754.

Logan, C.G., Steinmetz, J.E., Woodruff-Pak, D.S., & Thompson, R.F. (1985). Short-duration mossy fiber stimulation is effective as a CS in eyelid classical conditioning. *Society of Neuroscience Abstracts, 11*, 835.

Mackintosh, N.J. (1975). A theory of attention: Variations in the associability of stimuli with reinforcement. *Psychological Review, 82*, 276–298.

Madden, IV, J., Haley, D.A., Barchas, J.D., & Thompson, R.F. (1983). Microinfusion of picrotoxin into the caudal red nucleus selectively abolishes the classically conditioned nictitating membrane/eyelid response in the rabbit. *Society of Neuroscience Abstracts, 9*, 830.

Mamounas, L.A., Thompson, R.F., Lynch, G. & Baudry, M. (1984). Classical conditioning of the rabbit eyelid response increases glutamate receptor binding in hippocampal synaptic membranes. *Proceedings of the National Academy of Sciences 81,* 2548–2552.

Marr, D. (1969). A theory of cerebellar cortex. *Journal of Physiology, 202,* 437–470.

Mauk, M.D., Steinmetz, J.E., & Thompson, R.F. (1986). Classical conditioning using stimulation of the inferior olive as the unconditioned stimulus. *Proceedings of the National Academy of Science (USA), 83,* 5349–5353.

Mauk, M.D., & Thompson, R.F. (1987). Retention of classically conditioned eyelid responses following acute decerebration. *Brain Research, 403,* 89–95.

McCormick, D.A., Clark, G.A., Lavond, D.G., & Thompson, R.F. (1982). Intial localization of the memory trace for a basic form of learning. *Proceedings of the National Academy of Sciences 79,* 2731–2742.

McCormick, D.A., Guyer, P.E., & Thompson, R.F. (1982). Superior cerebellar peduncle lesions selectively abolish the ipsilateral classical conditioned nictitating membrane/eyelid response in the rabbit. *Brain Research, 244,* 347–350.

McCormick, D.A., Lavond, D.G., Clark, G.A., Kettner, R.E., Rising, C.E., & Thompson, R.F. (1981). The engram found? Role of the cerebellum in classical conditioning of nictitating membrane and eyelid responses. *Bulletin of the Psychonomic Society, 18*(3), 103–105.

McCormick, D.A., Steinmetz, J.E., & Thompson, R.F. (1985). Lesions of the inferior olivary complex cause extinction of the classically conditioned eyeblink response. *Brain Research, 359,* 120–130.

McCormick, D.A., & Thompson, R.F. (1984a). Cerebellum: Essential involvement in the classically conditioned eyelid response. *Science, 223,* 296–299.

McCormick, D.A., & Thompson, R.F. (1984b). Neuronal responses of the rabbit cerebellum during acquisition and performance of a classically conditioned nictitating membrane-eyelid response. *Journal of Neuroscience, 4,* 2811–2822.

Milner, B. (1966). Amnesia following operation on the temporal lobes. In C.W.M. Whitty & O.L. Zangwill (Eds.), *Amnesia,* (pp. 109–133). London: Butterworths.

Mishkin, M. (1978). Memory in monkeys severely impaired by combined but not by separate removal of amygdala and hippocampus. *Nature, 273,* 297–298.

Nagao, S., Ito, M., & Karachot, L. (1984). Sites in the rabbit flocculus specifically related to eye blinking and neck muscle contraction. *Neuroscience Research, 1,* 149–152.

Norman, R.J., Buchwald, J.S., & Villablanca, J.R. (1977). Classical conditioning with auditory discrimination of the eyeblink in decerebrate cats. *Science, 196,* 551–553.

Oakley, D.A., & Russell, I.S. (1972). Neocortical lesions and classical conditioning. *Physiology and Behavior, 8,* 915–926.

Pearce, J.M., & Hall, G. (1980). A model for Pavlovian learning: Variations in the effectiveness of conditioned but not unconditioned stimuli. *Psychological Review, 87,* 532–552.

Polenchar, B.E., Patterson, M.M., Lavond, D.G., & Thompson, R.F. (1985). Cerebellar lesions abolish an avoidance response in rabbit. *Behavioral and Neural Biology, 44,* 221–227.

Rescorla, R.A., & Wagner, A.R. (1972). A theory of Pavlovian conditioning: Variations in the effectiveness of reinforcement and non-reinforcement. In

A.H. Black & W.F. Prokasy (Eds.), *Classical conditioning. II: Current research and theory*. New York: Appleton-Century-Crofts.

Rosenfield, M.E., Devydaitis, A., & Moore, J.W. (1985). *Brachium conjunctivum and rubrobulbar tract: Brainstem projections of red nucleus essential for the conditioned nictitating membrane response. Physiology and Behavior, 34*, 751–759.

Rumbaugh, D.M., Rumbaugh, S.S., and McDonald, K. (1985). Language learning in two species of apes. *Neuroscience and Biobehavioral Reviews 9:* 653–665.

Schull, J. (1979). A conditioned opponent theory of Pavlovian conditioning and habituation. In G.H. Bower (Ed.), *The psychology of learning and motivation* (Vol. 13). New York: Academic Press.

Seyfarth, R.M., Cheney, D.L., and Marler, P. (1980). Monkey responses to three different alarm calls: Evidence of predator classification and semantic communication. *Science, 210*, 801–803.

Shambes, G.M., Gibson, J.M., & Welker, W. (1978). Fractured somatotopy in granule cell tactile areas of rat cerebellar hemispheres revealed by micromapping. *Brain, Behavior and Evolution 15*, 94–140.

Solomon, R.R., Lewis, J.L., LoTurco, J.J., Steinmetz, J.E., & Thompson, R.F. (1986). The role of the middle cerebellar peduncle in acquisition and retention of the rabbits classically conditioned nictitating membrane response. *Bulletin of the Psychonomic Society, 24*(1), 75–78.

Steinmetz, J.E., Lavond, D.G., & Thompson, R.F. (1985a). Classical conditioning of the rabbit eyelid response with mossy fiber stimulation as the conditioned stimulus. *Bulletin of the Psychonomic Society, 23*(3), 245–248.

Steinmetz, J.E., Lavond, D.G., & Thompson, R.F. (1985b). Classical conditioning of skeletal muscle responses with mossy fiber stimulation CS and climbing fiber stimulation US. *Society of Neuroscience Abstracts, 11*, 982.

Steinmetz, J.E., Rosen, D.L., Chapman, P.F., Lavond, D.G., & Thompson, R.F. (1986). Classical conditioning of the rabbit eyelid response with a mossy fiber stimulation CS. I. Pontine nuclei and middle cerebellar peduncle stimulation. *Behavioral Neuroscience, 100*, 871–880.

Steinmetz, J.E., Rosen, D.J., Woodruff-Pak, D.S., Lavond, D.G., & Thompson, R.F. Rapid transfer of training occurs when direct mossy fiber stimulation is used as a conditioned stimulus for classical eyelid conditioning. *Neuroscience Research, 3*, 606–616.

Sutton, R.S., Barto, A.G., & Thompson, R.F. (1981). Toward a modern theory of adaptive networks. *Psychological Review, 88*, 135–170.

Thompson, R.F. (1986). The neurobiology of learning and memory. *Science, 233*, 941–947.

Thompson, R.F., Berger, T.W., & Madden IV, J. (1983). Cellular processes of learning and memory in the mammalian CNS. *Annual Review of Neuroscience, 6*, 447–491.

Thompson, R.F., Clark, G.A., Donegan, N.H., Lavond, D.G., Madden IV, J., Mamounas, L.A., Mauk, M.D., & McCormick, D.A. (1984). Neuronal substrates of basic associative learning. In L. Squire & N. Butters (Eds.), *Neuropsychology of memory* (pp. 424–442). New York: Guilford Press.

Thompson, J.K., Lavond, D.G., & Thompson, R.F. (1986). Preliminary evidence for a projection from the cochlear nucleus to the pontine nuclear region. *Society of Neuroscience Abstracts, 12*, 754.

Wagner, A.R. (1981). SOP: A model of automatic memory processing in animal behavior. In N.E. Spears & R.R. Miller (Eds.), *Information processing in animals: Memory mechanisms.* Hillsdale, NJ: Lawrence Erlbaum Associates.

Weiss, C., McCurdy, M.L., Houk, J.C., & Gibson, A.R. (1985). Anatomy and physiology of dorsal column afferents to forelimb dorsal accessory olive. *Society of Neuroscience Abstracts, 11,* 182.

Weisz, D.J., Clark, G.A., & Thompson, R.F. (1984). Increased activity of dentate granule cells during nictitating membrane response conditioning in rabbits. *Behavioural Brain Research,* 12, 145–154.

Woodruff-Pak, D.S., Lavond, D.G., Logan, C.G., Steinmetz, J.E., & Thompson, R.F. (1985). The continuing search for a role of the cerebellar cortex in eyelid conditioning. *Society of Neuroscience Abstracts, 11,* 333.

Woodruff-Pak, D.S., Lavond, D.G., & Thompson, R.F. (1985). Trace conditioning: Abolished by cerebellar nuclear lesions but not lateral cerebellar cortex aspirations. *Brain Research 348,* 249–260.

Yeo, C.H., Hardiman, M.J., Glickstein, M. (1985a). Classical conditioning of the nictilating membrane response of the rabbit: I Lesions of the cerebellar nuclei. *Experimental Brain Research 60,* 87–98.

Yeo, C.H., Hardiman, M.J., & Glickstein, M. (1985b). Classical conditioning of the nictitating membrane response of the rabbit. II. Lesions of the cerebellar cortex. *Experimental Brain Research, 60,* 99–113.

CHAPTER 3

Modulation of Memory Storage Processes

James L. McGaugh

It seems most fitting that the first of a series of symposia commemorating G. Stanley Hall's contribution to psychology is devoted to the topic of memory. Memory processes are central to all aspects of psychological functioning: Our consciousness and our actions are shaped by our experiences. And our experiences shape us only because of their lingering consequences, which we term, collectively, *memory*. Memory is, of course, not the sole determiner of our experience and behavior. But in bridging the past and the present, memory serves a central coordinating role. Thus, understanding of the nature and bases of memory is essential for understanding of the broad range of problems that interested G. Stanley Hall. An analysis of memory processes seems appropriate as a beginning.

Critical Questions in the Study of Memory

The title of this inaugural symposium is also most appropriate. The study of memory requires an interdisciplinary—or multidisciplinary—approach, since the major questions must be addressed at several levels of analysis. Fundamentally, we wish to learn how experiences alter brain cells and systems in ways that enable us to acquire and use information. It is perhaps worth noting that our language has tended to constrain our research and our analyses. The word *memory* is singular. Thus, there has been, and to some extent still is, a tendency to study or to develop theories about memory as though memory involves but a single mechanism, process, or system, or as though there is a specific, unique, and perhaps static structure in the brain that correspond to our memory of a person, an event, or a skill. Collectively, our "memories linger," and if they seem not to linger we try to "dredge them up" or "retrieve them"—as though memories are preserved by tossing them into some sort of murky cerebral pool. Our conscious experiences of attempting to recall, as well as the language we use to describe the experience of recalling, serve to reinforce the notion that specific memories are stored as individual neural units subject to recall, much as defective automobiles are recalled by automobile manufacturers. Matters are not that simple; such metaphors, however useful in language, are of litle use in our effort to understand the nature and bases of memory.

Memory is, of course, not a "thing": Rather, memory is an outcome of the functioning of a complex set of neurobiological processes. Thus, the quest to understand the bases of memory encompasses a number of critical questions. If we are to understand the bases of memory we will need to know, at the very least, (a) how information is selected for storage, (b) how the storage process is modulated, (c) the loci and organization of the changes, (d) the bases of the changes underlying memory, and (e) how the neural changes mediate the cognitive changes seen in complex as well as simple forms of learning. I will touch briefly on each of these questions before returning to a more detailed discussion of my own research, which addresses the question of the modulation of storage.

Selection for Storage

A priori it seems to me unlikely that every sensory input leaves its trace somewhere in the nervous system. After all, our sensory systems are constantly stimulated, and the pattern of stimulation varies from moment to moment throughout our lives. As you read this are you recording in some way *all* that you see, hear, touch, taste, and smell as well as *all* of the positions and movements of your body? Do we store information to which we do not attend? Presumably, the capacity of the nervous system is not the limiting factor in information storage: The number of changes to be recorded should not necessarily be limited by the number of brain cells or even the number of synapses, since the number of possible interconnections is virtually limitless. Thus, the possibility that all sensory experience is recorded cannot be ruled out. Moreover, the fact that repetition of experiences results in learning, that is, that the effects of experiences accumulate, would seem to argue that each experience, alone, must produce some lasting change in the nervous system. This is the view taken by William James (from whom G. Stanely Hall received the first doctorate of philosophy in psychology granted in America):

Every smallest stroke of virtue or of vice leaves its never so little scar. The drunken Rip Van Winkle, the Jefferson's play excuses himself for every fresh dereliction by saying, "I won't count this time!" Well! he may not count it, and a kind Heaven may not count it; but it is being counted none the less. Down among his nerve-cells and fibres the molecules are counting it, registering and storing it up to be used against him when the next temptation comes. (James, W., *Principles of Psychology* 1890, p. 127)

Whether or not each experience is recorded in some way, it is clear from studies of animal learning (e.g., from experiments on "overshadowing" and "blocking") that the occurrence of an experience is not a sufficient condition for the experience to become associated with other experiences occurring at the same time (Mackintosh, 1983). Thus, any neurobiological account of memory needs to provide an explanation of how the nervous system selects, from sensory events, the specific information that is to be preserved.

Modulation of Storage

As we all know from our own experiences, some events are remembered well while other, perhaps comparable, events are remembered poorly if at all. What accounts for the differences in retention? In extreme cases, such as that of the well-studied patient H. M. (Scoville & Milner, 1957), the ability to acquire new information may be largely intact. In monkeys, lesions of the hippocampus and amygdala appear to produce effects on memory that are similar to those found in H. M. (Mishkin, Malamut & Bachevalier, 1984; Zola-Morgan & Squire, 1985). These findings suggest that limbic structures may be involved in processing recently acquired information. The finding that patients who have had head injury or who have received electroconvulsive therapy (ECT) typically have retrograde amnesia indicates that memory processes remain susceptible to modulating influences after information has been acquired (Russell & Nathan, 1946; Squire, 1986). Consolidation (Mueller & Pilzecker, 1900) of the newly acquired information appears to be based on time-dependent processes. It is now well known that, in animals, retention can be impaired or enhanced by a variety of treatments, including electrical stimulation of the brain, drugs, and hormones, if the treatments are administered shortly after learning takes place (Bloch & Laroche, 1984; Gold & Zornetzer, 1983; Kesner, 1982; McGaugh, 1983). Such findings have suggested that retention may be modulated or regulated by the endogenous activity of hormonal and brain systems (Gold & McGaugh, 1975; Kety, 1972). That is, information that is selected for storage appears to be regulated or modulated by physiological systems that do not themselves serve as the locus of the lasting changes underlying memory. Thus, if we are to understand the bases of memory we need to know what brain and hormonal systems are involved in the endogenous modulation of memory storage and how these systems act to influence the storage of information at a cellular level. I will return to these issues later.

Locus of Change

The search for the locus of the changes underlying learning constitutes a major portion of the history of physiological psychology. Lashley's search for the "engram" and the outcome of his search are well known (Lashley, 1950). His failure to find the engram did not cause the search to be abandoned. On the contrary, much current research continues to be guided by the assumption that the changes underlying memory must in some sense be localized—and localizable. The fact that changes in single unit activity associated with learning are readily recorded in many brain regions (John, 1967; Weinberger, Diamond, & McKenna, 1984) seems to suggest that the changes induced by learning may involve large numbers of neurons widely distributed throughout many brain regions. If this is the case, is it true for all forms of learning? The finding of Thompson and his colleagues (1986; chap. 2 this volume) that, in rabbits, retention of a conditioned eyelid response is abolished by a small lesion in a nucleus of the cerebellum strongly suggests that this region of the brain is an essential part of circuitry underlying the learning of the specific conditioned response. Thus, the basis of this form of conditioning appears to be, at least in part, highly localized rather than widely distributed. This finding leaves open the question of the function of changes in neural activity in other brain regions that are not critical for the performance of the learned response. Are different types of information held in a series of different neural circuits? That is, is there a circuit for the learned fear produced in a conditioning task, as well as one for the animal's knowledge of its spatial location, and others for the animal's memory of the researchers who provide the daily training? Does the storage of an event or skill consist of a collection of parallel circuits, each mediating a portion of the information? While this possibility is consistent with other recent evidence suggesting that the learning of facts and skills may be mediated by different neural systems (Mishkin et al., 1984; Squire, 1986), it remains to be determined whether forms of learning other than conditioned response learning will readily yield to a circuit analysis.

Bases of the Changes

The central feature of memory is that experiences alter subsequent experience and behavior. There must, then, be specific alterations in the central nervous system that underlie the behavioral changes. Recent findings from many laboratories have provided compelling evidence that the brain is changed by experience. Extensive evidence from animal studies indicates that, in rats, changes in brain morphology are induced by experience (Greenough, 1985; Rosenzweig & Bennett, 1976) and that, in mollusks, the functioning of individual neurons is altered in highly specific ways by conditioning (Alkon, 1985; Hawkins & Kandel, 1984). Further, electrophysiological studies of long-term potentiation (LTP) in vivo as well as in vitro have shown that activation of hippocampal synapses by brief stimulation of presynaptic fibers produces lasting changes in responsiveness to subsequent stimulation and that such changes are accompanied by morphological as well as neurochemical changes

(Greenough, 1985; Lee, Schottler, Oliver, & Lynch, 1980; Lynch & Baudry, 1984). Thus, there is accumulating and convincing evidence that sensory stimulation and direct neural stimulation, as well as specific training, induce lasting changes in the morphology and physiology of brain cells. Understanding of the biochemical basis (or bases) of the functional changes in cellular activity induced by experience will, of course, be a highly significant step in gaining understanding of the neural basis of memory.

When understanding of the cellular changes induced by experience is eventually achieved, the focus of inquiry will shift to the question of how such changes link neurons in ways that mediate learning. It is not sufficient simply to know that training alters the connections between cells. We need to know how the interactions among networks of cells provide a basis for memory and performance based on memory (cf. Lynch, 1986).

Cells, Systems, and Cognition

It is abundantly clear that learning does not consist of the linking of movements to sensory stimulation. Theories that made that claim in either simple (Watson, 1919) or sophisticated (Hull, 1943) ways were rejected by the evidence (Tolman, 1932) that animals acquire information which they then use in subsequent performance. Or, as Tolman put it, "Behavior reeks of cognition." The fact that proximal visual cues are poor predictors of our perception of objects (Brunswik, 1943; Tolman & Brunswik, 1935) argues that sensory information requires extensive processing to produce object constancy. Similarly, the fact that animals can and do vary their responses while learning to go to places in their environment (Lashley, 1930; Morris, 1984; Tolman, 1932) demonstrates that learning consists of the acquisition of information, not the acquisition of specific movements. Selection of movements appropriate for the particular environment requires processing based on the acquired information. The fact that the major evidence bearing on this issue is now ancient (as the brief history of psychology goes) does not make it any less valid or less important. Theories of the mechanisms of learning and memory must incorporate these facts. This challenge is the major one faced and failed by the baroque learning theories of several decades past. It remains the major problem for current neurobiological theories attempting to derive cognition from synapses.

Memory-Modulation: Experimental and Endogenous

I return now to the issue of modulation of memory. As I briefly indicated above, this area of research has its origins in studies of retrograde amnesia in humans. The findings of early studies of retrograde amnesia in rats and hamsters (Duncan, 1949; Gerard, 1949) were remarkably comparable to those from human studies: Electroconvulsive shock produced a selective loss of retention of information acquired shortly before the treatments. While the interpretation of the basis (or bases) of the retrograde amnesia has been a matter of considerable controversy (McGaugh & Herz, 1972), the conclusion that the retention of experiences is influenced by treatments administered following training and that the degree of the influence decreases with the time between the training and posttraining treatment is well documented. Susceptibility to posttraining modulating influences appears to be a common feature of human as well as animal memory: Posttraining treatments readily alter memory in rodents and monkeys as well as in fish, birds, and bees (Agranoff, 1980; Bowman, Heironimus, & Harlow, 1979; Cherkin, 1969; Menzel, 1983).

The fact that posttraining susceptibility to modulating influences is seen in so many species argues that this feature of memory has been conserved in evolution. But why should evolution conserve a process that enables memory impairment? The answer to this question may lie in findings indicating that retention can also be *enhanced* by a variety of treatments if the treatments are administered shortly after training (McGaugh, 1983; McGaugh & Herz, 1972). Lashley reported 70 years ago that rats' maze learning was enhanced by low doses of a stimulant drug (strychnine) given shortly before day's training trials. Petrinovich and I subsequently replicated Lashley's finding (McGaugh & Petrinovich, 1959); we published our findings in the *American Journal of Psychology*— which was founded by G. Stanley Hall. I then found that strychnine as well as other stimulant drugs would enhance retention if the drugs were administered shortly *after* training (see McGaugh, 1973, for a review). Subsequently, Bloch (1970) found that retention could be enhanced by posttraining electrical stimulation of the mesencephalic reticular formation. More recent findings indicate that retention can be enhanced by stimulation of other brain structures as well (Kesner, 1982; McGaugh & Gold, 1976).

The fact that retention can be enhanced or impaired by treatments administered after training suggests that possibility that the storage of experiences may be regulated by *endogenous* physiological systems, including peripheral hormones as well as brain systems activated by the experiences (Gold & McGaugh, 1975; Kety, 1972). From this perspective, modulation is seen as an integral part of the physiology of memory rather than as evidence that our brains, as well as those of other animals, may have been badly designed. And according to this view, neurobiological theories of memory will need to incorporate a central role for endogenous modulatory processes. The ultimate aim of studies using posttraining treatments to modulate memory storage is to understand the physiological systems involved in modulating storage as well as the cellular mechanisms underlying the modulation. Thus, research on memory modulation converges with other current attempts to answer critical questions in the study of memory.

Involvement of Hormones and Neurotransmitters in Memory Modulation

Extensive evidence indicates that hormones that are normally released by experiences influence memory storage (de Wied, 1984; McGaugh, 1983; McGaugh & Gold, in press). The hormonal systems studied most extensively include adrenocorticotropic hormone (ACTH), vasopressin, epinephrine, and opioid peptides. The research in my laboratory has focused on the involvement of adrenergic and opioid peptide systems. Briefly, our findings, as well as those of other investigators, provide strong evidence that these systems are involved in the endogenous modulation of memory. Figure 3.1 summarizes our view of the involvement of hormones in memory modulation, as suggested by recent findings. First, we assume that sensory stimulation activates cells in a memory system that provides the basis for lasting changes. We also assume that the same stimulation activates brain systems that serve to modulate the storage occurring in the memory system. Finally, we assume that the stimulation also influences the release of hormones that affect the central modulation system. In recent research we have attempted to determine the brain systems underlying the memory-modulating influences of adrenergic and opioid peptide systems. I turn now to a discussion of our recent findings.

Effects of Epinephrine on Memory

Numerous studies conducted over the past dozen years have shown that, in rats and mice, posttraining administration of the adrenal medullary hormone epinephrine alters subsequent retention (Borrell, de Kloet, Versteeg, & Bohus, 1983; Gold & van Buskirk, 1975; McGaugh & Gold, in press). Since epinephrine is known to be released from the adrenal medulla by the kind of stimulation typically used in animal memory experiments (Gold & McCarty, 1981), the findings have been interpreted as supporting the general view that endogenously released epinephrine

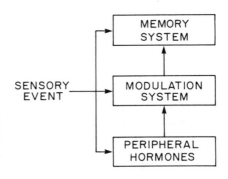

FIGURE 3.1. Interaction of peripheral hormones with central modulating and memory systems. From Liang et al., 1986.

modulates the processes underlying the storage of recently acquired information.

Most studies of the effects of epinephrine on memory have used one-trial inhibitory (passive) avoidance tasks. The findings shown in Figure 3.2 are typical: Retention is enhanced by low doses of epinephrine and impaired by high doses. If it is assumed that epinephrine effects on memory are due to a general modulating effect on memory storage, then epinephrine should affect retention in other tasks as well. That is, the effects should not be restricted to inhibitory avoidance tasks or, for that matter, to training tasks using aversive stimulation. There is clear evidence that epinephrine affects learning in a variety of aversively motivated tasks. Previously we found that epinephrine also affects retention of an active avoidance task (Liang, Bennett, & McGaugh, 1985), and Weinberger, Gold, and Sternberg (1984) reported that epinephrine enhances classically conditioned fear in deeply anesthetized rats.

In recent experiments we have found that posttraining epinephrine

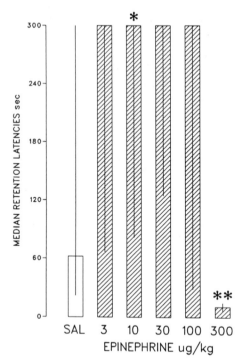

FIGURE 3.2. Dose-response effects of posttraining epinephrine on retention of an inhibitory avoidance response. Mice received saline or epinephrine (ip) immediately after training in a straight-alley inhibitory avoidance task (median ± interquartile range). Retention was tested 24 hours later. *P<0.05 and **P<0.01 compared with saline controls. N=12 mice per group. From Introini-Collison & McGaugh, 1987.

administration affects retention of a shock-motivated visual discrimination task as well as of a water-motivated discrimination task. Mice in the shock-motivated discrimination experiment (Introini-Collison & McGaugh, 1986) were trained to escape from a mild foot shock by entering the left, lighted arm of a Y maze (criterion of three successive correct choices). They were then immediately injected intraperitoneally with saline or epinephrine. On retention tests given to different groups 1 day, 1 week, or 1 month later, the location of the correct alley was reversed. The mice were given six trials on which they could escape from the shock only by entering the right, dark alley. As Figure 3.3 shows, at all retention intervals the mice given the posttraining low dose of epinephrine made more errors than did saline controls on the reversal training, while mice given the high dose made fewer errors. We interpret these findings as indicating that the low dose of epinephrine enhanced retention of original discrimination and that the high dose of epinephrine impaired retention of the original discrimination. These findings are highly comparable to those that we and other investigators have obtained with inhibitory avoidance tasks. These findings also indicate that both the enhancing and impairing effects of a single posttraining injection of epinephrine as lasting: Comparable effects are seen at retention intervals of 1 day, 1 week, and 1 month following the training.

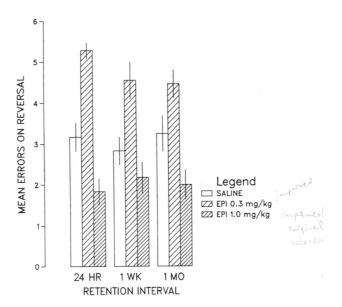

FIGURE 3.3. Effects, in mice, of immediate posttraining epinephrine (ip) on discrimination reversal training 1 day, 1 week, or 1 month following original training (mean ± SE). Retention of the original discrimination is indexed by errors made on the discrimination reversal. $N=18$ for 1-day group and $N=12$ for 1 week and 1-month groups. From Introini-Collison & McGaugh, 1986.

In the appetitively motivated discrimination learning study (Sternberg, Isaacs, Gold, & McGaugh, 1985) water-deprived mice were placed in a Y maze and allowed to explore until they found and drank water from a spout located at the end of a lighted alley. They were then given posttraining injections of saline or epinephrine and tested for retention 24 hours later. As Figure 3.4 shows, the animals given immediate posttraining epinephrine entered significantly fewer alleys prior to finding the water spout than did controls. These findings clearly indicate that the effects of posttraining epinephrine on retention are not restricted to tasks using aversive motivation. As Figure 3.4 also shows, the enhancing effect of epinephrine on retention was blocked by injections of the β-antagonist dl-propranolol and the α-antagonist phenoxybenzamine administered 30 minutes prior to training. These findings are consistent with findings from our laboratory indicating that both α- and β-antagonists also block the enhancing effects of epinephrine on retention of an inhibitory avoidance response (Sternberg, Korol, Novack, & McGaugh, 1986). These findings are of particular interest in view of other evidence, discussed below, suggesting that, in the brain, memory-modulating influences of several treatments selectively involve β-adrenergic receptors.

Thus, our findings indicate that epinephrine has highly similar effects in a variety of learning tasks involving different motivation and different response measures. They strongly support the view that epinephrine has a

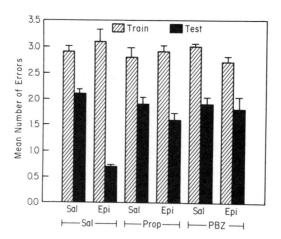

FIGURE 3.4. Effect of posttraining epinephrine on retention in a one-trial appetitively motivated task (mean ± SE). Mice received saline, propranolol, or phenoxybenzamine 30 minutes prior to training and saline or epinephrine immediately posttraining. For all conditions, errors made on the 24-hour retention test were lower ($P<0.05$) than errors on the training. Retention errors of posttraining epinephrine group were lower ($P<0.05$) than those of the saline group and of all groups given phenoxybenzamine or propranolol. $N=14$–19 per group. From Sternberg et al., 1985.

general role in the modulation of memory storage. With this evidence in place, the major question now is that of the basis or bases of the effects of epinephrine on memory. The available evidence (Weil-Malherbe, Axelrod, & Tomchick, 1959) indicates that epinephrine does not readily pass the blood-brain barrier. If this is the case, then its central effects must be initiated by its effect on peripheral receptors. Evidence that peripheral epinephrine stimulates the release of ACTH by activating pituitary adrenergic receptors (Reisine et al., 1983) suggested the possibility that the effects of epinephrine on memory might be mediated by ACTH. To examine this possibility, we studied the effect of posttraining epinephrine on 24-hour retention of rats given dexamethasone (to block ACTH release) 24 and 4 hours prior to inhibitory avoidance training. Dexamethasone did not attenuate the enhancing effects of epinephrine. Thus, epinephrine effects on memory appear not to be mediated by pituitary ACTH (McGaugh et al., 1987). The locus of the peripheral adrenergic receptors involved in epinephrine effects on memory remains to be determined.

Studies of the Involvement of Opiate Receptors

There is also extensive evidence that memory, as assessed in a variety of types of training tasks, is modulated by posttraining treatments affecting opiate receptors. Retention is generally impaired by posttraining administration of opiate receptor agonists (e.g., morphine, β-endorphin) and enhanced by opiate receptor antagonists such as naloxone and naltrexone (Castellano, 1975, 1981; Gallagher, 1985; Introini-Collison & Baratti, 1986; Izquierdo, 1979; Messing et al., 1979). The findings in Figure 3.5 show the effects of posttraining naloxone and β-endorphin on the Y-maze discrimination reversal task described above.

The memory-enhancing effect of opiate receptor antagonists appears to be based on central effects, since retention is not affected by posttraining intraperitoneal administration of naltrexone methyl bromide (MR2263), an opiate receptor antagonist that does not readily pass the blood-brain barrier. Further, the effects of β-endorphin as well as morphine also appear to be centrally mediated, since MR2263 does not antagonize the memory-impairing effects of these treatments (Introini, McGaugh, & Baratti, 1985).

Interaction of Adrenergic and Opiate Systems

Any brain system is, of course, subject to interactions with other systems. Recent evidence suggests that epinephrine effects on retention may involve interactions with a brain opioid peptide system. For example, recent findings indicate that the memory-impairing effect of high doses of epinephrine is blocked by naloxone (Introini-Collison & McGaugh, 1987;

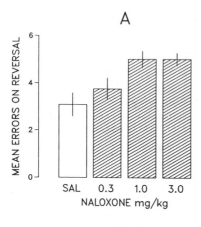

A

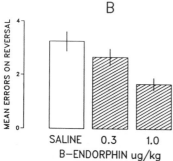

B

FIGURE 3.5. Effects of posttraining (A) naloxone and (B) β-endorphin on discrimination reversal training tested 24 hours following original training. Retention of the
original discrimination is indexed by errors
made on the discrimination reversal (mean
± SE). *P<0.05 and **P<0.01 compared
with saline controls. N = 12 mice per group.
From Introini-Collison & McGaugh, 1987.

Izquierdo & Dias, 1985). Such findings are consistent with other evidence
indicating that epinephrine releases brain β-endorphin (Carrasco et al.,
1982). However, the memory-enhancing effects of low doses of epinephrine clearly do not involve the release of β-endorphin, since low doses of
epinephrine block the memory impairment produced by posttraining
β-endorphin (Izquierdo & Dias, 1985; Introini-Collison & McGaugh,
1987). Further, as is shown in Figure 3.6, the effects of naloxone and
epinephrine on memory are additive: Low doses of naloxone and
epinephrine, which do not affect memory when administered alone,
significantly enhance memory when administered together. Other findings
discussed below suggest that both naloxone and epinephrine may affect
retention through influences on brain norepinephrine.

In a series of studies, Izquierdo and his colleagues have shown that
hypothalamic β-endorphin immunoreactivity is reduced for several hours
following novel training experiences (Izquierdo et al., 1984). These
findings, considered together with the evidence that posttraining administration of β-endorphin impairs retention, suggest that naloxone may
enhance retention by blocking the posttraining effects of endogenously
released β-endorphin. If this is the case, then naloxone should not be

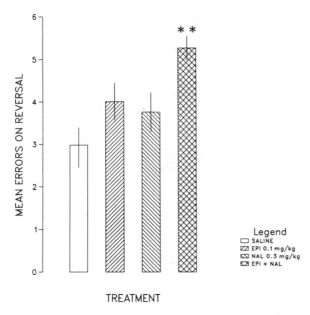

FIGURE 3.6. Effect of combined posttraining administration of low doses of epinephrine and naloxone on discrimination reversal training tested 24 hours following original training. Retention of the original discrimination is indexed by errors made on the discrimination reversal (mean ± SE). **$P<0.01$ compared with saline controls. $N=12$ per group. From Introini-Collison & McGaugh, 1987.

expected to enhance retention to animals given a novel experience prior to training. That is, if β-endorphin is not released by the training, then posttraining naloxone should be ineffective.

To examine this implication, mice were given either a 10-minute novel exploratory experience or intraperitoneal injections of β-endorphin or saline 1 hour prior to training on an inhibitory avoidance task. Immediately following training, the mice were given saline, naloxone, or a low dose of epinephrine. As is shown in Table 3.1, neither the novel experience nor β-endorphin given prior to training affected retention (tested 24 hours later) in animals given posttraining saline. Posttraining naloxone enhanced retention in mice given either β-endorphin or saline 1 hour prior to training. However, naloxone did not enhance retention in mice given the novel experience prior to training, as was expected on the assumption that naloxone effects on retention are due to blocking of the effects of β-endorphin released by training. In agreement with other evidence discussed above (Introini-Collison & McGaugh, 1987), the enhancing effects of low doses of epinephrine on retention appear to be independent of the effects of β-endorphin: Neither the novel experience nor β-endorphin given prior to training attenuated the enhancing effects of posttraining epinephrine (Izquierdo & McGaugh, 1985).

TABLE 3.1. Effect in mice of novel experience or intraperitoneal injection of
β-endorphin given before training in inhibitory avoidance task on 24-hr
retention after posttraining ip injection of saline, naloxone HCl, or epinephrine
HCl. N = 12 per group.

Treatment 1 hr before training (dose)	Posttraining treatment (dose) (N = 12/group)	Median (interquartile range) test minus training latency difference
Saline	Saline (0.1 ml)	19.1 (6.8/43.8)
Novel experience	Saline (0.1 ml)	41.1 (16.0/48.2)
βendorphin (0.1 μg)	Saline (0.1 ml)	30.8 (17.4/45.1)
Saline	Naloxone (0.1 mg)	270.9 (115.5/300.0)*
Novel experience	Naloxone (0.1 mg)	17.4 (7.1/32.9)
β-endorphin (0.1 μg)	Naloxone (0.1 mg)	133.5 (68.7/142.4)*
Saline	Epinephrine (0.3 μg)	139.2 (47.4/167.2)*
Novel experience	Epinephrine (0.3 μg)	101.1 (94.2/300.0)*
β-endorphin (0.1 μg)	Epinephrine (0.3 μg)	117.1 (93.0/241.1)*

*Significantly different (P <0.002) from other groups not asterisked.

The interpretations offered above are based on the assumption that the
effects of naloxone and the novel experience are due to the release of
β-endorphin and not to other effects, including the effects of other opioid
peptides. This interpretation is supported by our findings indicating that
the effects of two other classes of opioid peptides on memory are different
from those found with β-endorphin. For example, while posttraining
administration of the opioid peptide dynorphin impairs retention of
inhibitory avoidance training in mice, the peptide has no effect on
retention of the visual discrimination reversal task (Introini-Collison et
al., 1987 data). The effects of β-endorphin also differ from those of
Met-enkephalin and Leu-enkephalin. We have found, for example, that
the peripherally acting opioid antagonist naltrexone methyl bromide
(MR2263) blocks the memory impairment produced by posttraining
Met-enkephalin and Leu-enkephalin but does not block the amnestic
effects of β-endorphin or morphine (Introini, McGaugh, & Baratti, 1985).
This suggests that the enkephalins act through influences initiated peripherally. Since the effects of both enkephalins on retention are also blocked
by naloxone and naltrexone, it is possible that Met-enkephalin and
Leu-enkephalin impair retention by stimulating the release of central
β-endorphin.

Interaction of Noradrenergic and Opiate Systems

It is clear from the findings reviewed above that memory storage is
modulated by treatments affecting adrenergic opiate receptors. I turn now
to the question of the basis or bases of the memory-modulating influences

of these treatments. There is substantial evidence that opiates and opioid peptides exert an inhibitory influence on norepinephrine (NE) neurons (Walker, Khachaturian, & Watson, 1984). Electrophysiological studies have shown that, in neurons of the locus coeruleus, systemically as well as iontophoretically administered morphine and opioid peptides depress spontaneous as well as stimulation-induced firing rates and produce hyperpolarization of the neuronal membrane. The effects are naloxone reversible (Bird & Kuhar, 1977; Korf, Bunney, & Aghajanian, 1974; Pepper & Henderson, 1980; Strahlendorf, Strahlendorf, & Barnes, 1980; Young, Bird, & Kuhar, 1977). Morphine and β-endorphin depress the potassium-stimulated release of NE from rat cerebral cortex slices (Arbilla & Langer, 1978; Montel, Starke, & Weber, 1974). Nakamura, Tepper, Young, Ling, and Groves (1982) have reported that infusion of morphine into the cortical terminal fields of locus coeruleus neurons depresses excitability to direct stimulation. The finding that opiate receptor binding sites are reduced in NE terminal regions following 6-hydroxydopamine destruction of NE cell bodies suggests that opiate receptors are located presynaptically on NE cells (Llorens, Martres, Baudry, & Schwartz, 1978).

Evidence from a number of studies strongly suggests that adrenergic as well as opioid peptidergic systems may interact with central NE in their effects on memory. In the first study suggesting that opiate antagonists may affect memory through effects involving NE, Izquierdo and Graudenz (1980) reported that propranolol (a $\beta_{1,2}$ antagonist) blocked the enhancing effects of naloxone on memory. They interpreted their findings as suggesting that opioid antagonists may enhance retention by releasing brain NE neurons from the inhibitory effects of opioid peptides. Other recent evidence has provided additional support for the view that opioid effects on memory involve NE. For example, naloxone potentiates the memory-enhancing effects of clenbuterol, a centrally acting β-adrenergic agonist (Introini-Collison & Baratti, 1986). Moreover, the findings that the memory-enhancing effects of naloxone are not blocked by a peripherally acting β-antagonist (sotalol), or by α-antagonists (phenoxybenzamine or phentolamine) suggest that naloxone effects on memory involve central β-adrenergic receptors (Introini-Collison & Baratti, 1986).

In other recent studies, Gallagher and her colleagues have obtained further evidence that naloxone effects on memory involve brain NE. Their findings indicate that the enhancing effects of naloxone on retention are blocked in animals with 6-OHDA lesions of the dorsal noradrenergic bundle (Fanelli, Rosenberg, & Gallagher, 1985; Gallagher, Rapp, & Fanelli, 1985). These findings fit well with Introini-Collison and Baratti's finding (1986) that the memory-enhancing effects of naloxone are blocked in animals treated with DSP4, a neurotoxin that produces a relatively specific reduction in brain NE.

Involvement of the Amygdala in Noradrenergic and Opioid Modulation of Memory

The evidence presented above indicates that retention is modulated by posttraining treatments affecting opiate, adrenergic, and noradrenergic systems and suggests that opiate and adrenergic systems modulate memory through interactions involving the release of central NE. While the findings of studies using DSP4 and 6-OHDA, which reduce brain levels of NE, indicate that naloxone effects on memory require an intact NE system, they do not reveal whether NE in any specific brain region is of particular importance. Other recent findings suggest that effects of naloxone and epinephrine on memory may involve, in particular, the activation of NE receptors within the amygdaloid complex. These recent findings are of interest in view of the extensive evidence suggesting that the amygdaloid complex plays a role in memory storage (Sarter & Markowitsch, 1985a,b).

Involvement of the Amygdaloid Complex

It is well known that in humans as well as monkeys, lesions of the amygdala and hippocampus produce deficits in learning (Milner, 1966; Saunders, Murray, & Mishkin, 1984; Squire & Zola-Morgan, 1983) and that, in monkeys, amygdala lesions alone can impair learning (Mishkin & Aggleton, 1981; Murray & Mishkin, 1985). We have found that, in rats, retention is impaired by bilateral lesions of the amygdala produced shortly after training but not by lesions produced several days after training (Liang et al., 1982). These findings argue that it is unlikely that the amygdala is a site of memory storage. Rather, it seems more likely that the amygdala is involved in mediating or modulating the integration of recently acquired information (e.g., Sarter & Markowitsch, 1985b).

Many studies have shown that posttraining low-intensity (subseizure) electrical stimulation can modulate retention (Kesner, 1982; McGaugh & Gold, 1976). The effects of amygdala stimulation on retention are blocked by lesions of the stria terminalis, a major amygdala pathway, as well as by administration of naloxone, either parenterally or directly into the bed nucleus of the stria terminalis, immediately prior to the stimulation (Liang & McGaugh, 1983; Liang, Messing, & McGaugh, 1983). Such findings suggest that amygdala stimulation affects retention by modulating storage processes at sites in other brain regions.

Extensive evidence indicates that there are noradrenergic receptors in the amygdala (U'Prichard, Reisine, Masion, Fibiger, & Yamamura, 1980). The innervation is particularly dense in the central and basolateral nuclei (Fallon, 1981). Opiate receptors are also found throughout the amygdaloid complex. Immunohistochemical studies indicate that enkephalin fibers and cell bodies are located in the central nucleus and that

β-endorphin in located in the medial and central nuclei (Bloom & McGinty, 1981). Tanaka and his colleagues (Tanaka et al., 1982a,b) have reported that stress increases NE turnover in the amygdala and that the turnover is enhanced by naloxone. These findings suggest that endogenous opioid peptides in the amygdala attenuate stress-induced NE turnover.

Thus, the pharmacological, physiological, and anatomical evidence suggests that the amygdaloid complex is a likely candidate for a locus of the effects of treatments affecting opiate and noradrenergic receptors. This possibility is strongly supported by recent findings. We have found, for example, that lesions of the stria terminalis block the memory-enhancing effects of posttraining peripheral injections of both epinephrine and naloxone as well as of β-endorphin (Liang & McGaugh, 1983; McGaugh, Introini-Collison, Juler, & Izquierdo, 1986). Figure 3.7 shows the effects of stria terminalis lesions on retention (in the Y-maze discrimination task described above) of rats given posttraining naloxone and β-endorphin. We have also found that peripheral epinephrine alters the memory-modulating effects of posttraining electrical stimulation of the amygdala. Amygdala stimulation that produces retrograde amnesia in normal rats enhances retention in adrenal demedullated or denervated rats. However, if epinephrine is administered shortly before the amygdala stimulation, the stimulation produces amnesia (Bennett, Liang, & McGaugh, 1985; Liang et al., 1985).

Involvement of Intraamygdala Norepinephrine

It is generally assumed that epinephrine does not pass the blood-brain barrier and thus does not directly affect the brain. However, it is clear from the studies discussed here that epinephrine has central effects. Moreover, Gold and van Buskirk (1978) have reported that telencephalic NE level is significantly lowered shortly after peripheral injections of epinephrine in doses found to affect retention. The effects of peripheral epinephrine might be mediated by activation of visceral afferents projecting to central noradrenergic systems that are known to activate the amygdala (via the stria terminalis and the ventral amygdalo-fugal pathway). If this is the case, interference with the activation of central NE receptors would be expected to block the effect of peripheral epinephrine on memory. Evidence summarized below strongly supports this implication: Posttraining intraamygdala injections of β-adrenergic antagonists block the effects of systemic injections of epinephrine (as well as naloxone) on retention. Futher, since NE systems project to the amygdala in part via the stria terminalis, our findings that the effects of peripherally administered epinephrine as well as naloxone on retention are blocked by lesions of the stria terminalis are consistent with the view that such lesions attenuate NE release in the amygdala.

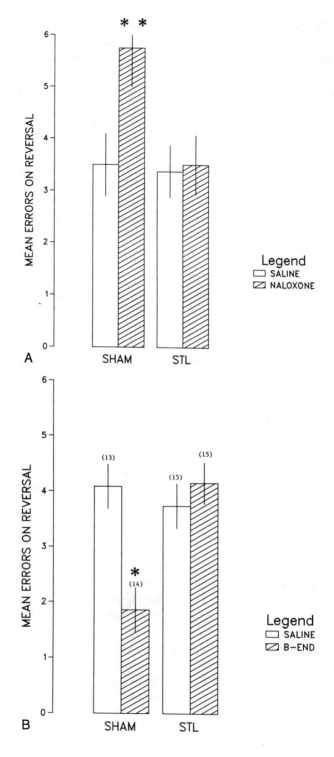

If modulation of memory storage processes involves noradrenergic activation within the amygdala, it should be possible to influence retention with posttraining intraamygdala injections of noradrenergic agonists and antagonists. Extensive recent evidence supports this implication. For example, Gallagher and her colleagues have reported that retention of an inhibitory avoidance response is impaired by posttraining intraamygdala injections of the β-antagonists propranolol and alprenolol. The effect is time dependent and stereo specific and is attenuated by concurrent intraamygdala administration of NE (Gallagher, Kapp, Pascoe, & Rapp, 1981). Kesner and his colleagures found that retention is impaired by posttraining intraamygdala injections of NE (Ellis, Berman, & Kesner, 1983; Ellis & Kesner, 1981,1983).

In recent experiments using doses of NE much lower than those used by Kesner and his colleagues, we have found that posttraining intraamygdala injections of NE enhance retention in an inhibitory avoidance task (Liang, Juler, & McGaugh, 1986). Rats in these studies were implanted bilaterally with amygdala cannulae. They were then trained on an inhibitory avoidance task and given immediate or delayed intraamygdala injections. As Fig. 3.8 shows, when administered immediately posttraining, low doses of NE enhanced retention on a 24-hour retention test, while higher doses were ineffective. Delayed injections of NE were also ineffective. Further, it seems clear that the effects are due specifically to influences on memory of the training experience, since intraamygdala NE administration did not affect the retention performance of animals that were not given foot shock on the training trial. The effect of NE was blocked by concurrent intraamygdala injections of propranolol. Posttraining intraamygdala injections of NE also attenuated the retention deficit produced by adrenal demedullation.

Further, as is shown in Fig. 3.9, we have found that posttraining intraamygdala injections of propranolol block the retention-enhancing effects of *peripherally* administered epinephrine. This finding provides strong evidence for our view that epinephrine affects memory by influencing the release of NE within the amygdala. Thus, considered together, these findings are consistent with the view that activation of noradrenergic receptors in the amygdaloid complex may be involved in endogenous as well as experimental modulation of memory storage.

FIGURE 3.7. Effects of (A) posttraining naloxone and ($N = 12$ per group) and (B) posttraining β-endorphin (number per group given in parentheses) on retention (Y-maze discrimination reversal) in sham-operated and stria terminalis lesioned (STL) rats. Retention of the original discrimination is indexed by errors made on reversal training (mean ± SE). *$P<0.05$ and **$P<0.01$ compared with saline controls. From McGaugh et al., 1986.

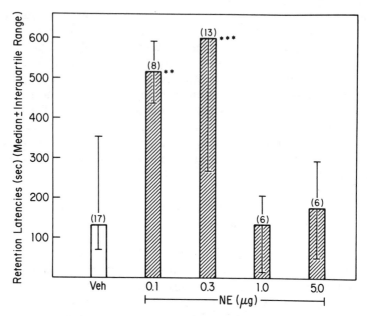

FIGURE 3.8. Effects of posttraining intraamydgala administration of norepinephrine on retention of an inhibitory avoidance response (median < interquartile
range). **$P<0.01$, ***$P<0.002$ compared with vehicle (Veh) controls. Number
per group is shown in parentheses. From Liang, Juler, & McGaugh, 1986.

Interaction of Noradrenergic and Opiate Systems

The findings of numerous recent studies indicate that retention can also be
modulated by intraamygdala injections of opioid agonists and antagonists.
Gallagher and her colleagues reported that posttraining intraamygdala
injections of the opiate agonist levorphanol produced a retention deficit
that was blocked by naloxone. Further, posttraining intraamygdala
naloxone administered alone enhanced retention (Gallagher & Kapp,
1978; Gallagher et al., 1981). As discussed above, the findings of studies
using peripheral injections of opioid antagonists have suggested that
effects of these compounds on memory may be due to blocking of opioid
inhibition of NE release. In further support of this interpretation,
Gallagher and her colleagues (1985) have found that 6-OHDA lesions of
the dorsal noradrenergic bundle block the effects of posttraining intraamygdala injections of naloxone on retention. These findings argue that
the NE projections to the amygdala may be critical for the memory-
modulating effects of naloxone.

Recent findings from my laboratory provide additional evidence suggesting that the modulating effects of naloxone on retention may also
involve activation of noradrenergic receptors within the amygdala
(McGaugh & Introini-Collison, unpublished data). Rats in these experi-

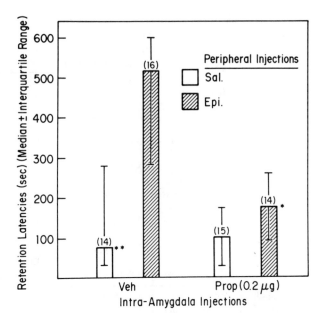

FIGURE 3.9. Effects of posttraining intraamygdala administration of propranolol and intraperitoneal administration of epinephrine on retention of an inhibitory avoidance response (median ± interquartile range). Number per group is shown in parentheses. *P<0.05, **P<0.02 compared with group given vehicle intra-amygdally and epinephrine ip (Veh). From Liang, Juler, & McGaugh, 1986.

ments received immediate posttraining intraamygdala injections of α- and β-adrenergic blockers or of a buffer control solution, through implanted cannulae, followed by intraperitoneal injections of naloxone. The experiments examined the effects of these treatments on 1-week retention of an inhibitory avoidance task as well as on Y-maze discrimination reversal task. Higher similar results were obtained with both training tasks. Tables 3.2 through 3.4 show findings obtained in the discrimination reversal task. The memory-enhancing effect of posttraining naloxone (as indexed by increased error scores on the reversal training) was blocked by propranolol (a β-1,2-antagonist), atenolol (a β-1-antagonist), and zinterol (a β-2-antagonist), in doses that did not affect retention when administered alone. However, the α-antagonist prazosin did not block the effect of naloxone. Moreover, the effects of naloxone were not blocked by propranolol injected into either the cortex or caudate nucleus immediately above the amygdala injection site. These findings are consistent with other evidence (Introini-Collison & Baratti, 1986) suggesting that naloxone affects memory through influences selectively involving central β-adrenergic receptors.

To date, our experiments have been restricted to studies of the effects

54 James L. McGaugh

TABLE 3.2. Effects in rats of posttraining intraamygdala injection of buffer solution, of β-adrenergic antagonists (propranolol, $\beta_{1,2}$; atenolol, β_1; or zinterol, β_2), or of α-antagonist (prazosin, α_1) plus intraperitoneal naloxone or saline administration on retention in Y-maze discrimination reversal task.

Immediate intraamygdala injection (dose)	2-min posttraining intraperitoneal injection (dose)	Retention[a] (mean ± SE)	
Buffer	Saline	3.44	0.18
Buffer	Naloxone (3.0 mg/kg)	5.22*	0.32
Propranolol (0.3 μg)	Saline	3.88	0.55
Propranolol (0.3 μg)	Naloxone (3.0 mg/kg)	3.89	0.44
Buffer	Saline	3.48	0.27
Buffer	Naloxone (3.0 mg/kg)	5.29*	0.18
Atenolol (1.0 μg)	Saline	3.50	0.33
Atenolol (1.0 μg)	Naloxone (3.0 mg/kg)	3.43	0.37
Zinterol (0.3 μg)	Saline	3.30	0.60
Zinterol (0.3 μg)	Naloxone (3.0 mg/kg)	2.50	0.46
Prazosin (1.0 μg)	Saline	3.64	0.24
Prazosin (1.0 μg)	Naloxone (3.0 mg/kg)	5.73*	0.14

[a] Indexed by errors made on discrimination reversal training 1 week after training.
*Significantly different ($P <0.05$) from other groups.

of adrenergic and opiate agonists and antagonists administered either parenterally or directly into the amygdala, caudate putamen, or overlying cortex. Consequently, we do not yet know whether the kinds of interactions we have found are restricted to the amygdala. It it clear, however, from other recent studies that opiate, adrenergic, and noradrenergic systems also interact with other neurohormonal systems involved in memory modulation. Gallagher and her colleagues (Gallagher, Fanelli, & Bostock, 1985) have found, for example, that retention is altered by administration of opiate antagonists into the medial septal area, a cholinergic brain region. And, Borrell and his colleagues have shown that the memory-enhancing effects of vasopressin are blocked by adrenal demedullation and that epinephrine effects on memory require the

TABLE 3.3. Effects in rats of posttraining injection of propranolol into caudate putamen plus intraperitoneal saline or naloxone administration on retention in Y-maze discrimination reversal task

Immediate caudate-putamen injection (dose)	2-min posttraining intraperitoneal injection (dose)	Retention[a] (mean ± SE)	
Buffer	Saline	2.00	0.43
Buffer	Naloxone (3.0 mg/kg)	5.50*	0.26
Propranolol (0.3 μg)	Saline	2.08	0.29
Propranolol (0.3 μg)	Naloxone (3.0 mg/kg)	5.58*	0.26

[a] Indexed by errors made on discrimination reversal training 1 week after training.
* Significantly different ($P < 0.05$) from other groups.

TABLE 3.4. Effects in rats of posttraining injection of propanolol into cortex plus intraperitoneal injection of naloxone on retention in Y-maze discrimination reversal task

Immediate cortex injection (dose)	2-min posttraining intraperitoneal injection (dose)	Retention[a] (mean ± SE)	
Buffer	Saline	2.50	0.33
Buffer	Naloxone (3.0 mg/kg)	5.71*	0.13
Propranolol (0.3 μg)	Saline	2.71	0.40
Propranolol (0.3 μg)	Naloxone (3.0 mg/kg)	5.57*	0.17

[a] Indexed by errors made on discrimination reversal training 1 week after training.
* Significantly different ($P < 0.05$) from other groups.

presence of vasopressin (Borrell, del Cerro, Guaza, Zubiaur, & de Wied, 1985). Obviously, there is research yet to be done to gain understanding of the complexity of the interactions of neurohormonal systems in the modulation of memory storage.

Modulation and Consolidation

Considered together, the findings that retention is influenced by treatments affecting opiate and β-adrenergic receptors within the amygdala provide additional evidence for the view that the amygdaloid complex is part of a brain system involved in processing recently acquired information. It is possible that the amygdala modulates memory storage through influences on other brain regions involved in the processing of recent information as well as on regions involved as storage sites. The nuclei of the amygdaloid complex have extensive connections with other brain regions that are thought to have important functions in learning and memory (Coyle, Price, & DeLong, 1983; Mishkin et al., 1984; Price, 1981; Squire & Cohen, 1984). The basolateral nucleus has direct projections to the neocortex as well as to the dorsomedial thalamus and the subiculum. The basal nucleus of Meynert receives projections from both the central nucleus and the basal nucleus of the amygdala. The lateral nucleus influences the hippocampus via projections to the entorhinal cortex. The central nucleus also projects to the hypothalamus, midbrain, pons, and medulla. Thus, activation of amygdaloid nuclei can produce widespread influences in many brain regions.

It seems unlikely that the amygdala is involved as a locus of changes underlying memory. The fact that recent memory was relatively intact in Milner's patient H.M. (Milner, 1966) argues that the amygdala is not involved as a site of storage of recent memory. Moreover, the fact that H.M.'s remote memory was largely intact, as well as our finding that, in rats, bilateral lesions of the amygdala do not impair retention if the lesions are produced several days after training (Liang et al., 1982), indicates that the amygdala is not a site for storage of long-term memory. It seems most likely, on the basis of available data, that the amygdala is involved in the modulation and processing of recently acquired information in ways that alter the long-term storage of the information. The alteration might consist, as Mishkin, Malamut, and Bachevalier (1984) have suggested, by adding affective qualities to sensory stimulation, that is, by altering of the nature of the stored information. Or, as we have suggested (McGaugh, Liang, Bennett, & Sternberg, 1984), the amygdala might influence memory by modulating cellular storage mechanisms at storage sites. These possibilities are, of course, not mutually exclusive.

The basic assumption underlying research on memory storage, or consolidation, is that it is possible to alter memory processes in transition from temporary to permanent storage. In most studies that use posttraining treatments to alter retention, the treatments are administered within a few minutes or hours. Generally, the effectiveness of the treatments diminishes within several hours. In our experiments using intraamygdala injections, for example, we found that the treatments were ineffective when administered several hours following training. Comparable findings are obtained with posttraining systemic injections in studies of the memory-enhancing effects of drugs and hormones (McGaugh, 1973,1983).

Thus, it has seemed reasonable to assume that such treatments act by modulating posttraining processes underlying the establishment of the neural representation or trace of the training experience. This view requires a prior assumption that recent or short-term memory is based on a different mechanism from that subserving long-term memory. It might be, as Hebb (1949) suggested, that the lasting trace of an experience develops from the strengthening of synapses in the network of neurons that provide a basis for recent memory. Alternatively, it could be that recent and remote memory are based on different neural systems (McGaugh, 1968). This issue has been difficult to address experimentally.

Studies of retrograde amnesia have shown that, in rats and mice, retention can be impaired by treatments, such as electroconvulsive shock, administered even a day or two following training (Mah & Albert, 1973; Squire & Spanis, 1984). Such findings would seem to indicate that the temporary memory processes bridging the transition to lasting processes remain active for a rather extensive period—certainly longer than a few seconds or minutes—and that the processes of memory consolidation also occur over a relatively long period following training. Squire and his colleagues (Squire, Emanuel, Davis, & Deutsch, 1975) have found that human patients given ECT have retrograde amnesia for events occurring up to 2 years prior to the treatments. On the basis of these findings, Squire has suggested that consolidation may proceed for several years (Squire, 1986). Since it seems highly unlikely that temporary memory processes last for months or years, this stage of consolidation would appear to be somewhat different from that occurring shortly after training. The fact that older memories remain relatively intact following a series of ECT does suggest that the more recent memories are more susceptible to disruption. But the fact that patients eventually recover from the ECT-induced amnesia argues that the treatments do not disrupt the storage of information learned a year or two earlier. In contrast, evidence from animal studies indicates that amnesia induced by posttraining treatments does not lessen with time (McGaugh & Herz, 1972).

It does seem likely that memory consolidation, in the broader sense of continually increasing resistance to disruption of the availability of information, occurs, as Squire has suggested, ". . . over a significant portion of the lifetime of the memory" (Squire, 1986, p. 1616). It remains to be determined whether the storage of traces of experiences is subject to modulating influences of drugs and hormones over such long periods of time following the experiences leading to their establishment. Evidence to date indicates that such memory-modulating influences are effective only for a short period following training. These findings are consistent with the view that modulation of memory storage by endogenous processes activated by an experience occurs at an early stage in the consolidation of a memory trace (Gold & McGaugh, 1975; McGaugh et al., 1984), while subsequent changes in the stability of the trace seen at longer intervals of time following learning may result, as Squire (1986) has suggested, from continuous reorganization of the neural ensembles mediating stored information.

Research attempting to provide answers to the critical questions concerning memory discussed earlier in this chapter has, in recent years, provided the beginning of an understanding of the neurobiological processes enabling the creation and subsequent lingering of memory. I have emphasized here the view that the process of storing information must be examined in broad physiological perspective. Understanding of the physiology of memory will, it seems, require knowledge of how neurohormonal systems shape changes in the interactions among neurons that serve as the bases of our memories. Such knowledge can only be gained by interdisciplinary research aimed at integrating the facts of behavior and experience with those of cells and systems.

Acknowledgment. The research reported in this chapter was supported by USPHS Research Grant MH12526 and Contract N00014-84-k-0319 from the Office of Naval Research.

References

Agranoff, B.W. (1980). Biochemical events mediating the formation of short-term and long-term memory. In Y. Tsukada & B.W. Agranoff (Eds.), *Neurobiological basis of learning and memory*. New York: John Wiley.

Alkon, D.L. (1985). Conditioning-induced changes of hermissenda channels: Relevance to mammalian brain function. In N.M. Weinberger, J.L. McGaugh, & G. Lynch (Eds.), *Memory systems of the brain: Animal and human cognitive processes* (pp. 9–26). New York: Guilford Press.

Arbilla, S., & Langer, S.Z. (1978). Morphine and beta-endorphin inhibit release of noradrenaline from cerebral cortex but not of dopamine from rat striatum. *Nature, 271,* 559–561.

Bennett, C., Liang, K.C., McGaugh, J.L. (1985). Depletion of adrenal catecholamines alters the amnestic effect of amygdala stimulation. *Behavioural Brain Research, 15,* 83–91.

Bird, S.J., & Kuhar, M.J. (1977). Iontophoretic application of opiates to the locus coeruleus. *Brain Research, 122,* 523–533.

Bloch, V. (1970). Facts and hypotheses concerning memory consolidation. *Brain Research, 24, 561–575.*

Bloch, V., & Laroche, S. (1984). Facts and hypotheses related to the search for the engram. In G. Lynch, J.L. McGaugh, & N.M. Weinberger (Eds.), *Neurobiology of learning and memory* (pp. 249–260). New York: Guilford Press.

Bloom, F.E., & McGinty, J.F. (1981). Cellular distribution and function of endorphins. In J.L. Martinez, Jr., R.A. Jensen, R.B. Messing, H. Rigter, & J.L. McGaugh (Eds.), *Endogenous peptides and learning and memory processes* (pp. 199–230). New York: Academic Press.

Borrell, J., de Kloet, E.R. Versteeg, D.H.G. & Bohus, B. (1983). The role of adrenomedullary catecholamines in the modulation of memory by vasopressin. In E. Endroczi, D. de Wied, L. Angelucci, & V. Scapagnini (Eds.), *Integrative neurohumoral mechanisms: developments in neuroscience* (pp. 85–90). Amsterdam: Elsevier/North Holland.

Borrell, J., del Cerro, S., Guaza, C., Zubiaur, M., & de Wied, D. (1985). Interactions between adrenaline and neuropeptides on modulation of memory processes. In J.L. McGaugh (Ed), *Contemporary psychology: biological processes and theoretical issues* (pp. 17–36). Amsterdam: North Holland.

Bowman, R.E., Heironimus, M.P., & Harlow, H.F. (1979). Pentylenetetrazol: Posttraining injection facilitates discrimination learning in rhesus monkeys. *Physiological Psychology, 7,* 265–268.

Brunswik, E. (1943). Organismic achievement and environmental probability. *Psychological Review, 50,* 255–272.

Carrasco, M.A., Dias, R.D., Perry, M.L.S., Wofchuk, S.T., Souza, D.O., & Izquierdo, I. (1982). Effect of morphine, ACTH, epinephrine, Met-, Leu- and des-Tyr-Met-enkephalin on beta-endorphin-like immunoreactivity of rat brain. *Psychoneuroendocrinology, 7,* 229–234.

Castellano, C. (1975). Effects of morphine and heroin on discrimination learning and consolidation in mice. *Psychopharmacology, 42,* 235–242.

Castellano, C. (1981). Strain-dependent effects on naloxone on discrimination learning in mice. *Psychopharmacology, 73,* 291–295.

Cherkin, A. (1969). Kinetics of memory consolidation: Role of amnesic treatment parameters. *Proceedings of the National Academy of Sciences, 63,* 1094–1101.

Coyle, J.T., Price, D.L., & DeLong, M.R. (1983). Alzheimer's disease: A disorder of cortical cholinergic innervation. *Science, 219, 1184–1189.*

de Wied, D. (1984). Neurohypophyseal hormone influences on learning and memory processes. In G. Lynch, J.L. McGaugh & N.M. Weinberger (Eds.),

Neurobiology of learning and memory (pp. 289–312). New York: Guilford Press.

Duncan, C.P. (1949). The retroactive effect of electroshock on learning. *Journal of Comparative and Physiological Psychology, 42,* 32–44.

Ellis, M.E., Berman, R.F., & Kesner, R.P. (1983). Amnesia attenuation specificity: Propranolol reverses norepinephrine but not cycloheximide-induced amnesia. *Pharmacology, Biochemistry and Behavior, 19,* 733–736.

Ellis, M.E., & Kesner, R.P. (1981). Physostigmine and norepinephrine: Effects of injection into the amygdala on taste association. *Physiology and Behavior, 27,* 203–209.

Ellis, M.E., & Kesner, R.P. (1983). The noradrenergic system of the amygdala and aversive memory processing. *Behavioral Neuroscience, 97,* 399–415.

Fallon, J.H. (1981). Histochemical characterization of dopaminergic, noradrenergic and serotonergic projections to the amygdala. In Y. Ben-Ari (Ed), *The amygdaloid complex* (pp. 175–184). Amsterdam: Elsevier/North Holland.

Fanelli, R.J., Rosenberg, R.A., & Gallagher, M. (1985). Role of noradrenergic function in the opiate antagonist facilitation of spatial memory. *Behavioral Neuroscience, 99,* 751–755.

Gallagher, M. (1985). Re-viewing modulation of learning and memory. In N.M. Weinberger, J.L. McGaugh & G. Lynch (Eds.), *Memory systems of the brain: Animal and human cognitive processes* (pp. 311–334). New York: Guilford Press.

Gallagher, M., Fanelli, R.J., & Bostock, E. (1985). Opioid peptides: Their position among other neuroregulators of memory. In J.L. McGaugh (Ed), *Contemporary psychology: Biological processes and theoretical issues* (pp. 69–94). Amsterdam: North Holland.

Gallagher, M., & Kapp, B.S. (1978). Manipulation of opiate activity in the amygdala alters memory processes. *Life Sciences, 23,* 1973–1978.

Gallagher, M., Kapp, B.S., Pascoe, J.P., & Rapp, P.R. (1981). A neuropharmacology of amygdaloid systems which contribute to learning and memory. In Y. Ben-Ari (Ed), *The amygdaloid complex* (pp. 343–354). Amsterdam: Elsevier/North Holland.

Gallagher, M., Rapp, P.R., & Fanelli, R.J. (1985). Opiate antagonist facilitation of time-dependent memory processes: Dependence upon intact norepinephrine function. *Brain Research, 347,* 284–290.

Gerard, R.W. (1949). Physiology and psychiatry. *American Journal of Psychiatry, 106,* 161–173.

Gold, P.E., & McCarty, R. (1981). Plasma catecholamines: Changes after footshock and seizure-producing frontal cortex stimulation. *Behavioral and Neural Biology, 31,* 247–260.

Gold, P.E., & McGaugh, J.L. (1975). A single-trace, two process view of memory storage processes. In D. Deutsch & J.A. Deutsch (Eds.), *Short-term memory* (pp. 355–378). New York: Academic Press.

Gold, P.E., & van Buskirk, R. (1975). Facilitation of time-dependent memory processes with posttrial epinephrine injections. *Behavioral Biology, 13,* 145–153.

Gold, P.E., & van Buskirk, R. (1978). Posttraining brain norepinephrine concentrations: Correlation with retention performance of avoidance training with peripheral epinephrine modulation of memory processing. *Behavioral Biology, 23,* 509–520.

Gold, P.E., & Zornetzer, S.F. (1983). The mnemon and its juices: Neuro-modulation of memory processes. *Behavioral and Neural Biology, 38,* 151–189.

Greenough, W.T. (1985). The possible role of experience-dependent synaptogenesis, or synapses on demand, in the memory process. In N.M. Weinberger, J.L. McGaugh & G. Lynch (Eds.), *Memory systems of the brain: Animal and human cognitive processes* (pp. 77–106). New York: Guilford Press.

Hawkins, R.D., & Kandel, E.R. (1984). Steps toward a cell-biological alphabet for elementary forms of learning. In G. Lynch, J.L. McGaugh & N.M. Weinberger, (Eds.), *Neurobiology of learning and memory* (pp. 385–404). New York: Guilford Press.

Hebb, D.O. (1949). *The organization of behavior.* New York: John Wiley.

Hull, C.L. (1943). *Principles of behavior.* New York: Appleton-Century-Crofts.

Introini, I.B., McGaugh, J.L., & Baratti, C.M. (1985). Pharmacological evidence of a central effect of naltrexone, morphine and beta-endorphin and a peripheral effect of Met- and Leu-enkephalin on retention of an inhibitory response in mice. *Behavioral and Neural Biology, 44,* 434–446.

Introini-Collison, I.B., & Baratti, C.M. (1986). Opioid peptidergic systems may modulate the activity of β-adrenergic mechanisms during memory consolidation processes. *Behavioral and Neural Biology, 46,* 227–241.

Introini-Collison, I., & McGaugh, J.L. (1986). Epinephrine modulates long-term retention of an aversively motivated discrimination task. *Behavioral and Neural Biology, 45,* 358–365.

Introini-Collison, I., & McGaugh, J.L. (1987). Naloxone and beta-endorphin alter the effects of posttraining epinephrine on retention of an inhibitory avoidance response. *Psychopharmacology, 92,* 229–235.

Introini-Collison, I.B., Cahill, L., Baratti, C.M., McGaugh, J.L. (1987). Dynorphin induces task-specific impairment of memory. *Psychobiology, 15,* 171–174.

Izquierdo, I. (1979). Effect of naloxone and morphine on various forms of memory in the rat: Possible role of endogenous opiate mechanisms in memory consolidation. *Psychopharmacology, 66,* 199–203.

Izquierdo, I., & Dias, R.D. (1985). Influence on memory of posttraining and pretest injections of ACTH, vasopressin, epinephrine, or β-endorphin, and their interaction with naloxone. *Psychoneuronedocrinology, 10,* 165–172.

Izquierdo, I., & Graudenz, M. (1980). Memory facilitation by naloxone is due to release of dopaminergic and beta-adrenergic systems from tonic inhibition. *Psychopharmacology, 67,* 265–268.

Izquierdo, I., & McGaugh, J.L. (1985). Effect of a novel experience prior to training or testing on retention of an inhibitory avoidance response in mice: Involvement of an opioid system. *Behavioral and Neural Biology, 44,* 228–238.

Izquierdo, I., Souza, D.O., Dias, R.D., Carrasco, M.A., Wolkmer, N., Perry, M.L.S., & Netto, C.A. (1984). Effect of various behavioral training and testing procedures on brain B-endorphin-like immunoreactivity, and the possible role of B-enodorphin in behavioral regulation. *Psychoneuroendocrinology, 9,* 381–389.

John, E.R. (1967). *Mechanisms of memory* (p. 468). New York: Academic Press.

Kesner R.P. (1982). Brain stimulation: Effects on memory. *Behavioral and Neural Biology, 36,* 315–367.

Kety, S. (1972). Brain catecholamines, affective states and memory. In J.L. McGaugh, (Ed.), *The chemistry of mood, motivation and memory* (pp. 65–80). New York: Raven Press.

Korf, J., Bunney, B.S., & Aghajanian, G.K. (1974). Noradrenergic neurons: Morphine inhibition of spontaneous activity. *European Journal of Pharmacology, 25,* 165–169.

Lashley, K.S. (1930). Basic neural mechanisms in behavior. *Psychological Review, 37,* 1–24.

Lashley, K.S. (1950). In search of the engram. In *Symposium, Society of Experimental Biology* (pp. 454–482). Cambridge, MA: Cambridge University Press.

Lee, K., Schottler, F., Oliver, M., & Lynch, G. (1980). Brief bursts of high frequency stimulation produce two types of structural changes in rat hippocampus. *Journal of Neurophysiology, 44,* 247–258.

Liang, K.C., Bennett, C., & McGaugh, J.L. (1985). Peripheral epinephrine modulates the effects of posttraining amygdala stimulation on memory. *Behavioral Brain Research, 15,* 93–100.

Liang, K.C., Juler, R., & McGaugh, J.L. (1986). Modulating effects of posttraining epinephrine on memory: Involvement of the amygdala noradrenergic system. *Brain Research, 368,* 125–133.

Liang, K.C., & McGaugh, J.L. (1983). Lesions of the stria terminalis attenuate the enhancing effect of posttraining epinephrine on retention of an inhibitory avoidance response. *Behavioural Brain Research, 9,* 49–58.

Liang, K.C., McGaugh, J.L., Martinez, Jr., J.L., Jensen, R.A., Vasquez, B.J., & Messing, R.B. (1982). Posttraining amygdaloid lesions impair retention of an inhibitory avoidance response. *Behavioural Brain Research, 4,* 237–249.

Liang, K.C., Messing, R.B., & McGaugh, J.L. (1983). Naloxone attenuates amnesia caused by amygdaloid stimulation: The involvement of a central opioid system. *Brain Research, 271,* 41–49.

Llorens, C., Martres, M.P., Baudry, M., & Schwartz, J.C. (1978). Hypersensitivity to noradrenaline in cortex after chronic morphine: Relevance to tolerance and dependence. *Nature, 274,* 603–605.

Lynch, G. (1986). *Synapses, circuits, and the beginnings of memory* (p. 122). Cambridge, MA: MIT Press.

Lynch, G., & Baudry, M. (1984). The biochemistry of memory: A new and specific hypothesis. *Science, 224,* 1057–1063.

Mackintosh, N.J. (1983). *Conditioning and associative learning.* Oxford, England: Oxford University Press.

Mah, C.J., & Albert, D.J. (1973). Electroconvulsive shock-induced retrograde amnesia: An analysis of the variation in the length of the amnesia gradient. *Behavioral Biology, 9,* 517–540.

McGaugh, J.L. (1968). A multi-trace view of memory storage. In D. Bovet, F. Bovet-Nitti, and A. Oliverio (Eds.), *Recent advances in learning and retention.* (pp. 13–24). Rome: Roma Academia Nazionale dei Lincei.

McGaugh, J.L. (1973). Drug facilitation of learning and memory. *Annual Review of Pharmacology, 13,* 229–241.

McGaugh, J.L. (1983). Hormonal influences on memory. *Annual Review of Psychology, 34,* 297–323.

McGaugh, J.L., Bennett, M.C., Liang, K.C., Juler, R.G., and Tam, D. (1987). Retention-enhancing effects of posttraining epinephrine is not blocked by dexamethasone. *Psychobiology, 15,* 343–344.

McGaugh, J.L., & Gold, P.E. (1976). Modulation of memory by electrical stimulation of the brain. In M.R. Rosenzweig & E.L. Bennett (Eds.), *Neural mechanisms of learning and memory* (pp. 549–560). Cambridge, MA: MIT Press.

McGaugh, J.L., & Gold, P.E. (in press). Hormonal modulation of memory. In R.B. Brush & S. Levine (Eds.), *Psychoendocrinology.* New York: Academic Press.

McGaugh, J.L., & Herz, M.J. (1972). *Memory consolidation* (p. 204). San Francisco: Albion Publishing.

McGaugh, J.L., Introini-Collison, I.B., Juler, R.G., & Izquierdo, I. (1986). Stria terminalis lesions attenuate the effects of posttraining naloxone and b-endorphin on retention. *Behavioral Neuroscience, 100,* 839–844.

McGaugh, J.L., Liang, K.C., Bennett, C., & Sternberg, D.B. (1984). Adrenergic influences on memory storage: Interaction of peripheral and central systems. In G. Lynch, J.L. McGaugh & N.M. Weinberger (Eds.), *Neurobiology of learning and memory.* (pp. 313–333). New York: Guilford Press.

McGaugh, J.L., & Petrinovich, L. (1959). The effect of strychnine sulphate on maze-learning. *American Journal of Psychology, 72,* 99–102.

Menzel, R. (1983). Neurobiology of learning and memory: The honeybee as a model system. *Naturwissenschaften, 70,* 504–511.

Messing, R.B., Jensen, R.A., Martinez Jr., J.L., Spiehler, V.R., Vasquez, B.J., Soumireu-Mourat, B., Liang, K.C., & McGaugh, J.L. (1979). Naloxone enhancement of memory. *Behavioral and Neural Biology, 27,* 266–275.

Milner, B. (1966). Amnesia following operation on the temporal lobes. In C.W.M. Whitty & O.L. Zangwill (Eds.), *Amnesia* (pp. 109–133). London: Butterworths.

Mishkin, M., & Aggleton, J. (1981). Multiple functional contributions of the amygdala in the monkey. In Y. Ben-Ari (Ed), *The amygdaloid complex* (pp. 409–420). Amsterdam: Elsevier/North Holland.

Mishkin, M., Malamut, B., & Bachevalier, J. (1984). Memories and habits: Two neural systems. In G. Lynch, J.L. McGaugh & N.M. Weinberger (Eds.), *Neurobiology of learning and memory,* (pp. 65–77). New York: Guilford Press.

Montel, H., Starke, K., & Weber, F. (1974). Influence of morphine and naloxone on the release of noradrenaline from rat brain cortex slices. *Naunyn-Schmiedeberg's Archives of Pharmacology, 283,* 357–369.

Morris, R.G.M. (1984). Is the distinction between procedural and declarative memory useful with respect to animal models of amnesia? In G. Lynch, J.L. McGaugh & N.M. Weinberger (Eds.), *Neurobiology of learning and memory* (pp. 119–124). New York: Guilford Press.

Mueller, G.E., & Pilzecker, A. (1900) Experimentelle Beitrage zur Lehre vom Gedachtnis. Zeitschrift für Psychologie, 1, 1–288.

Murray, E.A., & Mishkin, M. (1985). Amygdala impairs crossmodal association in monkeys. *Science, 228,* 604–606.

Nakamura, S., Tepper, J.M., Young, S.J., Ling, N., & Groves, P.M. (1982). Noradrenergic terminal excitability: Effects of opioids. *Neuroscience Letters, 30,* 57–62.

Pepper, C.M., & Henderson, G.H. (1980). Opiates and opioid peptides hyperpolarize locus coeruleus neurons in vitro. *Science, 209,* 394–396.

Price, J.L. (1981). The efferent projections of the amygdaloid complex in the rat, cat and monkey. In Y. Ben-Ari (Ed), *The amygdaloid complex* (pp. 121–132). Amsterdam: Elsevier/North Holland.

Reisine, T.D., Heisler, S., Hook, V.Y.H., & Axelrod, J. (1983). Activation of B2-adrenergic receptors on mouse anterior pituitary tumor cells increases cyclic adenosine 3 prime: 5 prime-monophosphate synthesis and adrenocorticotropin release. *Journal of Neuroscience, 32,* 174–178.

Rosenzweig, M.R., & Bennett, E.L. (1976). Enriched environments: Facts, factors, and fantasies. In L. Petrinovich & J.L. McGaugh (Eds.), *Knowing, thinking and believing* (pp. 179–214). New York: Plenum.

Russell, W.R., & Nathan, P.W. (1946). *Traumatic amnesia. Brain, 69,* 280–300.

Sarter, M., & Markowitsch, H.J. (1985a). Involvement of the amygdala in learning and memory: A critical review, with emphasis on anatomical relations. *Behavioral Neuroscience, 99*(2), 342–380.

Sarter, M., & Markowitsch, H.J. (1985b). The amygdala's role in human mnemonic processing. *Cortex, 21,* 7–24.

Saunders, R.C., Murray, E.A., & Mishkin, M. (1984). Further evidence that the amygdala and hippocampus contribute equally to recognition memory. *Neuropsychologia, 22,* 786–796.

Scoville, W.B., & Milner, B. (1957). Loss of recent memory after bilateral hippocampal lesions. *Journal of Neurology, Neurosurgery, and Psychiatry, 20,* 11–21.

Squire, L., Emanuel, C.A., Davis, H.P., Deutsch, J.A. (1975). Inhibitors of cerebral protein synthesis: Dissociation of aversive and amnesic effects. *Behavioral Biology, 14,* 335–341.

Squire, L.R. (1986). Mechanisms of memory. *Science, 232,* 1612–1619.

Squire, L.R., & Cohen, N.J. (1984). Human memory and amnesia. In G. Lynch, J.L. McGaugh, & N.M. Weinberger (Eds.), *Neurobiology of learning and memory* (pp. 3–64). New York: Guilford Press.

Squire, L.R., & Spanis, C.W. (1984). Long gradient of retrograde amnesia in mice: Continuity with the findings in humans. *Behavioral Neuroscience, 98,* 345–348.

Squire, L.R., & Zola-Morgan, S. (1983). The neurology of memory: The case for correspondence between the findings of man and non-human primate. In J. Anthony Deutsch (Ed.), *Physiological basis of memory.* New York: Academic Press, 199–268.

Sternberg, D.B., Isaacs, K., Gold, P.E., & McGaugh, J.L. (1985). Epinephrine facilitation of appetitive learning: Attenuation with adrenergic receptor antagonists. *Behavioral and Neural Biology, 44,* 447–453.

Sternberg, D.B., Korol, D., Novack, G., McGaugh, J.L. (1986). Epinephrine-induced memory facilitation: Attenuation by adrenergic receptor antagonists. *European Journal of Pharmacology, 129,* 184–193.

Strahlendorf, H.K., Strahlendorf, J.C., & Barnes, C.D. (1980). Endorphin-mediated inhibition of locus coeruleus neurons. *Brain Research, 191,* 284–288.

Tanaka, M., Kohno, Y., Nakagawa, R., Ida, Y., Ilimori, K., Hoaki, Y., Tsuda, A., & Nagasaki, N. (1982a). Naloxone enhances stress-induced increases in noradrenaline turnover in specific brain regions in rats. *Life Sciences, 30,* 1663–1669.

Tanaka, M., Kohno, Y., Nakagawa, R., Ida, Y., Takeda, S., & Nagasaki, N. (1982b). Time-related differences in noradrenaline turnover in rat brain regions by stress. *Pharmacology, Biochemistry and Behavior, 16,* 315–319.

Thompson, R.F. (1986). The neurobiology of learning and memory. *Science, 233,* 941–947.

Tolman, E.C. (1932). *Purposive behavior in animals and men.* New York: Appleton-Century-Crofts.

Tolman, E.C., & Brunswik, E. (1935). The organism and the causal texture of the environment. *Psychological Review, 42,* 43–77.

U'Prichard, D.C., Reisine, T.D., Masion, S.F., Fibiger, H.C., & Yamamura, H.I. (1980). Modulation of rat alpha- and beta-adrenergic receptor populations by lesions in the dorsal noradrenergic bundle. *Brain Research, 187,* 143–154.

Walker, J.M., Khachaturian, H., & Watson, S.J. (1984). Some anatomical and physiological interactions among noradrenergic systems and opioid peptides. In M.G. Ziegler & C.R. Lake (Eds.), *Norepinephrine* (pp. 74–91). Balitmore: Williams and Wilkins.

Watson, J.B. (1919). *Psychology from the standpoint of a behaviorist.* Philadelphia: J.B. Lippincott.

Weil-Malherbe, H., Axelrod, J., & Tomchick, R. (1959). Blood-brain barrier for adrenalin. *Science, 129,* 1226–1228.

Weinberger, N.M., Diamond, D.M., & McKenna, T.M. (1984). Initial events in conditioning: Plasticity in the pupillomotor and auditory systems. In G. Lynch, J.L. McGaugh, & N.M. Weinberger (Eds.), *Neurobiology of learning and memory* (pp. 197–230). New York: Guilford Press.

Weinberger, N.M., Gold, P.E., Sternberg, D.B. (1984). Epinephrine enables Pavlovian fear conditioning under anesthesia. *Science, 223,* 605–607.

Young, W.S., Bird, S.J., & Kuhar, M.J. (1977). Iontophoresis of methionine-enkephalin in the locus coeruleus area. *Brain Research, 129,* 366–370.

Zola-Morgan, S., & Squire, L.R. (1985). Medial temporal lesions in monkeys impair memory on a variety of tasks sensitive to human amnesia. *Behavioral Neuroscience, 99,* 22–34.

Part II   Perspectives from Cognitive Psychology

CHAPTER 4

Domains of Memory

Ulric Neisser

It is especially appropriate to consider the topic of memory at a Williams College synposium convened in honor of G. Stanley Hall. Hall himself, who spent his boyhood in the Massachusetts countryside not far from Williamstown, would have been keenly interested in both what we are doing and where we are doing it. In the middle of a busy professional life, Hall took time out for an extended geographical exploration of his own memory. He revisited the farms and homes where he had grown up, rewalked many once-familiar paths and trails, and reexamined the surviving memorabilia of childhood. His own account of that exploration, published in an 1899 issue of *The Pedagogical Seminary,* is a charming evocation of 19th century boyhood. More than that, it is also a rich source of illustrations for hypotheses about memory. In particular, it is consistent with a hypothesis that I will explore in some detail below: that personal memory and sense of place are intimately connected. Although Hall knew nothing of "cognitive maps" or "spatial modules" in their modern forms, he knew perfectly well that familiar places bring back old memories.

Almost everyone agrees that the study of memory has made great progress in the last decade or two. Some of that progress has been in our understanding of the neuroanatomy and physiology underlying memory, but I will leave the discussion of neurophysiological discoveries to other contributors. My task here is to review the accomplishments of the modern *psychology* of memory, which are numerous and impressive in their own right. That review will be presented in the first part of this chapter. (The second part will be devoted to more speculative hypotheses.) I believe that the most important result of recent studies of memory—more fundamental than the discovery of any single phenomenon or the emergence of any particular theory—has been the development of a broader and more responsible view of our subject matter itself. And in this broader view, the everyday uses of memory and the memory demands of the natural and social environment have come to occupy an increasingly prominent place.

Since I am known to be an advocate of studying memory in natural contexts (Neisser, 1982), my decision to characterize recent research achievements in this manner may not come as a surprise. But in fact I do *not* mean that progress began only with the recent surge of interest in naturalistic methods, or with the even more recent focus on recall of the experiences of daily life. As we shall see, the first steps in the new direction were taken by psychologists who were and are firmly committed to standard laboratory procedures. What has happened to all of us— regardless of our preferred research paradigms—is not just that we have come to prefer different methods but that we have adopted a new notion of what kinds of things are remembered at all.

The New *Memoria*

Twenty years ago, the principal function of memory was assumed to be the storage of individual experiences and actions. The strings of specific words or syllables that subjects had to remember in the laboratory were intended as surrogates for the sequences of specific stimuli (or percepts, responses, or ideas, etc.) that they presumably remembered in the outside world. What has been developing lately is not just a new skepticism about the "representativeness" of such experiments, but a broader notion of what memory experiments should be trying to represent in the first place. People don't just remember specific occasions, it turns out: They also remember facts, skills, scripts, places, story grammars, and all sorts of other temporally and spatially extended entities. Borrowing a useful word from Reiff and Scheerer (1959), I will call all of these things *memoria*,[1] a term that simply means "things we remember." Different kinds of memoria define different domains of memory.

Semantic Memory

The extension of the study of memory to these new domains began to gather momentum in the early 1970s. The first significant manifestation was probably Endel Tulving's (1972) contrast between episodic and semantic memory. Episodic memory, for Tulving, was what we had been studying all along: memory for specific and personally experienced events (including, of course, stimulus presentations in standard experiments). Semantic memory, however, was something new. The term *semantic memory* had originally been introduced by Ross Quillian (1966) to refer to

---

[1] My definition of memoria is different from that of Reiff and Scheerer (1959), who meant something roughly like Tulving's (1972) semantic memory. I use it—by analogy with Tolman's (1932) "manipulanda" and "discriminanda"—to refer to objectively existing entities rather than to mental structures; in particular, to every sort of thing that is remembered.

stored knowledge about word meanings, as that knowledge might be organized for a language-using computer. Tulving broadened it to include every kind of stable, nonpersonal fact that people could know—that the chemical formula for salt is NaCl, for example, or that summers are hot in Katmandu.

Most cognitive psychologists today, including Tulving himself (1985), think of semantic memory as an information-processing system in the head. Many specific models of that system have been proposed, most of them based on hypothetical networks of labeled associations. In my view, however, the vitality of Tulving's concept does not derive from any of these models—not even from his own. Tulving's major contribution was to introduce an entirely new domain into the study of memory, that is, to recognize the existence of a vast new class of memoria. People don't just remember experiences, they also remember *facts*.

Schematic Structures

It was also in the 1970s that Bartlett's old term *schema* began to acquire the new popularity that it continues to enjoy today. The first modern schema theorists (Mandler & Johnson, 1977; Rumelhart, 1975) were concerned with memory for stories just as Bartlett (1932) had been. Their research suggested that people have stable mental representations (*schemata*) of how a typical story is organized. Since then, a number of different models of these mental representations have been proposed. Once again, I believe that the major contribution of this work does not lie in the formulation of any particular theoretical model; rather, it lies in the recognition of the new domain itself. Every culture has stories. Taken together, those stories share a set of structural characteristics that is somewhat analogous to the grammar of a particular language. This *story grammar,* which transcends the details of any particular story or myth, is apparently something that people can remember. What's more, having this abstract entity in mind helps us to understand and remember particular stories as we encounter them.

Before extending my list of new memoria still further, it may be wise to restate the main difference between the way I am describing these developments and the interpretations of other theorists. The researchers who introduced the new developments—Quillian and Tulving in the case of semantic memory; David Rumelhart, Jean Mandler, and others for story grammars—thought of themselves as engaging in two roughly parallel enterprises. First, they were introducing (or reintroducing) a new subject matter into psychology: the study of memory for *facts* and *stories*, respectively. Second, they were developing theories to explain how that subject matter is actually remembered. It was with this theoretical end in view that they postulated the new mental structures that have now become so familiar—semantic memory, story schema, and so on. Because the formulation of mental models is widely supposed to be the principal aim of cognitive psychology, the development of those concepts has often been taken as the more important achievement. It seems to me, however, that the lasting contribution may have been the introduction of the new memoria themselves. Psychologists of the year 2000 will probably be working with brand new mental models, but I would wager good money that they will still be studying memory for facts and for stories.

I am not the first psychologist to try to distinguish among different domains of learning or memory. Edward Tolman, for example, listed six different kinds of learning in 1949. As one might expect, his list included such Tolmanian categories as "field expectancies," "drive discriminations," and "cathexes." Fifteen years later Arthur Melton (1964) proposed a set that included "conditioning," "rote verbal learning," and "conceptualization." Unfortunately, neither Tolman nor Melton was much concerned with what people actually learn and remember in the course of a day. Except for an occasional hazy intuition, their proposals made no reference to ecological considerations of any kind. That was not their aim; instead, they hoped to clarify the processes involved in familiar laboratory paradigms such as maze learning, classical conditioning, and concept attainment. Because lists of this kind become irrelevant when we have lost interest in the paradigms themselves, no one cites them today.

It seems to me that it is almost impossible to be right about cognitive processes without first having a good analysis of the information on which those processes must operate. This principle is particularly obvious in the case of perception (Neisser, 1977), but I believe that it is equally useful in the study of memory. Certainly it applies to what students of animal behavior call "learning": A generation of ethologists and behavioral biologists have established that point beyond any possible doubt. Their work has made it exquisitely clear that we must understand the fit between any given behavior and its environment before we can hope to understand the internal processes underlying the behavior itself. The list of memoria presented here is intended to help move the study of memory in a somewhat similar direction—or rather, to suggest that such a movement has been well under way (though not always explicitly recognized) for more than a decade.

Stories were only the beginning. Analogous schema concepts were soon developed in many other domains. It has been suggested that there are schemata for scenes (Mandler & Parker, 1976), for the self (Markus, 1977), for goal-directed events (Lichtenstein & Brewer, 1980), for other people (Fiske & Linville, 1980), for rooms (Brewer & Treyens, 1981), and so on. The fate of these theories themselves is still in doubt. (It is not obvious that postulating, say, room schemata adds much to the observation that one can remember rooms.) What is *not* in doubt is that we do remember such things. Although rooms and people and such are not episodes or momentary experiences—they exist over extended periods of time and have enduring properties—they must be included on any list of currently accepted memoria.

Scripts

Scripts (Schank & Abelson, 1975) came along at about the same time as schemata. Everyone's cultural experience includes certain familiar sequences of events. In America, visiting a restaurant or going to the doctor are familiar examples. In the mid-1970s psychologists began to explore (and students of artificial intelligence began to model) people's knowledge of these sequences and to define a class of mental representations for them called "scripts." Initial accounts of those scripts ("first you sit down at a table, then you consult the menu, then you give your order to the waiter or waitress. . .") had an almost ethnographic flavor: Each script was a description of the sequence of actions that usually takes place in a certain situation. Again, it seems to me that the most important contribution of the early script theorists was just to treat these event sequences as memoria in their own right. Because the study of scripts has prospered, no one now doubts that routines, both personal and cultural, are among the things we remember.

In the case of scripts, there has been a further development. A series of important studies by Katherine Nelson and her associates (see chap. 7 in this volume) have shown that young children are quite good at remembering such routines. Indeed, they often know the routines better than they remember even the most recent of the individual episodes in which a given routine is exemplified. This finding, too, is usually described in terms of mental representations. In particular, the child is assumed to convert the stored memories of several single episodes into a general script that represents their common features. I would prefer to describe the same phenomenon in a more ecological way: The memories of young children are more closely attuned to one class of objectively existing memoria (repeated sequences) than they are to another (unique episodes).

This way of describing scripts may seem rather odd. Is a repeated sequence really something that exists objectively in the world? Although we find it natural enough to treat a single time-bounded event as something that really happens, we do not always extend the same courtesy to sequences of such events. Psychologists, especially, tend to assume that a series of separate episodes does not exist in its own right, that it only has whatever unity is conferred on it by someone's mental representation. This is not a necessary assumption. From the ecological point of view, the single concrete event and the sequence of events are both things that happen in the world. Either of them can be selected as an object of memory or of thought.

An example from a different domain may help to clarify the notion that sequences of events can be objects of cognition in their own right. It seems likely that young children notice and learn reduplicated syllables ("ma-ma") more easily than they would notice and learn the component syllables occurring alone ("ma"). It would be awkward to explain such a difference in terms of the integration of two separate "ma- representations," one stored in short-term memory and the other perceived a moment later. It seems more natural to assume that the repetitive stimulus structure ("ma-ma") is picked up in its own right. I am simply suggesting that something similar occurs—over a much longer span of time—when the child notices a repeated routine.

School Learning

Another important recent development is also worth mentioning. Cognitive psychology has finally begun to consider a class of memoria that we should have been studying all along: material learned in school and college. Some years ago (Neisser, 1978) I complained rather vigorously about the absence of research on this important problem. How can we be so indifferent (I asked rhetorically) about whether our students remember what we teach them? Happily, it turned out that not everyone was as indifferent as I had supposed. Harry Bahrick's (1984) careful and statistically sophisticated study of memory for Spanish has now shed a good deal of light on this problem. Indeed, Bahrick's research has produced a surprising discovery: Some of the material learned in Spanish classes is essentially immune to forgetting! Retest scores do decline for the first few years after learning, but after that they level off and nothing more is forgotten for decades.

In his published article, Bahrick (1984) described this discovery in terms of the fate of individual "responses." After enough practice, some learned responses are said to move into *permastore*—a sort of special forgetting-proof state. I prefer to put it differently (Neisser, 1984). Students of Spanish do not merely learn responses; they acquire structured knowledge. Aspects of that structure that are sufficiently unique (for a given subject) will suffer little interference in subsequent years because there is nothing with which they can be confused. Some aspects of the cognitive structure of Spanish were evidently still represented in the minds of the subjects at the time of Bahrick's retest. These surviving "mental representations" were residues of the much richer knowledge structures that the subjects had acquired when they first took Spanish. (Reassuringly, students who had received A's in their courses remembered substantially more than those who had earned lower grades!) The originally acquired knowledge structures, in turn, were at least rough representations of what I take to have been the real memoria in Bahrick's study, that is, the structure of the Spanish language and its relation to English.

Generic Memories and Skills

My survey of the new memoria is not complete even yet, but it is worth noting that those considered up to this point have one characteristic in common. All of them are based on *repeated* rather than *unique* experiences. People discover story grammars by hearing many different stories, they acquire the restaurant script by going to many different restaurants (or to one restaurant many times), they learn Spanish by attending many classes and doing lots of homework. What is remembered in these cases is an underlying structure that has become "manifest" on different occasions; the occasions themselves may not be recalled at all. Typically we do not remember the individual stories from which we learned the grammar, the restaurant experiences from which we learned the script, or the class meetings in which we learned the Spanish. Generic memories can persist even when the individual episodes that gave rise to them have been entirely forgotten.

A very similar effect has recently been obtained under laboratory conditions by Watkins and Kerkar (1985). They conducted a list-learning experiment in which some words were presented twice, in two different colors of print. Subjects often remembered that a given word had occurred (generic memory) without remembering either one of its colors of presentation (which would have been a specific-occasion memory). Moreover, the level of generic recall was so high that it could not have been based on just the recall of either specific presentation alone, or even of both of them. In short, the subjects were not remembering the *experience* of seeing a given word; they remembered the *fact* that the word had been on the list.

Memory for generic characteristics rather than for specific occasions is typical of still another currently important domain: acquisition of skill. I cannot count motor skills as entirely "new" memoria; psychologists have been studying them too long for that. Nevertheless, the same principle applies. Bartlett said it as well as anyone:

Suppose I am making a stroke in a quick game, such as tennis or cricket. . . . When I make the stroke I do not, as a matter of fact, produce something absolutely new, and I never merely repeat something old." (Bartlett, 1932, pp. 201–202)

Recent findings have highlighted the generic character of skill learning in a new and dramatic way. I refer, of course, to the discovery that amnesic patients can acquire an entirely new skill—or can learn a new piece on the piano—without any episodic memory of the occasions on which that learning occurred (Hirst, 1982; Starr & Phillips, 1970). Moreover, the independence of accumulated skill from cumulating occasions is not restricted to motor activity alone. It also appears in more strictly perceptual skills such as reading mirror-reversed text (Cohen &

Squire, 1980). This discovery, which was made simply by studying the memories of amnesics in a wider range of domains, is already beginning to change our conceptions of amnesia in a fundamental way.

Similar phenomena have recently been demonstrated in entirely normal subjects. In Larry Jacoby's ingenious experiments (Jacoby, 1988), a subject who fails to recognize that a given word was among those recently presented on a memory list (i.e., who seems to have forgotten the word entirely) may nevertheless exhibit behavior that shows effects of the word's earlier presentation. The subject may *see* the word more easily than control words when it is briefly flashed, for example, or *think of it* more readily in a fragment-completion experiment. These studies use the traditional materials and paradigms of the psychology of memory, but they are very important. They imply that the "personal index" of an experience—the fact that you yourself saw a given word on a given occasion—is separable from other memoria that were noted at the same time and can have an independent fate.

Autobiographical Memory

Such findings suggest that we may have to reexamine the links between the recall of individual life experiences and other kinds of memory. So far, that reexamination has only begun, and it is sure to produce a good many surprises in the years ahead. One especially interesting link of this kind is the relation between memory for an individual episode and the *contexts* of that episode, both temporal and spatial. Things do not happen to us in isolation; they are embedded in larger activities and they occur at particular places. One way or another, the rest of this chapter will be primarily concerned with those embeddings.

To begin with, any individually remembered event is embedded in our life experience as a whole, in what is called "personal" or "autobiological" memory. David Rubin's recently published book (*Autobiographical Memory*, 1986) is only the latest sign of an interest that has been increasing for over a decade. In that time we have developed a number of new systematic methods for the study of personal memory, especially including diary studies (Barclay & DeCooke, 1988; Linton, 1975,1982; Wagenaar, 1986) and the cued recall of personal events (Crovitz & Shiffman, 1974 Robinson, 1976). The use of these methods has led to significant discoveries. Rather than reviewing those findings, however, I will consider a preliminary issue that grows directly out of the analysis presented earlier in this chapter: What are the *memoria* of autobiographical memory?

At one level the answer is given by definition: Autobiographical memory is memory for "the events of one's own life." But what shall we count in that category? "Hearing the news that President Kennedy had been shot" was unquestionably an event, but how shall we treat more extended experiences like "going to college" or "the year we spent in

California?'' On the evening when I presented this address to my fellow conferees in Williamstown, everyone in the room was experiencing the G. Stanley Hall Symposium on Memory. Conferences are ''events''; they are certainly among the kinds of things included in autobiographical memory. But a conference is a complex event: A whole host of other events—talks, discussions, dinners, and many other things—were nested ''inside'' the Williamstown meeting. This is not an unusual situation; events almost always have a nested structure (Gibson, 1979).

The memoria of autobiographical memory include many events that are just as long as conferences, and many others that are longer still. In a recent study, Lawrence Barsalou (1988) has found that extended memories are both common and important. He simply asked a number of undergraduates to tell him—in 5 minutes or so—what they had done the previous summer. In the upshot, only 21% of the subjects' responses described specific events like seeing a play or going on a picnic. They were much more likely to summarize recurrent patterns of activity—''I watched a lot of TV''—or to report extended events—''I worked there for 2 weeks'' or ''I went on a diet.'' Indeed, other subjects who were explicitly asked to confine their responses to brief concrete events found it very difficult to do so. The request appeared to disturb their normal mode of recall. In short, brief individual life experiences are remembered, but they may have no unique and privileged status in memory. The study of autobiographical memory has forced us to realize that generic events, extended situations, and typical patterns of behavior are remembered too (see Brewer, 1986, for more on this point.)

The G. Stanley Hall Conference was a real event, taking place in Williamstown in the first week of October 1986. My talk was a real event too, ''nested'' in the conference. We perceive real events at many levels of analysis. There are conferences, talks, and sentences; personal relationships, special evenings, and pregnant moments; graduate school years, particular seminars, memorable remarks. Events have a hierarchical structure, and it seems likely that our memories of those events are organized in some similar way. On this hypothesis, the mental representations of events would be functionally nested in one another just like the events themselves: We have memories of conferences as well as memories of particular talks given at those conferences and of particular ideas expressed in those talks. Lossely speaking, at least, the structure of autobiographical memory seems to be hierarchical.

Spatial Orientation and Memory

It seems to me that we experience the temporal nesting of events somewhat in the way that we experience the analogous geographical nesting of *places*. Places, too, are defined at many embedded levels of analysis. J.J. Gibson put it this way:

A *place* is a location in the environment as contrasted with a point in space. . . . Whereas a point must be located with reference to a coordinate system, a place can be located by its inclusion in a larger place (for example, the fireplace in the cabin by the bend of the river in the Great Plains. (Gibson, 1979, p. 34)

It seems, then, that the structure of events and of places (i.e., of ecologically defined time and space) can be described in rather similar terms. Our *experiences* of these two domains also have much in common. Although there are important differences, we think of events as nested in a way that is somewhat analogous to the way we think of places as nested. Why is this so? There are at least three possibilities. First, of course, the similarity between these two kinds of cognitive structure may just be a coincidence. (After all, any two entities are bound to have at least some similarities.) Second, the similarity of the two cognitive domains may just follow from a deeper similarity between the corresponding real domains: Since both times and places really have nested structures, we naturally think of them in that way. That is an entirely plausible view, and I will not be dismayed if it turns out to be adequate, that is, if no additional hypothesis about cognitive structure is necessary. Nevertheless, the rest of this chapter will explore a third possibility: that the similarity between personal memory and sense of place may arise from their common use of a single underlying mechanism. On this hypothesis, people have adapted a neural/psychological system originally evolved for purposes of spatial orientation to a new purpose, as the fundamental organizing structure for personal memory.[2]

Human beings, like many other animal species, are very good at finding their way around. But that ability—*spatial orientation*, as it is usually called—necessarily involves the storage of lots of highly structured information. It follows, then, that we can remember a lot about places. Because places are intrinsically quite different from the other memoria we have considered, and because spatial orientation seems more or less independent of other kinds of mental activity, I will treat place as a separate domain of memory. What do we know about it?

Cognitive Maps

The domain of place seems to include several distinct types of memoria. One of these, obviously, is the permanent layout of the environment itself. All of us can find our way around our own homes and home towns, as well as a good many other places. There is now an enormous literature on this ability and on its development (Evans, 1980; Lynch,1960; Pick & Acredolo, 1983). Much of that literature assumes that spatial or orientation depends on special mental representations called *cognitive maps* (O'Keefe & Nadel, 1978; Tolman, 1948); the term *image* is occasionally

---

[2] I provide a more extensive justification of this hypothesis in Neisser (1987).

used in the same sense (Boulding, 1956; Lynch, 1960). Unfortunately, such terms inevitably suggest that people and animals find their way around by aiming some kind of inner eye at some kind of inner display. That doesn't seem right, even introspectively. While I may *sometimes* experience something rather like a mental image of a map, such images are by no means constantly present as I move purposefully about. I usually look at the environment itself, not at an internal representation of it. The model of an individual examining a map does not seem plausible for an ability that is so directly driven by stimulus information, or for one so widely distributed in the animal kingdom and so phylogenetically old. For this reason, my own use of the term cognitive map (Neisser, 1976) has always been carefully qualified. I have suggested that we should not use the term to denote some hypothetical inner object of regard, but to stand for the "orienting schemata" that function to direct our pickup of environmental information. Whatever the value of this distinction,[3] there is no doubt that human beings retain impressive amounts of spatial information.

Developmental and Comparative Studies

We remember not only the permanent layout of the environment—the positioning of furniture in a room, the rooms and doors and hallways of a house, the streets and rivers and bridges and buildings of a city—but also the temporary positions of objects *in* that environment. This ability appears very early. It can be demonstrated in 2-year-olds, using an experimental task devised by Judy DeLoache and her collaborators (DeLoache & Brown, 1978; DeLoache, Cassidy, & Brown, 1985). In this task, the child watches an experimenter hide a favorite toy and then, after a delay, must retrieve it. The results are clear: The children can easily remember a hidden toy's location overnight, and often for very much longer.

It seems likely that DeLoache's young subjects could have remembered even more than was required of them in these experiments. I must turn to the animal literature here, for lack of relevant data on our own species. (There are surprisingly few human studies of memory for the locations of real things in the real environment, and I know of none that have systematically varied the number of stimuli as well as the delay.) Emil Menzel has shown, for example, that a chimpanzee who has just watched an experimenter hide up to 16 food items (the experimenter carries the chimp around during the hiding process) can then go and find

---

[3] Sholl (1987) has recently demonstrated that both kinds of cognitive maps may exist. The mental structures that underlie spatial orientation are sometimes imagined maps and sometimes orienting schemata, depending on both the subject's experience and the task at hand.

every one of them (Menzel, 1973; Menzel, 1987). The chimp does not do this by retracing the experimenter's steps in a rote manner, but by following a new "least effort" path from one hiding place to another. Larry Sherry (1987) has shown that the marsh tit, a bird found in Great Britain, keeps track of over a hundred different locations where it has cached bits of food—in stumps, in holes in trees, and so on. The birds do not return to a cache once it has been emptied.

Although these findings might be taken to mean that chimpanzees and marsh tits have very good memories, that is not quite the interpretation I propose. Such performances probably do not depend so much on a general memory system as on one that is highly specialized for spatial orientation. Such a system necessarily stores a good deal of information about the permanent environmental layout. Why not suppose that it preserves information about more temporary locations as well? This would mean that the marsh tit knows that there is a seed in a given hole in much the same way as it knows that the hole is in a particular tree, or for that matter that the tree itself stands in a certain position in the grove. Similarly, your own memory of where the aspirin bottle stands in your medicine cabinet (temporary location) depends on the same spatial system by virtue of which you can find the medicine cabinet itself in the bathroom (permanent layout). Indeed, it is the same system by which you find your way to the bathroom when you are elsewhere in the house, and to the house when you are elsewhere in town. Spatial memory, like the environment itself, is replete with nested structure.

The Mnemonic Use of Places

It is a very effective way to store information. Indeed, it is so effective that people have been using it as a deliberate mnemonic device for some 2,000 years. The famous *method of loci,* in which arbitrary lists of items are remembered by mentally "placing" images of them at successive locations along a well-known path, is just a way of getting the spatial system to do a nonspatial job. We can remember indefinitely many items in this way, because our spatial systems are capable of learning about indefinitely many real layouts to an arbitrary level of detail. So far as anyone now knows, there is no capacity limitation on this kind of learning.

The method of loci is sometimes described as a matter of "associating" objects with places—a usage so convenient that I occasionally adopt it myself. But what is involved is not an association in the classical sense of that word—a one-point bond between two otherwise unrelated items. Objects are not merely "associated" with locations. They are *in* particular locations, in a spatial sense that implies that they have some particular position and orientation, whether that position is actually remembered or not. Similarly, our knowledge of the layout of the environment is not a matter of associations between items but of structured, *nested* spatial relationships. It is just such relationships to which the spatial cognitive system is tuned, and which it enables us to remember.

Objects are not the only things linked with places. Even more impressive, perhaps, are the memories of events and feelings that often come flooding back when we revisit some once-familar spot. Dozens of such experiences are recorded in Hall's memoir of revisiting his boyhood Massachusetts homes—visits that he undertook as an explicit mnemonic exercise. At a farm where he had spent a number of months each year from age 8 to 13, for example, Hall had this experience:

On entering the cellar, the first though was of a pitcher of cider I had fallen with and broken; the next of an old apple parer, the next of a relative I had often heard of, who long ago fell down the stairs of the old house and broke her neck; then of a musk rat I once caught at the mouth of the cellar drain, next of. . . . (Hall 1899, p. 499)

Revisiting another farm where Hall had lived earlier and longer (from age 2 1/2 to 11 1/2) produced a great variety of recollections, especially of memorable moments:

Very many square rods of ground where I had mowed and raked I could recall nothing of, while another no better marked spot shone out like a star of the first magnitude as a place where I had caught a mink, built a willow booth, slid in winter, learned to skate, pushed over my little brother, had a long fight after school with another boy, made my first effort to smoke, built a bonfire, played fox and geese in winter, etc." (p. 490)

Some of the memories aroused at this earlier farm were generic rather than particular: "There was a hallow maple tree where I fancied monkeys lived, and I took pleasure in hunting for them there" (p. 493) evidently refers to a repeated experience, as does "where I . . . slid [sledded] in winter." Moreover, many of them were primarily memories of mood and feeling tone: "A kind of open glen in the woods, for instance, recalled nothing but gave a very extraordinary and unwonted sense of pleasure and of previousness" (p. 491). Or again "A crooked tree seemed tense, dissatisfied, unhappy, and another with low branches always invited us to climb and took pleasure in having us in its limbs" (p. 494).

Almost everyone has had experiences like these; they show that remembered events and feelings, like remembered objects, can be vividly associated with places in the environment. Taken by themselves, they do not necessarily indicate that the spatial system has a unique role in memory; perhaps it merely provides a convenient set of distinctive and dissimilar stimuli, that is, different places, to which memories can be associated. After all, floods of memory can also be released by other kinds of stimuli: by the taste of the "petite madeleine" in Proust's famous example, or in Hall's case by objects familiar from childhood:

. . . the little red and lettered cup, my penny banks, a curious old firkin—of a good many of these I could write a brief treatise were I to characterize all the incidents and especially the feelings which they brought to mind." (p. 506)

If the spatial system plays a special role in memory, that role is not merely to mediate the recollections that come to mind so readily in old and familiar places. On the contrary, it may be to mediate recall on occasions when we are safely at home sitting in our own armchair and have no travel plans at all. Even then we can remember distant places, coherently nested one within the other—say, the kitchen of a house we lived in on a certain street in a distant city. Similarly we can recall distant events, and they are nested in much the same way—say, the look she gave you at a certain moment, in that memorable conversation long ago when you finally understood one another.

Future Directions

Is it likely that this hypothesis is true—that spatial and autobiographical memory are linked in some fundamental way? I must admit that there is no direct psychological evidence for the hypothesis as yet. (Positive correlations between spatial skill and some kind of nonspatial recall would be relevant evidence, but so far no such correlations have been reported.[4]) On the other hand, certain clinical and neurological findings may be relevant. As a complete amateur in neuropsychology, I cannot help being impressed with how frequent the *hippocampus* turns up in discussions of both space and memory. The evidence that this subcortical structure is critical for spatial orientation was already strong in 1978, when O'Keefe and Nadel published *The Hippocampus as a Cognitive Map*; so far as I know, that evidence is even stronger today. The evidence that it also plays a major role in autobiographical memory begins with the famous case of H.M., the unfortunate man who has been almost completely unable to remember any new personal experiences since the two sides of his hippocampus were surgically removed many years ago. That evidence has also become stronger, so far as I know. But the fit is not an obvious one: H.M. apparently does not have the acute problems with orientation in familiar environments that this hypothesis seems to require. So far, then, we cannot tell whether the similarity between the nested structures of spatial knowledge and personal memory reflects their

---

[4] Cheryl Lorenz and I have recently completed a factor-analytic study of individual differences in spatial ability (Lorenz & Neisser, 1986). We found several factors relevant to orientation and spatial memory in the normal environment (interestingly, these ecological factors were unrelated to scores on traditional paper-and-pencil tests of "visualization"), but no correlations between these factors and measures of personal memory.

dependence on a common neural structure. I look forward to the time when the progress of neuropsychology has made it possible to answer this question.

This is an auspicious time in the history of the study of memory. The opening up of half a dozen new kinds of memoria to systematic research has coincided with several other significant advances, for example, new methods for the study of memory in infancy (cf. chap. 7 in this volume). And thanks to the astonishing rate of progress in contemporary neuroscience, we are beginning to develop a whole array of new hypotheses about the biological basis of memory—hypotheses that may soon lead us to unravel one of the brain's most tangled puzzles (cf. chap. 2 and 3). If we are lucky, we may soon find that some of these movements are beginning to converge, for example, as in my conjecture about personal knowledge, spatial memory, and the hippocampus. But even if we are not that lucky, we can still look forward to continued rapid progress in all areas of memory represented in the symposium, progress that will bring the understanding of memory as a whole steadily closer.

References

Bahrick, H.P. (1984). Semantic memory content in permastore: Fifty years of memory for Spanish learned in school. *Journal of Experimental Psychology: General, 113,* 1–29.

Barclay, C.R., & DeCooke, P.A. (1988). Ordinary everyday memories: some of the things selves are made of. In Neisser, U., & Winograd, E. (Eds.). *Real events remembered: Ecological and traditional approaches to the study of memory.* New York: Cambridge University Press.

Barsalou, L.W. (1988). The content and organization of autobiographical memories. In Neisser, U., & Winograd, E. (Eds.), *Real events remembered: Ecological and traditional approach to the study of memory.* New York: Cambridge University Press.

Bartlett, F.C. (1932). *Remembering.* Cambridge, England: Cambridge University Press.

Boulding, K.E. (1956). *The image.* Ann Arbor, MI: University of Michigan Press.

Brewer, W.F. (1986). What is autobiographical memory? In D.C. Rubin (Ed.), *Autobiographical memory.* Cambridge, England: Cambridge University Press.

Brewer, W.S., & Treyens, J.C. (1981). Role of schemata in memory for places. *Cognitive Psychology, 13,* 207–230.

Cohen, N.J., & Squire, L.R. (1980). Preserved learning and retention of pattern-analyzing skill in amnesia: Dissociation of knowing how and knowing that. *Science, 210,* 207–210.

Crovitz, H.F., & Schiffman, H. (1974). Frequency of episodic memories as a function of their age. *Bulletin of the Psychonomic Society, 4,* 517–518.

DeLoache, J.S., & Brown, A.L. (1979). Looking for big bird: Studies of memory in very young children. *Quarterly Newsletter of the Laboratory of Comparative Human Cognition, 1,* 53–57.

DeLoache, J.S., Cassidy, D.J., & Brown, A.L. (1985). Precursors of mnemonic strategies in very young children's memory. *Child Development, 56,* 125–137.

Evans, G.W. (1980). Environmental cognition. *Psychological Bulletin, 88*, 259–287.

Fiske, S.T., & Linville, P.W. (1980). What does the schema concept buy us? *Personality and Social Psychology Bulletin, 6*, 543–557.

Gibson, J.J. (1979). *The ecological approach to visual perception.* Boston: Houghton Mifflin.

Hall, G.S. (1899). Note on early memories. *Pedagogical Seminary, 6*, 485–512.

Hirst, W. (1982). The amnesic syndrome: Descriptions and explanations. *Psychological Bulletin, 91*, 435–460.

Jacoby, L.L. (1988). Memory observed and memory unobserved. In Neisser, U., & Winograd, E. (Eds.), *Real events remembered: Ecological and traditional approaches to the study of memory.* New York: Cambridge University Press.

Lichtenstein, E.H., & Brewer, W.F. (1980). Memory for goal-directed events. *Cognitive Psychology, 12*, 412–455.

Linton, M. (1975). Memory for real-world events. In Norman, D.A., & Rumelhart, D.E. (Eds.), *Explorations in cognition.* New York: W.H. Freeman.

Linton, M. (1982). Transformations of memory in everyday life. In Neisser, U. (Ed.), *Memory observed: remembering in natural contexts.* New York: W.H. Freeman.

Lorenz, C.A., & Neisser, U. (1986). *Ecological and psychometric dimensions of spatial ability* (Emory Cognition Project report #10). Atlanta: Emory University Psychology Department.

Lynch, K. (1960). *The image of the city.* Cambridge, MA: MIT Press.

Mandler, J.M., & Johnson, N.S. (1977). Remembrances of things parsed: Story structure and recall. *Cognitive Psychology, 9*, 111–151.

Mandler, J.M., & Parker, R.E. (1976). Memory for descriptive and spatial information in complex pictures. *Journal of Experimental Psychology: Human Learning and Memory, 2*, 38–48.

Markus, H. (1977). Self-schemata and processing information about the self. *Journal of Personality and Social Psychology, 35*, 63–78.

Melton, A.W. (1964). *Categories of human learning.* New York: Academic Press.

Menzel, E. (1973). Chimpanzee spatial memory organization. *Science, 182*, 943–945.

Menzel E. (1987). Behavior as a locationist views it. In Ellen, P., & Thinus-Blanc, C. (Eds.), *Spatial orientation in animals and man.* Dordrecht, The Netherlands: Martinus Nijhoff.

Neisser, U. (1976). *Cognition and reality.* New York: W.H. Freeman.

Neisser, U. (1977). Gibson's ecological optics: Consequences of a different stimulus description. *Journal for the theory of social behavior, 7*, 17–28.

Neisser, U. (1982). *Memory observed: Remembering in natural contexts.* New York: W.H. Freeman.

Neisser, U. (1984). Interpreting Harry Bahrick's discovery: What confers immunity against forgetting? *Journal of Experimental Psychology: General, 113*, 32–35.

Neisser, U. (1987). A sense of where you are: Functions of the spatial module. In Ellen, P., & Thinus-Blanc, C. (Eds.), *Spatial orientation in animals and man.* Dordrecht, The Netherlands: Martinus Nijhoff.

O'Keefe, J., & Nadel, L. (1978). *The hippocampus as a cognitive map.* Oxford, England: Oxford University Press.

Pick Jr., H.L., & Acredolo, L.P. (Eds.), *Spatial orientation: Theory, research & application.* New York: Plenum Press.

Quillian, M.R. (1968). Semantic memory. In M. Minsky (Ed.), *Semantic information processing.* Cambridge, MA.: MIT Press.

Reiff, R., & Scheerer, M. (1959). *Memory and hypnotic age regression.* New York: International Universities Press.

Robinson, J.A. (1976). Sampling autobiographical memory. *Cognitive Psychology, 8,* 578–595.

Rubin, D.C. (1986). *Autobiographical memory.* New York: Cambridge University Press.

Rumelhart, D.E. (1975). Notes on a schema for stories. In Bobrow, D.G., & Collins, A.M. (Eds.), *Representation and understanding: Studies in cognitive science.* New York: Academic Press.

Schank, R.C., & Abelson, R. (1975). *Scripts, plans, goals, and understanding.* Hillsdale, NJ: Lawrence Erlbaum Associates.

Sherry, D.F. (1987). The function and organization of memory in food-storing birds. In Ellen, P., & Thinus-Blanc, C. (Eds.), *Spatial organization in animals and man.* Dordrecht, The Netherlands: Martinus Nijhoff.

Sholl, J. (1987). Cognitive maps as orienting schemata. *Journal of Experimental Psychology: Learning, Memory, and Cognition, 13,* 615–628.

Starr, A., & Phillips, L. (1970). Verbal learning and motor memory in the amnesic syndrome. *Neuropsychologia, 8,* 75–81.

Tolman, E.C. (1932). *Purposive behavior in animals and men.* New York: Century.

Tolman, E.C. (1948). Cognitive maps in rats and men. *Psychological Review, 55,* 189–208.

Tolman, E.C. (1949). There is more than one kind of learning. *Psychological Review, 56,* 144–155.

Tulving, E. (1972). Episodic and semantic memory. In Tulving, E., & Donaldson, W. (Eds.), *Organization of memory.* New York: Academic Press.

Tulving, E. (1985). How many memory systems are there? *American Psychologist, 40,* 385–398.

Wagenaar, W.A. (1986). My memory: A study of autobiographical memory over six years. *Cognitive Psychology, 18,* 225–252.

Watkins, M.J., & Kerkar, S.P. (1985). Recall of a twice-presented item without recall of either presentation: Generic memory for events. *Journal of Memory and Language, 24,* 666–678.

CHAPTER 5

Memory: Conscious and Unconscious

George Mandler

Introduction

Cognitive psychologists have begun to talk about consciousness, but they have frequently shied away from explicitly including conscious phenomena in their theories. The ambivalence toward consciousness probably arises in part out of the proscription of consciousness during the behaviorist interlude; in part it is a function of the drive for computational models. At the present time consciousness is not proscribed, but it is also not (yet) computable. I assert, though, that an understanding of the functions of consciousness is important for a complete cognitive psychology. My explorations of consciousness are offered, in part, to convince the cognitive community that it should try to come to grips with the problem.

I shall first present some general considerations about mental structures. The focus will be on the distinction between the activation and the elaboration of mental structures, as well as on three general types of mental structures—coordinate, subordinate, and proordinate. I shall then summarize some characteristics of human consciousness, with special emphasis on the selective effects of consciousness on the one hand, and its limited serial structure on the other. The functions of consciousness are then applied to a variety of different memorial phenomena. I shall go on to argue that a view of mental structures and their interaction with conscious mechanisms accounts for several dichotomies that have been proposed in recent years, generally under the rubric of automatic versus controlled systems. I shall argue that these distinctions are not dichotomous, but rather are continuous manifestations of the interactions of structures and consciousness. Next, I shall apply this argument to a proposal about the source of memorial disabilities in anterograde amnesia. Finally, I shall discuss some interpretations of the commonsense notions of reminding.

Mental Structures and Memory

In this section I describe several theoretical propositions about memory that have occupied me over the years. I stress these in particular because they are relevant to the application of conscious functions to memorial phenomena.

Activation/Integration and Elaboration

Briefly, activation/integration reflects the effects of environmental or intrapsychic input on previously established representations of knowledge. The effect of activation is of particular interest when such representations are well bounded, that is, are unitary, mental contents.[1] The presentation of information (objects, events, actions) activates relevant existing knowledge units. One of the consequences of such activation is that the constituent features of the representation preferentially activate the other features of the unit. Such mutual activation leads to increasing integration, that is, to the more compact, unitized availability of that mental unit. Consequences of this activation include the phenomenal experience of increased familiarity (Mandler, 1980) and the perceptual fluency described by Jacoby and his associates (e.g., Jacoby & Dallas, 1981). Activation also increases the accessibility of units that is observed in response bias (McKoon, Ratcliff, & Verwoerd, 1986). Activation/ integration operates on units that are already established or that are in the process of formation as a function of consistent inputs.

In contrast, elaboration is the process whereby existing mental contents (units) are related to one another. It is most evident in the establishment of new organizations that make possible subsequent access, retrieval, and successful "search" processes. The concept has been used at various points in the recent literature and it is generally assumed to be relevant to many of the phenomena we find in deliberate memory, such as recall, to be partially relevant in recognition, and, of course, to be important in memorial constructions. The distinction between activation and elaboration has been useful in a wide variety of areas, ranging from quasiperceptual phenomena (Jacoby, 1983) to representational theory (Hinton, 1981) and was used extensively in our work on the dual process theory of recognition (Mandler, 1980).

The Integration of Functional Units

The integration of the representations of actions, perceptions, and memories obviously varies in degree. Newly learned units will be initially

---

[1] For a review of the development of the distinction and a discussion of the interaction between integration and elaboration see Mandler (1979a, 1980, 1982, 1985).

variable, and the process whereby these representations become stable and invariant involves the formation of the units of mental life. At the highly integrated end of this continuum we encounter mental events that may be qualitatively different from less integrated ones. These representations have been discussed primarily in the context of expert knowledge. For example, chess masters can quickly recognize "good" and "bad" chess board positions. This phenomenon is not a function of the knowledge of the board and the pieces on it, since chess masters are not better than novices in reconstructing random chess positions. Recently, it has been shown that human face recognition is a similar (acquired) expertise (Diamond & Carey, 1986), rather than the "genetic" characteristic detailed in some sociobiological "just so . . ." stories. I want to extend these findings to all knowledge structures, whether actions, memories, or perceptions, in which the individual becomes expert. Once a particular instance or a canonical representation of a class has been encountered and used frequently enough, it acts autonomously and represents an independent mental unit that is quickly, and often automatically, accessed and used in conscious constructions.

Three Mental Structures

In following up the concept of organization and its operation in memory (e.g., Mandler, 1967), I proposed three kinds of mental organizations that subsume the vast majority of possible organizations that are used in memorial productions (Mandler, 1979b). These are (a) *subordinate* structures, which involve the hierarchical or heterarchical structure of mental contents and which provide access to a particular object or event via superordinate or subordinate levels; (b) *proordinate* structures, which are serial in nature and in which access to any one unit is provided automatically or deliberately by the serial organization of the material, as in many syntactic structures, some mnemonic devices, number series, event representations, and so on; (c) *coordinate* structures, in which two or more functional units are brought together to produce a new functional unit, and which are exemplified by mental imagery and compound words and phrases. I will be particularly concerned with these coordinate structures. Coordination of two or more previously distinct units into a new entity is a very general process that may occur within any of the three structures. It incorporates the process of *unitization,* which is a major economic tool of mental life.

Obviously, I do not wish to argue that these structures represent different memory "systems," but rather that there exist a variety of structures and representations and a variety of ways in which memories may be accessed. In addition, these structures rarely occur in isolation. Most tasks represent a mixture of all three kinds of structures (cf. Segal & Mandler, 1967).

An Approach to Consciousness

If we wish to relate memory phenomena to consciousness, we cannot do so in a theoretical vacuum, that is, by simple correlations between states of consciousness and memory phenomena. I start by summarizing and extending my own speculations, accumulated over more than a decade. I shall only list those aspects of (momentary) consciousness that are directly relevant to the issues at hand; for more extended discussions of these and other issues see Mandler (1985, chap. 3; 1986).

First, however, a word about "attention." Ever since the behaviorist period, "attention" has served as a synonym or hiding place for "consciousness," including such various terms as "focal attention," "working memory," "directed consciousness," and so on. To avoid confusion, I have suggested (1985) that it would be useful to restrict attention to spatiotemporal orientations, whereas the directive and conceptually selective aspects of the ordinary use of attention be delegated to the directive and constructive function of consciousness. In doing so I follow a trend in the use of attention which has been endorsed by students of attentional phenomena (e.g., Kahneman & Treisman, 1984; LaBerge, 1983).

The Functions of Consciousness

Consciousness is constructive, that is, the contents of consciousness are *constructed* out of available (activated) unconscious contents. A constructivist position asserts that conscious contents are created to respond to momentary needs, demands, and tasks; they are not the result of unconscious material being pushed, elevated, or illuminated into consciousness. Consciousness is not a threshold phenomenon—with unconscious contents becoming conscious when a threshold of excitation, strength and so on has been exceeded.

Customarily, we are conscious of the important aspects of the environs but not of all the evidence that enters the sensory gateways or of all our potential knowledge of the event. In the absence of any specific requirements (internally or externally generated), the current construction will be the most general (or abstract) available. As needs and requirements become more specific, conscious contents become more concrete. For example, when trying to remember a name or phrase, we may start with general specifications that often become very specific, eventually descending to the level of phonology and spelling. A current conscious state will be changed if it does not account for (make sense of) the available evidence. When the environment is constant, we respond to internal demands for conscious constructions.

While not all new learning is conscious, the acquisition or restructuring of knowledge and most complex skills requires conscious participation. In the adult, thoughts and actions are typically conscious before they become well integrated and subsequently automatic. Learning to drive a car is a conscious process, whereas the skilled driver acts automatically and unconsciously.

The function of conscious construction that I stress here is that it brings two or more previously separate mental contents into direct juxtaposition. The phenomenal experience of choice seems to involve exactly such an occurrence. We usually do not refer to a choice unless there is a consciousness of two or more alternatives. The attribute of "choosing" is applied to a decision process regarding, for example, items on a menu, television programs, or careers. Choices are determined by complex unconscious mechanisms, but we need the prior selective function of consciousness to determine the events or objects on which these mechanisms operate. The mechanisms that select certain actions or items among alternatives are not themselves conscious, but the range included in making the choice is created consciously, thus giving the appearance of conscious free choices and operations of the will. The simultaneity of objects and events in consciousness makes possible the formation of new associations.

Just as current perceptions are, within schema theory, seen as the result of both external evidence and internal processes (bottom up and top down), so is consciousness in general determined by activated higher order structures as well as by the evidence from the environment. Structures that represent intentions and interpretations of situational requirements are activated primarily "top down"; they depend on prior evaluations, on activations of situational identifications and interpretations, and on current needs and goals. They need not receive activation from the physical evidence of our surroundings. These structures depend primarily on interpreted evidence, on information about requirements and needs. In the normal course of events it is such more abstract and general structures that define what we are doing, what we want to do, and what we need to do. When task and intention are narrowed down to particulars, less general and more specific schemas determine conscious constructions.

One of the important characteristics of consciousness is that it can have effects on *subsequent* mental events and (physical) actions. In brief, events represented in consciousness are constructed from activated structures and, in turn, activate relevant underlying structures. Since active, conscious structures reflect current requirements of the situation, the process will selectively and preferentially activate those structures that are most likely to serve current goals. The possible alternatives and competing hypotheses that have been represented in consciousness (and their related structures) will receive additional activation and thus will be enhanced. The search for problem solutions and the search for memorial targets (as in recall) typically have a conscious counterpart, frequently expressed in "thinking aloud" protocols. What appears in consciousness in these tasks is likely to be those points in the course of the search when steps toward the solution have been taken and a choice point has been reached. At that point the current state of the world is reflected in consciousness. That state reflects the progress toward the goal as well as some of the possible steps that could be taken next. A conscious state is constructed that reflects those aspects of the current search that *do* (partially and often inadequately) respond to the goal of the search. Consciousness at these points depicts waystations toward solutions and serves to restrict and focus subsequent pathways by selectively activating those that are currently within the conscious construction.

In summary, conscious processing produces new knowledge that is independent of current stimulus-response contingencies. Such new learning responds to goals and concerns that are not exclusively a function of current situations and contexts. It is distinguished from new information that is acquired automatically, as in the case of many perceptual and motor skills and other simple "associations", which are stimulus driven rather than the result of deliberate (conscious) knowledge acquisition.

Limited Capacity and the Utility of Consciousness as a Serial Device

The limited capacity of consciousness serves to reduce the "blooming confusion" that the physical world potentially presents to the organism. Just as sensory end organs and central transducers radically reduce the world of physical stimuli to the functional stimuli that are in fact registered, so does the conscious process further reduce the available information to a small, manageable, and serial subset. The conscious state (being conscious of something) occurs when a relatively slow second-order serial representation of a small sample of mental events becomes useful or necessary in order to access the parallel and rapid activation of unconscious processes (Rumelhart & McClelland, 1986). Among the conditions that require such a process are the bringing of two or more previously unrelated mind contents together or into juxtaposition, the characterization of the most important aspects of the current state of the world, choosing among alternatives, and the encoding of new information. All of these require a system of representation that can function independently of, and in parallel with, the other current processes that our mental apparatus engages.

Memory and Consciousness

The commonsense notion of human memory intrudes into psychological discussions by its insistence on consciousness as a criterion. In the common language, memory and remembering usually refer to deliberately bringing into consciousness something that is absent or that has occurred in the past. Psychologists have, especially recently, also used the term *memory* to refer to any mental content that is produced, for example as a response to an incomplete stem of a word, regardless of whether the subject knows or recognizes the production as being "memorial," that is, as being relevant to some past or current intention or requirement. It is in this context that one speaks of unconscious memories.

Recall and Retrieval

The most frequent emergence of memorial consciousness is found in the act of recall. Both the commonsense notions of recalling and remembering and the experimental procedures for recall require a conscious construction that is seen to be responsive to some demand or requirement. Recall typically requires a retrieval process that is often, but not always, indexed by waystations that appear in consciousness. It is in recall that people describe such waystations, as well as conscious equivalents of search processes, and—at times—attempts at recognition of the retrieved material. In recall a higher order demand or task specifies what are and what are not acceptable conscious constructions. Errors in recall are constructions that, while factually erroneous, still respond to some higher order requirement, as, for example, in a recall that conveys the gist of the message but is not "correct" in the narrower sense.

Recognition

In recognition tasks in particular, different kinds of methods and instructions will produce different conscious constructions. The underlying activation, usually expressed phenomenally in terms of familiarity, will emerge in different forms in the conscious constructions.

   Consider first of all the most frequently used recognition task. Subjects are presented with materials, some of which have been previously shown and some of which are new, distractor items. As the subjects see or hear each of these items, they are required to say whether they have seen or heard this material before. In such a situation the presented material activates its representation and activation spreads to other related representations. If the "stored" material has also recently been activated, "old" items will have a greater total current activation (and will be more integrated) than will "new" items. If some criterion is set for such levels of activation, the old items will usually fall above it and new items below. This rather crude criterion of relative activation may be sufficient to trigger the "yes" and "no" responses. What is the current conscious construction? It will be in keeping with the instruction, "Tell me which one you think you have seen before." The highly activated items are more likely to be experienced as "having been seen before"—the subjects will, in keeping with the task and instructions, "have an 'old' experience." In actuality, the situation is more complicated, since retrieval processes also enter into the judgment (see Mandler, 1980).

Now consider the forced-choice recognition experiment. Here the subject is presented with an "old" and a "new" item at the same time; the instructions—explicit or implicit—are NOT to say which looks old (i.e., familiar), but rather to make a choice between the two items. The underlying process—of differential activations reaching a level above or below a crude criterion—is much the same.[2] The subject produces the same kind of action, but what is experienced is much more a sense of having made a choice. Thus, subjects may report that they are "judging familiarity" in one case and "making choices among alternatives" in the other.

Conscious and Unconscious Memories

Over the past decade intense interest has arisen in a type of "memory" research that strains the commonsense definition. The work on lexical decisions, priming, and spreading activation makes distinctions among memory and other cognitive categories, such as perception, rather tenuous (e.g., Greenwald & Liu, 1985; Marcel, 1983; Meyer & Schvaneveldt, 1971; Neely, 1977). The fact that people perceive words more easily after having seen related items, that they make lexical decisions faster after having been primed, or that they can identify higher order characteristics without being able to identify lower order ones raises (unnecessary) questions about the extent to which the use of prior experience constitutes memory or perception. As far as consciousness is concerned, little attention has been paid to whether subjects in these experiments are aware of the fact that some of their productions are related to prior experiences. In most cases they do not seem to be; they are unconscious of the connection. Activation may produce effects without any conscious registration when, for example, the indirect activation of words has comparable effects on a priming task and a recognition task (Mandler, Graf, & Kraft, 1986).

A rather startling, and deleterious, effect of conscious intervention was discovered by Graf and me (Graf & Mandler, 1984, exper. 3). Subjects were given one of two processing tasks with lists of 15 words. These were either semantic (each word was rated for how the subject liked it) or nonsemantic (the subject responded to purely physical aspects of the word). Following the presentation, subjects were given one of two tests: stem completion or cued stem completion. Both tests used three-letter

---

[2] See also the argument in signal detection theory that the yes/no method and the forced-choice method yield equivalent discrimination values (Green & Swets, 1966).

stems. Some could be completed with the words originally presented, while others were unrelated distractor stems (Warrington & Weiskrantz, 1970). The only difference between the two tests was the instruction. On the completion test subjects were asked to give the first word that came to mind, but on the cued completion test they were told that the list of stems contained the initial letters of the presented words and that they should complete the stems with the help of these cues.

The results are shown in Table 5.1, which shows percent stem completions that were "correct," that is, that were completed with the presented words. The effect is obvious: The completion test showed no difference as a function of type of processing, but the cued completion test showed a very large effect. Cueing instructions significantly improved performance following semantic processing, but they significantly *decreased* performance following nonsemantic processing. These data suggest that automatic stem completion, without deliberation or conscious intervention, is independent of type of initial processing; all that is needed is some activation of the target words. When the instructions require retrieval, that is, deliberate recovery of the original lists, prior semantic processing is very useful—the list is retrievable and helps in the completion task. However, when the instructions require retrieval and retrieval is not possible because of nonsemantic processing, the search process—the conscious intervention—impairs the completion process. The conscious search effort does not produce any useful retrievals; it intrudes into the limited capacity of consciousness and dramatically interferes with the automatic process. Under the nonsemantic conditions in cued completion, subjects complete what they can recall, which is very little.[3]

Different Memory Systems or Different Uses of Constructive Consciousness?

There has been an increasing tendency in recent years to assign different kinds of memorial functions to different, sometimes independent, systems. The number of such distinctions among systems is quite great, but on examination, most of these distinctions have one common characteristic. They refer to access to knowledge, which is in the one case achieved automatically, and in the other case achieved by the intervention of a limited-capacity serial consciousness. The most popular distinction has been between automatic and controlled (or deliberate) access.

---

[3] In fact, the cued completion data reflect a recall process. Free recall (on a 20-item list in exper. 2 in Graf & Mandler, 1984) was 36.0% and 8.9% following semantic and nonsemantic processing, respectively.

TABLE 5.1. "Correct" stem completion following semantic
and nonsemantic processing: normal subjects.

Type of test	Processing task	
	Semantic	Nonsemantic
Completion, not cued	23.3%	20.0%
Cued completion	40.6%	7.8%

Baseline (chance) completions of the stems with the target words
were 2.8%.

Automatic and Deliberate Memories

In discussions of the distinction between memories that are brought to
mind deliberately (consciously searched) and nondeliberate ones (uncon-
scious/automatic), a number of apparent dichotomies have been proposed
(Table 5.2).

The first seven attributes in Table 5.2 (originally published in Mandler,
1985, p. 93) describe characteristics of two poles of the various
automatic/nonautomatic distinctions. I have added the last three dichotomies, which have more often been ascribed to different systems. My
argument with respect to these "systems" should be obvious by now.
Among other characteristics, all of these distinctions refer to the use or
nonuse of the conscious processes to store or retrieve information. I am
specifically referring to the conscious or unconscious processes whereby
information is accessed; in all cases the final product is, of course, a
conscious content. The second column of Table 5.2 describes aspects of
access to information or action that involve consciousness. Conscious
intervention involves relatively *slow* processes, *mediated* or *controlled* by
other mental contents that are *indirect,* that depend on appropriate
contextual cues, and that are demanding of conscious *capacity* and have

TABLE 5.2. Distinctions between nonconscious and
conscious processing.

No conscious processing (Automatic)	Conscious processing (Nonautomatic)
Fast	Slow
Immediate	Mediated
Unconscious	Conscious
Uncontrolled	Controlled
No capacity demand	Capacity demanding
Direct access	Indirect access
Involuntary	Voluntary
Context free	Context dependent
PROCEDURAL	DECLARATIVE
SEMANTIC	EPISODIC
IMPLICIT	EXPLICIT

Adapted from Mandler, 1985, p. 93.

the phenomenal appearance of being *voluntary*. The same kinds of characteristics have been ascribed to the three "systems" at the bottom of the table. I shall discuss two of these systems in more detail.

Procedural and Declarative Knowledge

Whatever definition of "procedural" one uses, it is generally considered to be a system that runs without conscious intervention (cf. Cohen & Squire, 1980). The distinction is often coextensive with the more traditional distinction between knowing how and knowing that. Anderson (1982) claimed that automatic skills develop from declarative knowledge into procedural productions. Only declarative knowledge is available in working memory (a synonym for consciousness). There are some problems with this account, in particular with reference to the acquisition of skills by very small children. J. Mandler (1984) has noted that in the infant the original acquistion of skills (knowledge) is procedural and probably remains procedural, that is, unconscious. Just like children, adults acquire some skills procedurally—without conscious access to the components of the skill—though secondary structures that point to the procedures may be invoked, as in the case of learning to play tennis or ride a bicycle. We frequently know "that" we know "how" and may even know "how" we know "that." Whatever, the utility of the procedural/declarative distinction, it seems obvious that the intervention of consciousness is an alternative way of describing one of its primary features. The conscious/unconscious distinction has the additional advantage that various tasks and memorial accesses may be described as using conscious mechanisms only partially or occasionally: It is not dichotomous.

Semantic versus Episodic Memory

There has been much argument recently about the semantic/episodic distinction and its use as a theoretical device in psychological experiments (e.g., Mandler, 1985; McKoon, Ratcliff, & Dell, 1986; Ratcliff & McKoon, 1986; Tulving, 1986). The distinction has heuristic value in distinguishing between general semantic knowledge, which is often automatically available, context free, and "known" (Tulving, 1985) and autobiographical, episodic knowledge, which is deliberately and consciously accessed, context dependent, and "remembered." Semantic knowledge is unitized and often represents the kind of qualitatively different structure that I ascribed to expert knowledge in an earlier section. Episodic knowledge, on the other hand, may or may not be subject to such qualitative integration. Some episodic autobiographical knowledge seems to have automatic characteristics, and some general semantic knowledge requires contextual retrieval. In terms of the automatic/controlled dimension, the distinction between automatic knowing and deliberate remembering does not easily map into the distinction between semantic and episodic information. The distinction between semantic/general and episodic/autobiographical knowledge has obvious heuristic value, but little in the way of principled theoretical utility (Tulving, 1986). Whereas automatic and nonmediated access describes much of semantic knowledge, and conscious access much of episodic knowledge, the distinction between the two systems is far from clear.

In summary, the dichotomies advocated and the systems proclaimed may map fuzzily into one common characteristic—the use of consciousness in achieving access to information. There are of course a number of other distinctions that these dichotomies describe. My only concern here is their common characteristic. The use and intervention of conscious processes is the result of specific tasks, demands, and intentions. Conscious processing is usually invoked for some parts of most memorial activity—it is not an all-or-none function.

Primary and Short-Term Memories

An understanding of the role of consciousness in memorial functions also restructures the current confusion among various versions of short-term, working, primary, and scratch-pad memories. I start with consciousness as the common end point of all of these constructions.[4] William James used the term "primary memory" to refer to the current contents of consciousness that are immediately present and need no "retrieval." Given the limitation of conscious capacity, one would expect all such contents to be limited to some five to seven units—the limits usually imposed on "short-term" memories. Thus, one of the components of short-term memory involves current conscious contents. Instead of postulating an additional short-term memory system or "box," I use degree of activation to define other quickly accessible memorial contents. Assuming a rather steep initial decay of activation, material that has been presented or processed during preceding seconds can be quickly and efficiently brought into conscious constructions. Rehearsal may either maintain material within current conscious constructions or keep activation very high so that the material can quickly be brought into consciousness. In addition there are mental contents that are kept at relatively high levels of activation. I have referred to these as "state of the world" memories. They contain information about who and where we are, what we are doing, and what our currently effective goals and plans are. Finally, the executive functions of short-term memory (if any) are subsumed under the serial and prospective functions of consciousness

---

[4] I summarize here a discussion from Mandler (1985, chap. 4).

described above. This kind of approach eliminates the need for different short- and long-term systems and brings short-term and long-term phenomena into a common theoretical framework.

Amnesia: A Disease of Consciousness

Research and theory of the past 20 years have shown that the amnesic syndrome provides a superb natural laboratory for examining current theories of memory. The best recent summary of the current state of the art is found in Weiskrantz (1985), to whom I am indebted despite various disagreements. In fact, the intent of what follows is to respond to Weiskrantz's challenge to design the "new theoretical formulations and practical techniques necessary to approach the 'evaluative' or 'cognitive mediational system' damaged in [amnesic] patients . . ." (p. 411). Several of the "systems" in Table 5.2 have been proposed as explanatory devices for the amnesic syndrome. Given my view of these distinctions, I want to argue that an appeal to the functions of consciousness provides the theoretical formulation for an understanding of the memorial disability that we find in anterograde amnesia. For purposes of this discussion, I shall restrict myself to the kind of phenomena typically found in the performance of patients suffering from Korsakoff's syndrome. Whether the same arguments apply to other pathologies of the mind is left open.

Amnesia and Consciousness

The central proposition is that the amnesic patient suffers from an inability to consciously create new concatenations or new contexts for old knowledge, or to use access routes to information that is not available automatically. In short, the amnesic patient has a deficiency in conscious functioning that prevents the storage of new information or the retrieval of previously stored material, unless it can be done automatically and without the intervention of the conscious apparatus. What the amnesic patient cannot do is to encode and store "belongingness"—what goes with what—unless it is done automatically. Weiskrantz (1985) stressed, as have other writers, what it is that is *spared* in amnesic patients. An appeal to conscious functions describes what is *impaired* as well as what is spared. What is impaired is the ability to construct new conscious contents or to retrieve recently encoded information.

Various reports on patients with very dense amnesias have described the pathologies of consciousness. Patients describe themselves as being "prisoners of the present," as experiencing only "momentary consciousness." They appear to construct conscious contents only as a function of current activations, when there is bottom up activation, or in terms of pretraumatic automatically accessed memories. What they cannot do is to use or construct novel posttraumatic contents. Tulving (1985) has presented a case that illustrates this conscious inability, the failure to construct conscious contents. One extract from Tulving has the interviewer ask what the patient will be "doing tomorrow." The answer is that the patient "doesn't know" and his mind is "blank" when trying to think about it. He is living in a "permanent present."[5] He cannot remember particular episodes in the past or construct possible futures. In other words, he is unable to construct conscious contents about the past or present, that is, concatenations of new or imagined events or of the present and the past. On the other hand, knowledge that does not require novel constructions is generally unimpaired; the "semantic" memory is intact.

The variety of distinctions that have been used to describe the amnesic failures (cf. Weiskrantz, 1985) are all related to the use of novel conscious constructions. Rather than rehearse the argument I have made in that respect in the preceding pages, I shall address next some selected issues in the performance of anterograde amnesic patients.

The Acquisition of New Information in Amnesia

One of my disagreements with Weiskrantz is with the *general* claim that what is spared in amnesic patients is "the acquisition of new relationships (cf. Warrington and Weiskrantz, 1982)" (Weiskrantz, 1985, p. 403).[6] The problem is that the instances of the acquisition of new information or relationships are all examples of learning that requires little or no conscious intervention. This learning involves typically the acquisition of motor skills, perceptual relationships, or the achievement of new unitizations. All of these are, or can be, acquired automatically, without the intervention of consciousness. In fact, one can demonstrate the automatic acquisition of complex skills in the absence of conscious participation. For example, amnesic patients can acquire computer routines without knowing (consciously) that they have learned them (Glisky, Schacter, & Tulving, 1986).

I know of no instance in which amnesic patients have been shown equal to normal controls with respect to new declarative, episodic, or explicit information (the terms used to describe the acquisition of information that requires conscious intervention). It is the case, of course, that amnesic patients can at times engage in some limited conscious elaboration, because their amnesias are rarely so dense that they recall nothing on a

---

[5] It is interesting to speculate that living in the present may characterize some lower animals and very young infants as well (see G. Mandler, 1986; J.M. Mandler, 1988).

[6] The other characteristic that Weiskrantz says is spared is "facilitation through priming," and I have of course no disagreement on that topic. Priming operates without access to conscious mechanisms.

free recall test, for example. In other words, there is usually some "saved"function even in a recall test.

Whereas there is no argument about the acquisition of perceptual and motor skills, the claim of saved function is often made for new declarative knowledge learning in paired-associate tests (whether tests are called this or are designated context-target tasks or cued recall tests). One of the most extensive and recent such demonstrations has been provided by Graf and Schacter (1985).

In the Graf and Schacter study subjects were given word pairs (A-B pairs) and required to generate a meaningful sentence that included the pair. The word pairs were either related (e.g., RIPE-APPLE) or unrelated (e.g., KINDLY-STICK). Using the stem completion task, the subjects were tested on the B member of the pair by being given the initial letters of the words for completion. The performance of amnesic patients was essentially the same as that of normal controls when word completion of the B member was tested in the presence of a related, an unrelated, or a new A member. More important, the level of performance for patient and normal groups was significantly higher when the "context" was the same (i.e., the old A items) than it was when the context was different (new A items). Since the cued *recall* performance of the amnesic subjects was severely impaired, Graf and Schacter concluded that implicit and explicit memory for *new* associations "are mediated by different underlying processes" (p. 512).[7]

This study, and similar ones by the same and other authors, offers evidence that can be interpreted to show the importance of integrative processes for the performance of amnesic patients, but little evidence that underlying elaborative processes are operating adequately for these patients. The argument concerns the nature of the task and the processes that are involved in different tasks. The paired-associate task is an excellent example of unitization, the combination of two units into a new structure that acts as an independent unit.[8] I argue that the paired associate task used by Graf and Schacter draws on the ability to amnesic patients to perform an integrative (as opposed to an elaborative) task. In such a task the coordination of the pair produces the integration of the two constituent items into a single unit, as well as the activation of each of the items. One example of this process is found in their data on cued recall, that is, when the A member is presented and the B response

---

[7] Consistent with my arguments, Schacter and Graf (1986) have reported that the formation of "new associations" is actually found only in "mildly-to-moderately amnesic patients," and is absent in "severely amnesic patients."

[8] See Mandler, Rabinowitz, and Simon (1981) for an extensive demonstration that the recall, cued recall, and recognition of word pairs is based on the unitized, holistic representation of the pairs.

required. The "recall" by the amnesic subjects is indeed severely impaired, but it is significantly less impaired for the related than for the unrelated pairs. The percent cued recall for the amnesic subjects was 33.3 and 2.2 for the related and unrelated pairs; for the matched controls the means were 72.8 and 35.0, respectively. Thus, the amnesics performed at 46% of the level of their controls for related pairs but at only 6% for the unrelated pairs. The performance level for the related pairs is inconsistent with "recall' by amnesic subjects as generally reported in the literature. Six percent of normal performance (as for the unrelated pairs) is typical, but the 46% is not what one would get from any usual recall test. It would be surprising for amnesics to have that high a level of recall if by "recall" we mean deliberate search and retrieval. However, if the cued recall test is seen as another version of the completion test, which is performed "implicitly," then the result is neither surprising nor a demonstration of the acquisition of new associations in the usual sense of the term. Another piece of evidence also suggests that cued recall and completion are, in this experiment, based on similar processes. The probability of correctly completing a word given that it had been "recalled" on the cued recall test was essentially identical for the control and amnesic subjects (.69 and .68). Since we know that the usual recall test and completion performance are "dissociated" in amnesic patients, this similarity between patients and controls suggests that cued recall here is quite different from the usual test of new learning in amnesics. In other words, associated pairs are, under certain conditions, examples of coordination and successful unitization; they are accessed as single units and are not exemplars of new associations in the usual sense.[9]

I should note that Graf and Schacter did discuss notions of unitizing and redintegration in connection with their data, and the final interpretation is that "completion performance is mediated by implicit memory for new associations that is independent of explicit recollection." I would suggest that new units must form an integrated unit, a coordinated whole (such as an image or some other unitary memory unit), in order to be effective for amnesic patients. But that is different from the kind of new association that is found in typical free recall tasks, in which structures that provide pathways for new associations are formed. Apparently identical memory tests (such as recall) cannot be compared across tasks unless one understands what is processed under the conditions of the different tasks.

---

[9] Parenthetically, Schacter and Graf reported another study of idiomatic expressions in which both amnesics and controls performed equally well on giving the second member of a pair (e.g., SOUR-GRAPES) but both groups were essentially unable to give the response if new pairing was given (e.g., SOUR-POTATOES). In this case the preexisting unit was even stronger than the related pairs used in their main study, and amnesics and controls performed equally well.

Encoding Versus Retrieval in Amnesia

Given the assumption that novel conscious constructions are impaired in amnesic patients and that consciounsess is needed for new encodings and retrievals, the issue whether the central problem in the amnesic disability is one of encoding or one of retrieval becomes moot (Cermak, 1979; Weiskrantz, 1985). Amnesic patients should show deficits in *both* encoding and retrieval. Since nothing can be retrieved that has not been encoded first, one would expect that the major problem for amnesics would be one of encoding, for which the conscious concatenation is necessary. However, one equally would expect retrievals to be difficult, if they are of knowledge that has not been integrated and that cannot be automatically accessed.

In Mandler (1980) I suggested that stem completion should behave in a fashion similar to the familiarity component of recognition, and that normal subjects should behave similarly to amnesic patients if they were prevented from consciously elaborating material at input. That prediction was borne out in an experiment by Graf, Mandler, and Haden (1982). College students were given lists of words under two encoding conditions: perceptual/nonsemantic and conceptual/semantic. This was followed by recall or stem completion tests. Under these conditions, the normal population mirrored the amnesic pattern. Following nonsemantic processing, the subjects showed a large recall deficit compared with the semantic condition, but the stem completion performance of the two groups was equivalent. What this experiment shows is that an amnesic symptom can be simulated in normal subjects by changing only the condition of encoding (or storage). In a condition in which retrieval is demonstrably absent in the recall test because of the nonsemantic encoding at presentation, completion performance is unaffected. Granted that this simulation may mirror the performance of amnesics for reasons other than the actual etiology of amnesic symptoms, still it does provide support for the argument that faulty encoding may affect recall (retrieval) without affecting the stem completion test. Imperfect (nonelaborative) storage does not affect the completion task that depends primarily on the activation of the perceptual aspect of the target word, but it does provide a reasonable explanation for the recall deficit.

Further evidence for this position is found in a comparison between normal subjects and amnesic patients on the uncued and cued stem completion test. Table 5.3 shows the performance of amnesic patients and their controls, following semantic processing on cued and uncued stem completion tests. The pattern here can be compared with that shown in Table 5.1 for normal subjects. However since different materials and different populations were used, the absolute data are not comparable across Tables 5.1 and 5.3. We found no difference between the cued and the uncued tests for the amnesics but a significant improvement for the

Table 5.3. "Correct" stem completion following semantic processing: amnesic patients and matched controls[a]

Type of test	Percent correct	
	Controls	Amnesics
Completion, not cued	48.5%	57.2%
Cued completion	69.0%	57.6%

[a] The free recall performance was 37% and 13% for controls and amnesics, respectively.
[b] Data from Graf, Squire, & Mandler, 1984.

controls on the cued completion test. These data also argue for an encoding explanation, similar to that demonstrated in the Graf, Mandler, and Haden experiment. Except for the maintenance of performance following cuing instructions, the amnesic patients, following semantic processing, behaved like normal subjects following nonsemantic (nonelaborative) encoding. I have already pointed out that the deterioration in performance for the cued completion task in our college population following nonsemantic processing was due to conscious interference, because normal subjects attempt to recall items which they *cannot* retrieve. Following semantic processing, the control subjects improved when asked to produce items that they had seen before, just as the college students did in the first study (Table 5.1). Amnesic subjects, on the other hand, showed equivalent performance for both conditions. They did not benefit from reference to the cued target list (which they could not remember), nor did they suffer the deficit shown by normal subjects following nonsemantic encoding. The absence of both of these effects is due to the same factor: Amnesic subjects cannot remember the target list. Such a failure does not provide additional retrievals, nor does it produce interference due to failed or inaccurate retrievals.

Recognition in Amnesia

Evidence for the dual process theory of recognition is now fairly secure. To recapitulate: The experience of recognition is constructed out of two underlying processes, a context-free activation of the representation of the target which, under appropriate circumstances, gives rise to the phenomenal experience of familiarity, and a context-dependent retrieval/search process which identifies the target event as to *what* it is, not just whether it looks or sounds familiar. If, as I have maintained, in amnesics the activation process is intact and the retrieval process is impaired, some, but not complete, deterioration of recognition performance in amnesic patients could be expected.

Since it is important to understand what is required of an amnesic subject in a recognition task, we need to clarify the meaning of and requirements in tests of "familiarity." Squire, Shimamura, and Graf (1985) have claimed that amnesic patients "do not express feelings of familiarity" (p. 42).[10] It all depends on what you mean and what you test; these patients certainly do behave toward people and objects in a "familiar" way—they even learn to behave that way toward novel (e.g., hospital) environments. If asked whether something looks familiar, how do they interpret the question? Do they, as we all do at times, interpret it as a recognition task that requires a specification of who, where, and when? If so, then they surely will say that the event is not "familiar," because they are not able to engage the retrieval process that is needed for specificity. On the other hand, we often claim to recognize somebody because the person looks very familiar, without knowing who he or she is; we rely on a part of the full recognition process. In addition, queries about familiarity may be confusing. As I sit in my office, I don't think of my desk as looking familiar, unless I am asked, and then I will certainly agree—though with some perplexity at the nature of the question. It all depends on the way the question is asked and the way it is interpreted by the subject.

What are the data on recognition in amnesia? Given the problem of what the task is or might have been, the data are predictably variable. Sometimes you get recognition in amnesics and sometimes you don't. However, Johnson and Kim (1985) have shown that recognition performance by Korsakoff patients is generally above chance but below that of normal controls, which is consistent with the notion that the amnesics respond only to the familiarity (activation/integration) component of recognition. In Graf, Squire, and Mandler (1984) we have shown significant recognition performance by amnesics marching nicely in step with stem completion priming, both of which are produced by relevant activations.[11]

In calling amnesia a disease of consciousness I do not, of course, assert that all or even most conscious functions in amnesic patients are impaired. Rather, anterograde amnesia is a disease of the conscious functions involved in the acquisition and (sometimes) retrieval of newly elaborated knowledge and information.

Reminding: Conscious and Unconscious

Psychologists have generally ignored the suggestion that some memorial events occur without deliberate retrieval, and have focused on deliberate retrievals. However, much of everyday memory experiences are in fact

---

[10] They also claim to have demonstrated intact priming in the absence of recognition. However, since they base their conclusion on a single postelectroconvulsive therapy test, the generality of the claim is in doubt.

[11] See also Mandler, Graf, and Kraft (1986).

nondeliberate. Events and objects come to mind continuously without any deliberate/conscious effort. In fact, one can argue that most of our daily use of "memory" is of such a nature. As one speaks, converses, or contemplates, one accesses prior experiences and knowledge without obviously searching for or deliberately accessing that information. Deliberate retrieval of information seems to be the exception rather than the rule. One can argue that much of the nondeliberate access to previously stored/encoded information occurs automatically or as a result of higher order spreading activation. Thus, when I discuss the topic of making beef Wellington, of solving a particular equation, or of driving to my office, the relevant information seems to come to mind unbidden and automatically. At other times some chance remark or event may remind me of some other event or object, in which case a conscious construction occurs that is experienced as somehow relevant to the current state of affairs. That is, we usually find ourselves experiencing the relevance of the reminded mental content. In short, sometimes events come to mind that are simply accepted as fitting the stream of our productions, at other times they are specially noticed. At times we find ourselves saying or thinking things that do not seem to fit, events that are frequently referred to as "slips." Finally, there are cases in which we deliberately try to retrieve a name, word, or event and find ourselves unable to do so, only to discover the appropriate mental content coming to mind apparently unbidden at some time later.[12]

The study of reminding, of nondeliberate access to memorial contents, is in its infancy and the various cases I have described need extensive and analytical experimentation and analysis. It is a commonplace that much memorial material is generated without our specific recognition of our productions, as in ongoing conversation, for example. It has been demonstrated extensively in the laboratory. For example, subjects in the stem completion task are often not aware of the fact that their productions are relevant to the prior presentation of a list.[13]

The challenge of "reminding" phenomena, whether they occur apparently haphazardly, in continuous speech, or as pathological or normal slips or errors, suggests that much is still to be done in the study of memory. It also suggests, together with other evidence presented here, that there is no isolated problem of memory. Prior experiences affect practically everything we do, whether we consider the rubric of phenom-

---

[12] Presumably in this case, the prior activation and some happenstance but relevant later events combine to provide adequate activation and context for a conscious construction.

[13] Weiskrantz (1985) stressed that "[amnesic] subjects do not have an experienced 'memory' for items that are facilitated in a priming procedure" (p. 408). The same holds for normal subjects following nonsemantic processing and does not distinguish the amnesic syndrome.

ena to be perception, language, or memory. I have tried to suggest a variety of ways in which consciousness and other mental functions interact. I have also tried to avoid any suggestion that we are dealing with different "systems"—of memory or anything else. The power of human mentality lies in part in the availability of most of our mental apparatus to the large variety of activities in which we engage.

Acknowledgment. Preparation of this chapter has been supported by grant BNS 84-04228 from the National Science Foundation. I am indebted to Jean Mandler who, despite theoretical disagreements, commented on and improved an earlier draft.

References

Anderson, J.R. (1982). Acquisition of cognitive skill. *Psychological Review, 89,* 369–406.

Cermak, L.S. (1979). Amnesic patients' level of processing. In L.S. Cermak & F.I.M. Craik (Eds.), *Levels of processing in human memory.* Hillsdale, NJ: Lawrence Erlbaum Associates.

Cohen, N.J., & Squire L.R. (1980). Preserved learning and retention of pattern analyzing skill in amnesia: Dissociation of knowing how and knowing that. *Science, 210,* 207–209.

Diamond, R., & Carey, S. (1986). Why faces are and are not special: An effect of expertise. *Journal of Experimental Psychology: General, 115,* 107–117.

Glisky, E.L., Schacter, D.L., & Tulving, E. (1986). Computer learning by memory-impaired patients: Acquisition and retention of complex knowledge, *Neurospychologia, 24,* 313–328.

Graf, P., & Mandler, G. (1984). Activation makes words more accessible, but not necessarily more retrievable. *Journal of Verbal Learning and Verbal Behavior, 23,* 553–568.

Graf, P., Mandler, G., & Haden, P. (1982). Simulating amnesic symptoms in normal subjects. *Science, 218,* 1243–1244.

Graf, P., & Schacter, D.L. (1985). Implicit and explicit memory for new associations in normal and amnesic subjects. *Journal of Experimental Psychology: Learning, Memory, and Cognition, 11,* 501–518.

Graf, P., Squire, L.R., & Mandler, G. (1984). The information that amnesic patients do not forget. *Journal of Experimental Psychology: Learning, Memory, and Cognition, 10,* 164–178.

Green, D.M., & Swets, J.A. (1966). *Signal detection theory and psychophysics.* New York: John Wiley.

Greenwald, A.G., & Liu, T.J. (1985). Limited unconscious processing of meaning. *Bulletin of the Psychonomic Society, 23,* 292.

Hinton, G.E. (1981). Implementing semantic networks in parallel hardware. In G.E. Hinton, & J.A. Anderson (Eds.), *Parallel models of associative memory* (pp. 161–187). Hillsdale, NJ: Lawrence Erlbaum Associates.

Jacoby, L.L. (1983). Perceptual enhancement: Persistent effects of an experience. *Journal of Experimental Psychology: Learning, Memory, and Cognition, 9,* 21–38.

Jacoby, L.L., & Dallas, M. (1981). On the relationship between autobiographical memory and perceptual learning. *Journal of Experimental Psychology: General, 110,* 306–340.

Johnson, M.K., & Kim, J.K. (1985). Recognition of pictures by alcoholic Korsakoff patients. *Bulletin of the Psychonomic Society, 23,* 456–458.

Kahneman, D., & Treisman, A. (1984). Changing views of attention and automaticity. In R. Parasuraman, & R. Davis (Eds.), *Varieties of attention.* New York: Academic Press.

LaBerge, D. (1983). Spatial extent of attention to letters and words. *Journals of Experimental Psychology: Human Perception and Performance, 9,* 371–379.

Mandler, G. (1967). Organization and memory. In K.W. Spence, & J.T. Spence (Eds.), *The psychology of learning and motivation: Advances in research and theory* (Vol. 1). New York: Academic Press.

Mandler, G. (1979a). Organization and repetition: Organizational principles with special reference to rote learning. In L.-G. Nilsson (Ed.), *Perspectives on memory research.* Hillsdale, NJ: Lawrence Erlbaum Associates.

Mandler, G. (1979b). Organization, memory, and mental structures. In C.R. Puff (Ed.), *Memory organization and structure.* New York: Academic Press.

Mandler, G. (1980). Recognizing: The judgment of previous occurrence. *Psychological Review, 87,* 252–271.

Mandler, G. (1982). The integration and elaboration of memory structures. In F. Klix, J. Hoffmann, & E. van der Meer (Eds.), *Cognitive research in psychology.* Amsterdam: North Holland.

Mandler, G. (1985). *Cognitive psychology: An essay in cognitive science.* Hillsdale, NJ: Lawrence Erlbaum Associates.

Mandler, G. (1986). *The function of consciousness in psychological theory* (Paper delivered to symposium on "Aspects of consciousness and awareness"). Center for Interdisciplinary Studies, University of Bielefeld, Bielefeld, West Germany; December, 1986.

Mandler, G., Graf, P., & Kraft, D. (1986). Activation and elaboration effects in recognition and word priming. *The Quarterly Journal of Experimental Psychology, 38A,* 645–662.

Mandler, G., Rabinowitz, J.C., & Simon, R.A. (1981). Coordinate organization: The holistic representation of word pairs. *American Journal of Psychology, 94,* 209–222.

Mandler, J.M. (1984). Representation and recall in infancy. In M. Moscovitch (Ed.), *Infant memory.* New York: Plenum.

Mandler, J.M. (1988). How to build a baby: On the development of an accessible representational system. Cognitive Development, *3,* 113–136.

Marcel, A.J. (1983). Conscious and unconscious perception: An approach to the relations between phenomenal experience and perceptual processes. *Cognitive Psychology, 15,* 238–300.

McKoon, G., Ratcliff, R., & Dell, G.S. (1986). A critical evaluation of the semantic-episodic distinction. *Journal of Experimental Psychology: Learning, Memory, and Cognition, 12,* 295–306.

McKoon, G., Ratcliff, R., & Verwoerd, M. (1986). A bias interpretation of

facilitation in perceptual identification. *Bulletin of the Psychonomic Society,*
24, 323.

Meyer, D.E., & Schvaneveldt, R.W. (1971). Facilitation in recognizing pairs of
words: Evidence of a dependence between retrieval operations. *Journal of*
Experimental Psychology, 90, 227–234.

Neely, J.H. (1977). Semantic priming and retrieval from lexical memory: Roles of
inhibitionless spreading activation and limited-capacity attention. *Journal of*
Experimental Psychology: General, 106, 226–254.

Ratcliff, R., & McKoon, G. (1986). More on the distinction between episodic and
semantic memories. *Journal of Experimental Psychology: Learning, Memory,*
and Cognition, 12, 312–313.

Rumelhart, D.E., & McClelland, J.L. (1986). *Parallel distributed processing:*
Explorations in the microstructure of cognition. Vol. 1-*Foundations.* Cambridge, MA.: MIT Press.

Schacter, D.L., & Graf, P. (1986). Preserved learning in amnesic patients:
Perspectives from research on direct priming. *Journal of Clinical and Experi-*
mental Neuropsychology, 8, 727–743.

Segal, M.A., & Mandler, G. (1967). Directionality and organizational processes in
paired-associate learning. *Journal of Experimental Psychology, 74,* 305–312.

Squire, L.R., Shimamura, A.P., & Graf, P. (1985). Independence of recognition
memory and priming effects: A neuropsychological analysis. *Journal of Experi-*
mental Psychology: Learning, Memory, and Cognition, 11, 37–44.

Tulving, E. (1985). Memory and consciousness. *Canadian Psychology, 26,* 1–12.

Tulving, E. (1986). What kind of a hypothesis is the distinction between episodic
and semantic memory? *Journal of Experimental Psychology: Learning, Mem-*
ory, and Cognition, 12, 307–311.

Warrington, E.K., & Weiskrantz, L. (1970). Amnesia: Consolidation or retrieval?
Nature, 228, 628–630.

Weiskrantz, L. (1985). On issues and theories of the human amnesic syndrome. In
N. M. Weinberger, J.L. McGaugh, & G. Lynch (Eds.), *Memory systems of the*
brain: Animal and human cognitive processes (pp. 380–415). New York:
Guilford Press.

CHAPTER 6

The Uses of Working Memory

Alan Baddeley

G. Stanley Hall was a man of broad interests whose early theological training in no way blinded him to the exciting evolutionary ideas that were so influential at the time. For that reason, I like to think that he would approve of the topic I have chosen, working memory, since it touches on a wide range of other disciplines including developmental psychology, the psychology of education, and neuropsychology. My own involvement in the concept stems from a series of experiments carried out jointly with Graham Hitch on short-term memory, experiments that were aimed at answering the implicitly evolutionist question, "What is STM for?" I would like to describe some of the results of our pursuit, and to emphasize that it continues to be useful to bear in mind the question of evolutionary value in investigating the many phenomena that have been revealed by recent research on human memory.

Short-Term Versus Long-Term Memory

In his classic book, *Organization of Behavior,* Hebb (1949) argued among other things for a separation between short-term memory, a system based on temporary electrical activity, and long-term memory, a system depending on a durable change in the neural substructure of the brain. Active interest in the possible dissociation between short-term memory (STM) and long-term memory (LTM) became a much more live issue with the demonstration by Brown (1958) and by Peterson and Peterson (1959) that small amounts of material are rapidly forgotten if the subject is prevented from continuous rehearsal. These investigators interpreted their results in terms of a separate short-term store in which forgetting resulted from trace decay. This view was resisted in the early 1960s, notably by Melton (1963), who argued that a single theory based on classical interference principles was able to explain the data from both STM and LTM. This in turn led to a flurry of experimentation in the mid-1960s concerned with the question of whether it is necessary to assume separate STM and LTM systems.

Evidence in favour of a dichotomy came from the following phenomena:

1. *Limited storage capacity.* STM appears to have a capacity of about
seven items (Miller, 1956), whereas the storage capacity of LTM is clearly
enormous.

2. *Two-component tasks.* A number of tasks clearly comprise two
separable components, one relatively durable, the other showing rapid
forgetting if rehearsal is prevented. The most extensively studied example
of this is of course free recall, where retention of the last few items is
excellent if recall is immediate (the recency effect), but is severely
impaired by a brief filled delay. In contrast, performance on earlier items
is much more robust (see Glanzer, 1972, for a review).

3. *Differential coding.* Immediate serial recall of sequences of letters or
words appears to depend principally on a speech-based phonological
code, whereas the long-term learning of equivalent material appears to be
primarily based on semantic coding (Baddeley, 1966a,b).

4. *Neuropsychological evidence.* The classic amnesic syndrome involves grossly impaired LTM coupled with intact STM, as measured by the
recency effect in free recall or by immediate memory span (Baddeley and
Warrington, 1970; Milner, 1966). Shallice and Warrington (1970) showed
the converse pattern in the case of patients who have grossly impaired
digit span couped with normal long-term learning capacity. Both types of
patients suggest that STM and LTM depend on separate underlying
systems.

By the late 1960s, the evidence seemed strongly to favor a dichotomous
view of memory such as that reflected in the influential model proposed
by Atkinson and Shiffrin (1968). During the early 1970s, however, it
became increasingly clear that the picture was more complicated than that
suggested by the Atkinson and Shiffrin "modal model" of memory.

One particularly problematic aspect of the modal model was its
assumption about the role of STM in long-term learning. The model
assumed that to be registered in LTM, or indeed retrieved from LTM, an
item must pass through STM. It further assumed that the greater the time
spent in STM, the higher the probability of transfer, and hence the greater
the learning (Atkinson & Shiffrin, 1968). However, Craik and Watkins
(1973) showed that it is possible to set up a situation in which items are
maintained in STM for substantial periods of time, with relatively little
long-term learning and in the absence of any evidence for a positive
correlation between time in STM and probability of long-term retention.
A further problem was presented by the STM patients studied by Shallice
and Warrington (1970). Since such patients were shown to have grossly
defective STM, and long-term learning is crucially dependent on STM,
then LTM should also have been impaired. Yet the patients' long-term
learning capacity was quite normal.

The relationship between type of coding and duration of memory also proved to be more complex than at first suggested. In particular, it is clearly necessary to have phonologically based LTM as well as phonological STM if people are ever to learn to speak or understand a language. Even the two-component task evidence began to look questionable when it was demonstrated that recency effects could be demonstrated that were not obliterated by a period of backward counting (e.g., Tzeng, 1973), and indeed under certain circumstances could be shown to extend over a matter of days or even weeks, as in the demonstration of recency in the memory of players for rugby football games described by Baddeley and Hitch (1977).

One attempt to circumvent these growing problems was presented by Craik and Lockhart (1972) in their "levels of processing" approach to memory. This replaced the concept of structurally separate STM and LTM systems, each relying principally on a different type of coding, with the assumption that the coding itself was the principal factor in determining memory trace durability. The more deeply an item was encoded, the longer its trace was likely to last. Craik and Lockhart continued to view memory as dichotomous, with primary memory being responsible for the recoding of incoming stimuli. However, the point of emphasis of this approach was on the relationship between coding and durability in LTM, with the nature and characteristics of the short-term or primary memory system receiving little attention from Craik and Lockhart themselves, and even less from others who subsequently embraced the levels of processing approach.

The Role of Short-Term Memory

About the time that Craik and Lockhart were formulating their new approach, Graham Hitch and I were similarly dissatisfied with the current state of research on STM. We decided to tackle the problem by asking an apparently very simple question, "What is STM for?" We decided that if its only function was to keep experimental psychologists happy, then we would rather be kept happy in some other way. In fact there was no shortage of speculations as to the role of STM, although there was remarkably little direct evidence. The most common claim was that it served as a *working memory,* a system for temporarily holding information involved in such important cognitive skills as comprehending, reasoning, and learning. There was, however, little evidence in support of this view. Indeed, one might argue that the evidence from STM patients was diametrically against it, since such patients as had been described often appeared to have remarkably few problems in coping with everyday life. Shallice and Warrington's patient J.B., for example, was a very successful secretary, while P.V., a patient studied by Vallar and I, (1984) was able to run a small shop single-handedly as well as look after her family. The question, then, remained an open one.

One of the difficulties in asking questions about STM stemmed from the fact that there were many different models, each with its own set of assumptions. Fortunately, however, virtually all of the models made two central assumptions; that STM has a limited capacity and that immediate memory span is set by this capacity. We therefore decided to study the capacity of our subjects to perform tasks assumed to depend on short-term memory while at the same time they were retaining sequences of digits. If STM is used for immediate memory span, and STM is essential for reasoning, comprehending, and learning, then a concurrent memory span task should occupy all or most of the available STM capacity, and hence should grossly impair the capacity to reason, comprehend, and learn.

We carried out a range of experiments in which subjects were presented with sequences of digits for immediate recall at the same time as they were performing another cognitive task. In one such study, a concurrent digit load ranging from zero to nine items was combined with a reasoning task. This required the subject to verify sentences that varied in syntactic complexity. Each sentence described the order of two letters, A and B. The subject was required to process the sentence and letters and then press a "true" or "false" key as rapidly as possible. The sentences ranged from simple active declarative sentences such as *A follows B—BA* (true) to more complex items such as *A is not preceded by B—BA* (false). The results of our study are shown in Fig. 6.1, from which two things are clear. First, there is a tendency for verification time to increase systematically with concurrent digit span load. This is obviously consistent with the idea that a single limited-capacity system is involved in both immediate memory span and verbal reasoning. A second point to note, however, is that although the effects of concurrent span are clear, they are far from catastrophic. Even when the subject is given a memory load of nine items, beyond the span of most of our subjects, the increase in latency is only about 30%. Even more striking, however, is the absence of an effect of concurrent load on error rate, which remains at approximately 5% regardless of the length of the concurrent digit sequence. This is clearly inconsistent with the concept of a single unitary STM system acting as a working memory, since a sequence of nine digits should be more than sufficient to occupy the total capacity of the working memory, leaving no capacity for performing the verbal reasoning task.

Data from research on comprehension and learning produced a similar pattern, namely, that concurrent digit span produced a clear decrement in performance, but one that was far from catastrophic. Particularly problematic for the modal model of memory was our finding that the recency effect in free recall was quite unaffected by concurrent digit span

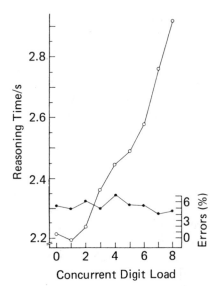

FIGURE 6.1. Speed and accuracy of verbal reasoning as a function of concurrent memory load.

(Baddeley & Hitch, 1977). This latter result rules out the classic interpretation of recency, which assumes it to reflect the output of the same limited-capacity short-term store as it responsible for verbal digit span (Atkinson & Shiffrin, 1968).

To explain our pattern of results, Hitch and I abandoned the idea that working memory reflects a single unitary system. We replaced this view with a model that assumes a controlling central executive of limited capacity that is aided by a number of subsidiary slave systems. Two such systems have been explored in some detail. The *visuospatial sketchpad* is assumed to be responsible for the temporary storage and manipulation of visuospatial information, while the *articulatory loop* is assumed to be a system for temporarily holding speech-based material. I will briefly describe the evidence for the two systems, and then say something about the purpose that each might serve.

The Visuospatial Sketchpad

This slave system is assumed to be involved in the setting up and temporary maintenance of visuospatial images. Hence, given the question "How many windows are there in your present home?," most people work out the answer by forming some kind of visual image of their house and then counting the windows. The visual image is assumed to be held in the sketchpad, while the running total involved in counting depends on the articulatory Loop (Logie & Baddeley, 1987). The distinction between visual and verbal coding is well represented by a recent as-yet unpublished study by Logie, Zucco, and myself (see Baddeley, 1988). This involved two memory tasks, one visuospatial and the other verbal, and two interference tasks. The visual memory task involved presenting the subject with a matrix of cells, half of which were filled and half unfilled at random. After a 2-second presentation and a 2-second delay, the matrix was presented again, with the exception that one of the previously occupied cells was now empty. The subject's task was to point to that cell. We began with a 2 × 2 matrix, adding two cells each time the subject was successful until a point occurred when performance broke down. This is a modification of the task used extensively by Phillips and his colleagues to study visual short-term memory (e.g., Phillips & Christie, 1977).

Our verbal span task also involved testing by recognition. In this case, consonants were presented one at a time in a certain sequence in the center of a visual display unit. Retention was then tested by presenting a sequence that was identical except for the change of one letter. We started with sequences of two consonants, incrementing the sequence length until the subject made three successive errors.

The visuospatial interference task involved the *auditory* presentation of information that allowed the subject to construct a *visual* digit by filling in the cells of the 3 × 5 matrix. Hence, if F represented a filled cell and U an unfilled cell, with the order of reporting of cells being left to right and top to bottom, the digit 7 would be represented by

$F F F$
$U U F$
$U U F$
$U U F$
$U U F$

The verbal interfering task required the subject to add a sequence of single digits, reported the running total after each new digit. An example might be (with the subject's response in parentheses): 7, 4(11), 8(19), 6 (25), 2(27). Subjects combined the two distracting tasks with the two memory tasks. The degree of decrement observed in the various conditions is shown in Figure 6.2.

While it is clear that both secondary tasks can create a certain amount of decrement in the case of both memory tasks, there is a very clear crossover interaction, as would be predicted by separable visuospatial and verbal memory systems. Needless to say, a single experiment is not sufficient to establish the need to assume a system as complex as working memory. A much more extensive and detailed justification is given in Baddeley (1986).

Suppose, for the sake of argument, we accept the case for a visuospatial sketchpad—what function does it serve? One obvious possibility is that it might underlie the enormously powerful effect of imagery in verbal learning. Paivio (1971) has shown that the rated imageability or con-

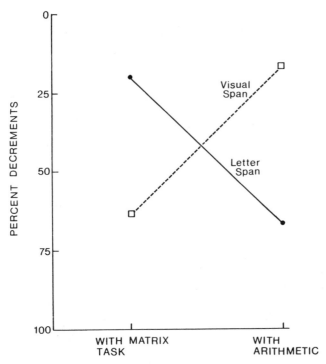

FIGURE 6.2. Disruption of visual and verbal span by concurrent imagery and counting tasks. Data from an unpublished study by Logie, Zucco, and Baddeley.

creteness of a word is a very effective predictor of ease of recall. It is possible that this effect is mediated by the sketchpad, with imageable words being represented not only in verbal memory but also in terms of a temporary visuospatial images. Such an image might allow the setting up of an additional supplementary encoding, which in turn enhances subsequent recall.

We tested this studying the effect on paired-associate learning of high and low imageability material of a task know to disrupt the operation of the visuospatial sketchpad. The task was tracking a spot of light following a circular path on a pursuit rotor, a task that we had previously shown to have a devastating effect on the use of a short-term visuospatial imagery mnemonic. We had our subjects learn and immediately recall pairs of items that were either highly imageable (e.g., *BULLET-GREY*) or low in imageability (e.g., *IDEA-ORIGINAL*), under either control conditions or while a visuospatial tracking task was performed. We obtained a very large effect of imageability and a small effect of tracking, but no trace of an interaction. It appears, then, that concurrent tracking does not interfere with the advantage enjoyed by high imageability items (Baddeley

& Lieberman, 1980). We interpret this as suggesting that the word-imageability effect is based on the already established characteristics of the word as represented in semantic memory; it does not depend on the recreation of an image for its effectiveness.

We went on from this to look at the effects of disruption of the sketchpad on the use of visual imagery mnemonics that might be assumed to demand the active manipulation of visuospatial images. In one study, we taught our subjects to use a location mnemonic in which a sequence of 10 objects were imaged at 10 locations along a walk through a university campus. We contrasted this with a condition in which the items were presented too rapidly to allow the formation of images but on several occasions, to equate total learning time. Our results showed a clear advantage to the imagery mnemonic under control conditions, but the advantage was totally abolished when the tasks were combined with visuospatial tracking (Baddeley and Lieberman, 1980).

Further evidence of the involvement of the visuospatial sketchpad in imagery mnemonics comes from a recent series of experiments by Logie (1986). Logie showed that performance on the well-known one-is-a-bun pegword mnemonic can be disrupted by concurrent visual stimulation, even when the subject is merely required to keep the eyes focused on a screen on which line drawings appear, with no requirement that the potentially disrupting material be processed or retained. As we shall see later, an equivalent effect occurs in the case of disruption of short-term phonological storage by unattended spoken material.

Apart from exploration of the role of the sketchpad in visual imagery, there has been relatively little investigation of its importance in other tasks. This is beginning to change, however: Recent studies have shown the importance of the system in a task involving simple spatial problem solving (Farmer, Berman, & Fletcher, 1986), its involvement in the early though not later stages of learning a complex computer game (Logie, Baddeley, Mane, Donchin, & Sheptak, 1988), and that some such system is probably involved in drivers' responding to verbal instructions about routes (Wright, Holloway, & Aldrich, 1974).

One area that would clearly to worth exploring further is the role of the system in reading and comprehension, where there is some evidence that visually imageable material may need some form of visuospatial storage (Eddy & Glass, 1981). A rather more low level but possibly even more important potential function for something equivalent to a sketchpad is involved in how a reader manages to keep his or her place while reading text presented on a crowded page. Clearly some form of relatively precise visual framework must be stored and used, although the nature of such a framework remains unclear (Kennedy, 1983).

The Articulatory Loop

Conrad (1964) observed that when subjects attempted the immediate serial recall of sequences of visually presented consonants, intrusion errors were far from random. In particular they tended to be similar in sound to the correct items, *B*, for example, being much more likely to be misremembered as *V* than as *S*, which was much more likely to occur as a substitution for a phonologically similar letter such as *F*. He suggested that STM might be acoustically based, a suggestion that subsequently attracted a good deal of support.

The working memory model reinterpreted these results by suggesting that they represent the operation of one of the slave systems of working memory, a system termed the *articulatory loop*. The system is assumed to comprise a short-term phonological store in which traces will decay unless refreshed by rehearsal. The process of rehearsal is analogous to that of subvocal speech, although it does not depend on the actual operation of the peripheral articulatory processes. This articulatory control process is useful in two ways: It is able to act as a rehearsal loop, hence maintaining the fading memory trace, and in addition it serves to allow visually presented material to be phonologically coded (provided, of course, that the items are phonologically codable). Although relatively simple, the assumption of a phonological store supported by an articulatory control process is capable of explaining a rich and complex range of data. Phenomena that can be explained include the following:

1. *The phonological similarity effect.* Similar items lead to poorer immediate serial recall than dissimilar items because the code of registration is phonological. Hence the items are potentially more confusable and harder to recall (Conrad & Hull, 1964). This is not simply a general similarity effect, since similarity of meaning does not impair immediate recall while similarity of sound has a dramatic effect (Baddeley, 1966a,b).

2. *The unattended speech effect.* Immediate serial recall of visually presented digits or words is impaired when presentation is accompanied by irrelevant spoken material (Colle & Welsh, 1976). The effect does not depend on the semantic characteristics of the unattended material, since nonsense syllables or the words of an unfamiliar language are just as disruptive as English, although the phonological characteristics of the unattended message are important (Salame & Baddeley, 1982). It is assumed that this effect occurs because the unattended material gains obligatory access to the phonological store and hence can interfere with the attempt to use this store to aid the remembering of the visually presented items.

3. *The word-length effect.* Immediate memory for word sequences is a direct function of the time it takes to say the relevant words. Span is

equivalent to the amount that can be spoken in approximately 1.5 s, and as such is greater for short words than for long (Baddeley, Thomson, & Buchanan, 1975). The effect depends on speaking duration rather than number of syllables, with span being better for disyllabic words with short vowel sounds such as *bishop* and *wicket* than for those involving long vowel sounds such as *harpoon* and *Friday*. The word-length effect is assumed to reflect the active process of articulatory rehearsal. Span is assumed to be a joint function of the time it takes a memory trace within the phonological store to fade, and the speed at which it can be refreshed by rehearsal. Short words can be rehearsed faster than long, hence more short items can be maintained, leading to a greater memory span.

4. *The articulatory suppression effect.* If the subject is prevented for subvocal rehearsal by having to repeatedly articulate some irrelevant sound such as the word *the,* immediate memory performance is impaired (Murray, 1968). With visual presentation of the memory material, suppression removes the effects of phonological similarity, unattended speech, or word length. This is presumably because suppression prevents the subject from transferring the visual material into a phonological code, and hence makes it impossible to use the phonological store to supplement memory performance. With auditory presentation, suppression does not remove either the phonological similarity or the unattended speech effects, since spoken stimuli gain direct access to the articulatory loop (Baddeley, Lewis, & Vallar, 1984). The word-length effect, however, is disrupted, since this is assumed to depend on the same articulatory control process as is required for performing the suppression task.

5. *Neuropsychological evidence.* Analysis of the performance of patients with a specific deficit of verbal STM indicates that the deficit can be accounted for by the articulatory loop model relatively easily. For example, patient P.V. studied by Vallar and Baddeley (1984a) proved to have impaired auditory STM coupled with the absence of a phonological similarity effect for visually presented material, and absence as well of a word-length effect. Her capacity to articulate rapidly, however, was unimpaired, suggesting that the articulatory control process was normal. The reason for her deficits probably stemmed from a very limited-capacity phonological store; subvocal rehearsal would offer few advantages, since it would simply result in feeding information into the defective component of the system.

To summarize, the concept of an articulatory loop comprising a phonologically based short-term store and an articulatory control process is able to explain a wide range of empirical results. I know of no equivalent model that can deal with this rich pattern of data, and regard this as strong evidence for the continued usefulness of the articulatory loop concept. However, while the concept may be very useful in accounting for laboratory data, it still leaves open the question of what function this system might serve from an evolutionary viewpoint.

What is the Articulatory Loop For?

As we have seen, laboratory evidence for some kind of system resembling the articulatory loop is relatively strong, and yet there is comparatively little evidence for the importance of this system outside the laboratory. In particular, as mentioned earlier, two of the most extensively studied STM patients appear capable of carrying on a normal everyday life with few signs of obvious handicap. There does appear to be considerable evidence for the involvement of short-term phonological storage in learning to read (Baddeley, 1986, chap. 9; Jorm, 1983), but on an evolutionary time scale, the development of reading is surely far too recent to support the claim that the loop evolved as a result of its role in reading. A more plausible suggestion is that is serves a crucial function in the comprehensive of spoken language. For example, Clark and Clark (1977) have suggested that the process of sentence comprehension demands the storage of the sentence in some temporary phonological code prior to its syntactic and semantic analysis. What is the evidence for this?

It is almost certainly the case that the strong version of the hypothesis as presented by Clark and Clark is incorrect. Indeed, a recent study by Butterworth, Campbell, and Howard (1986) claims to find no evidence of impaired comprehension in a subject who has a digit span of only three to four items. However, unlike the previously reported STM patients, this subject was apparently born with a reduced capacity for immediate memory, and appears to have developed techniques for coping with this rather effectively. She is able to read sufficiently well to obtain a good psychology degree, but nonetheless is a phonological dyslexic in that she is unable to read nonwords (Campbell & Butterworth, 1985). She appears by dint of careful tuition to have learned to read almost entirely through the visual route. It is therefore possible that her comprehension may also be highly atypical.

What of patients who have acquired their STM deficit as a result of brain damage? Vallar and I have studied in some detail the comprehension of spoken and written language by the previously described patient P.V. (Vallar & Baddeley, 1984b; Baddeley, Vallar, & Wilson, 1987). Our results can be briefly summarized as indicating that comprehension of both spoken and printed text is impaired, but not dramatically so. For example, we tested P.V.'s capacity to understand sentences of three types. *Simple sentences* described obvious aspects of the world (e.g., *Canaries have wings*). *Verbose sentences* were essentially equivalent to the simple items except that irrelevant verbiage was added (*It is com-*

monly believed and with some justification that canaries belong to the class of creatures that possess wings). We termed the third type *complex sentences;* in the use of these we assumed that it would be necessary to maintain the surface characteristics of the sentence in order to verify it. An example of this type is the sentence *The earth divides the equator into two halves, the northern and the southern.*

Out patient P.V. had no difficulty in comprehending sentences of the first two types, but was severely impaired relative to a control group in comprehending the third complex sentence type. On the other hand, when this type of sentence was compressed so as to ensure that is was within her memory span for sentential materials (six words), her performance was near normal.

Data from this and other paradigms therefore suggested that P.V. would encounter comprehension problems only with relatively complex material (Vallar & Baddeley, 1984b). Does this then suggest that the articulatory loop is of only marginal importance in speech comprehension, providing a backup for handling particularly complex material, or is some other explanation possible?

One possibility is to point out that although P.V.'s span is impaired, it is far from obliterated by her brain damage. Indeed, with sentential material she has a span of six words. If one assumes that the phonological store acts as a kind of mnemonic "window" allowing incoming items to be held simultaneously and interrelated, then it is conceivable that a window of six words is sufficient to understand all but complex material. The best way to test this is to attempt to find and test a patient who is intellectually as unimpaired as P.V. but who has an even shorter sentence span. Such a patient should show a much greater impairment in the comprehension of spoken language. A colleague, Barbara Wilson, and I recently studied such a patient, T.B. (Baddeley, Vallar, & Wilson, 1987).

T.B. is a highly intelligent man who was working as a professional mathematician until epileptic seizures and consequent memory problems forced him to retire. He coupled a very high I.Q. and normal speech with a grossly impaired immediate memory span, which even for sentential materials was limited to two words. We tested T.B. on a range of tasks including Bishop's (1982) Test for the Reception of Grammar (TROG). T.B.'s performance on this test steadily declined as the sentences became longer. This might of course reflect either his limited memory span or the fact that longer sentences tended to be syntactically more complex.

We tried to separate these two possibilities by means of a number of further experiments. In one study, we took sentences from the TROG that he was able to comprehend and extended their length by adding a number of redundant adjectives and adverbs. For example, the sentence *The pencil is above the knife* might be changed to *The long red pencil is directly above the sharp pointed knife.* Since all the pencils were red and of the same length, all knives were sharp, and all the pictured representations had one item directly above the other, the added material was entirely redundant. Nonetheless, it reduced his performance from 21/24 to a chance level of 6/24 items correct, supporting an interpretation in terms of sentence length rather than syntactic complexity.

In a further test, we allowed T.B. to read each sentence at his own speed. Under these conditions, his error rate dropped substantially, but only at the expense of a very substantial increase in reading time for certain of the longer sentences. The sentences of the TROG fell into three broad categories: (a) Some sentences were verified as rapidly and accurately as was the case for a control subject. These tended to be short, though not necessarily syntactically simple sentences, an example being *The boy is not running*. (b) A second type of sentence was one in which T.B. was able to respond correctly when reading the sentence, but not when hearing it. Typically his reading time was slow, as if he were performing the task as a verbal jigsaw puzzle, combining and permuting words until the correct solution was achieved. *The pencil is on the book that is yellow* is an example of this type of sentence. (c) Finally, certain sentences were still verified very poorly, despite a lengthy and determined attempt at comprehension. An example of such a sentence is *The book the pencil is on is red*. The sentences of the latter type tended to be characterized by some form of self-embedding, where comprehension required the simultaneous holding of sentence fragments exceeding two or three words. If one splits the sentence up into three-word chunks, none of the chunks is enough to disambiguate it. With the example just given, splitting yields *The book the, book the pencil, the pencil is, pencil is one, is on is, on is red*, in contrast to the earlier examples, where chunks of three items are usually sufficient for comprehension, for example, *The boy is, boy is not, is not running*.

In conclusion, then, when memory span is reduced to two or three words, comprehension is grossly impaired. Such results are consistent with the view that the phonological storage component of the articulatory loop plays a crucial role in the comprehension of spoken language.

Is this the only role of the articulatory loop system? As mentioned earlier, an impaired memory span appears to be one of the more striking characteristics of developmental dyslexia, a finding that has been reinforced by some recent work by Susan Gathercole and myself. We were interested in investigating the characteristics of a small group of 7- to 8-year-old children who were classified as having normal intelligence but delayed language development. When tested, a group of such children did indeed prove to have impaired performance on the type of immediate memory task that is assumed to reflect the operation of the articulatory loop. In fact, the most striking difference between these children and controls matched for general intelligence was their performance on a task that involved the simple repetition of nonwords varying in length and complexity. On this task they averaged no less than 42 months (range 38-61) below the performance of other children of their age.

It seems at least plausible that the incapacity to store incoming phonological information may have severe implications for the development of vocabulary (see chap. 8 in this volume). Subsequently, impaired articulatory loop capacity may well disrupt the acquisition of a skill such as reading in which it is necessary to map visually presented letter sequences onto phonologically based sounds. We are currently carrying out a prospective study in which we hope to follow up a cohort of children from their first arrival at school to the point at which they should have learned to read, correlating performance on this simple nonword repetition task with both vocabulary and reading development. We hope that this may allow us to predict which children will have difficulty, and possible subsequently to devise teaching methods that may alleviate this problem.

If the articulatory loop is needed for new phonological learning such as is involved in the acquisition of vocabulary, one might expect that learning new vocabulary would be difficult for STM patients. Vallar, Papagno, and I are exploring this in the case of our Italian STM patient P.V. In the first of our studies, we have compared her capacity for learning to associate pairs of familiar Italian words with her capacity to perform a word–nonword task equivalent to that of teaching her Russian vocabulary. We have studied her capacity for learning when presentation of both the Italian and the Russian words is verbal and when presentation is visual. Compared with a group of control subjects of equivalent age and intelligence, P.V. shows normal paired-associate learning when the items to be associated are familiar Italian words. However, when she has to learn to respond with a Russian word to an Italian stimulus, her performance is significantly impaired with visual presentation and is disastrously bad when presentation is auditory. Indeed, in the auditory condition, after 10 successive trails she failed to learn a single Italian-Russian associate.

It appears, then, that the articulatory loop plays a central role in new phonological learning, a task that is of course essential for learning one's native language. It is likely to be similarly important in the acquisition of secondary skills such as reading and second language learning. Finally, recent work demonstrating that articulatory suppression leads to a marked impairment in counting accuracy (Logie & Baddeley, 1987), coupled with Hitch's (1978) earlier evidence for the importance of working memory in mental arithmetic, suggests that the articulatory loop may prove to have a role in a much wider range of cognitive skills.

Conclusions

The research I have described stemmed from taking the concept of short-term memory, a concept central to the information-processing approach to cognition, and asking what function it serves, a question that is more frequently associated with biological approaches to behavior. The simple combination of these two has provided a good deal of new empirical information and has thrown light on problems of neuropsychology, education, and development that extend considerably beyond the boundaries of the initial experiments on STM. I like to think that such research on working memory is characteristic of a current trend in cognitive psychology, namely, that of serving as a link between fields that have in the past too often been seen as offering separate and competing views of psychology. As such, I trust that Stanley Hall with his range of interests and breadth of knowledge would perhaps have approved.

Acknowledgement. I am grateful to Karalyn Patterson and Robert Logie for comments on an earlier draft of his paper.

References

Atkinson, R.C., & Shiffrin, R.M. (1968). Human memory: A proposed system and its control processes. In Spence, K.W. (Ed.), *The psychology of learning and motivation: Advances in research and theory* (Vol. 2, pp. 89–195). New York: Academic Press.

Baddeley, A.D. (1966a). The influence of acoustic and semantic similarity on long-term memory for word sequences. *Quarterly Journal of Experimental Psychology, 18,* 302–309.

Baddeley, A.D. (1966b). Short-term memory for word sequences as a function of acoustic, semantic and formal similarity. *Quarterly Journal of Experimental Psychology, 18,* 362–365.

Baddeley, A.D. (198). *Working memory.* Oxford, England: Oxford University Press.

Baddeley, A.D. (1988). Imagery and working memory. In Denis, M., & Engelcamp, J., & Richardson, J.T.E. (Eds.) *Cognitive and neuropsychological approaches to mental imagery.* Boston, U.S.A: Martinus Nijhof. pp 169–180.

Baddeley, A.D., & Hitch, G.J. (1977). Recency re-examined. In Dornic, S. (Ed.), *Attention and performance* (Vol. 6, pp 647–667). Hillsdale, NJ: Lawrence Erlbaum Associates.

Baddeley, A.D., Lewis, V., & Vallar, G. (1984). Exploring the articulatory loop. *Quarterly Journal of Experimental Psychology, 36,* 233–252.

Baddeley, A.D., & Lieberman, K. (1980). Spatial working memory. In Nickerson, R.S. (Ed.), *Attention and performance* (Vol. 8, pp. 521–539). Hillsdale, NJ: Lawrence Erlbaum Associates.

Baddeley, A.D., Thomson, N., & Buchanan, M. (1975). Word length and the structure of short-term memory. *Journal of Verbal Learning and Verbal Behavior, 14,* 575–589.

Baddeley, A.D., Vallar, G., & Wilson, B. Comprehension and the articulatory loop: Some neuropsychological evidence. In Coltheart, M. (Ed.), *Attention and performance. XII The psychology of reading.* London: Lawrence Erlbaum Associates, (pp. 509–529).

Baddeley, A.D., & Warrington, E.K. (1970). Amnesia and the distinction between long- and short-term memory. *Journal of Verbal Learning and Verbal Behavior, 9,* 176–189.

Bishop, D. (1982). *T.R.O.G.: Test for reception of grammar*. Abingdon, Oxon, England: Thomas Leach (printed for the Medical Research Council).

Brown, J. (1958) Some tests of the decay theory of immediate memory. *Quarterly Journal of Experimental Psychology, 10*, 12–21.

Butterworth, B., Campbell, R., & Howard, D. (1986). The uses of short-term memory: A case study. *Quarterly Journal of Experimental Psychology, 38A*, 705–738.

Campbell, R., and Butterworth, B. (1985) Phonological dyslexia and dysgraphia in a highly literate subject: A developmental case with associated deficits of phonemic processing and awareness. *Quarterly Journal of Experimental Psychology, 37A*, 435–475.

Clark, H.H., & Clark, E.V. (1977). *Psychology and language*. New York: Harcourt Brace Jovanovic.

Colle, H.A., & Welsh, A. (1976). Acoustic masking in primary memory. *Journal of Verbal Learning and Verbal Behavior, 15*, 17–32.

Conrad, R. (1964). Acoustic confusion in immediate memory. *British Journal of Psychology, 55*, 75–84.

Conrad, R., & Hull, A.J. (1964). Information, acoustic confusion and memory span. *British Journal of Psychology, 55*, 429–432.

Craik, F.I.M., & Lockhart, R.S. (1972). Levels of processing: A framework for memory research. *Journal of Verbal Learning and Verbal Behavior, 11*, 671–684.

Craik, F.I.M., & Watkins, M.J. (1973). The role of rehearsal in short-term memory. *Journal of Verbal Learning and Verbal Behavior, 12*, 599–607.

Eddy, J.K., & Glass, A.L. (1981). Reading and listening to high and low imagery sentences. *Journal of Verbal Learning and Verbal Behavior, 20*, 333–345.

Farmer, E.W., Berman, J.V.F., & Fletcher, Y.L. (1986). Evidence for a visuo-spatial scratchpad in working memory. *Quarterly Journal of Experimental Psychology, 38A*, 675–688.

Glanzer, M. (1972). Storage mechanisms in recall. In Bower, G.H. (Ed.), *The psychology of learning and motivation: Advances in research and theory* (Vol. 5). New York: Academic Press.

Hebb, D.O. (1949). *Organization of behavior*. New York: John Wiley.

Hitch, G.J. (1978). The role of short-term working memory in mental arithmetic. *Cognitive Psychology, 10*, 302–323.

Jorm, A.F. (1983). Specific reading retardation and working memory: A review. *British Journal of Psychology, 74*, 311–342.

Kennedy, A. (1983). On looking into space. In Rayner, K. (Eds.), *Eye movements in reading: Perceptual and language processes*. New York: Academic Press.

Logie, R.H. (1986). Visuo-spatial processing in working memory. *Quarterly Journal of Experimental Psychology, 38A*, 229–247.

Logie, R.H., & Baddeley, A.D. (1987) Cognitive processes in counting. *Journal of Experimental Psychology: Learning, Memory, and Cognition. 13*, 310–326.

Logie, R.H., Baddeley, A.D., Mane, A., Donchin, E., & Sheptak, R. (1988). Visual working memory in the acquisition of complex cognitive skills. In Denis, M., Engelcamp, J., & Richardson, J.T.E. (Eds.), *Cognitive and neuropsychological approaches to mental imagery*. Boston, U.S.A: Martinus Nijhof (pp. 191–202).

Melton, A.W. (1963). Implications of short-term memory for a general theory of memory. *Journal of Verbal Learning and Verbal Behavior, 2,* 1–21.

Miller, G.A. (1956). The magical number seven, plus or minus two: Some limits on our capacity for processing information. *Psychological Review, 63,* 81–97.

Milner, B. (1966). Amnesia following operation on the temporal lobes. In Whitty, C.W.M., & Zangwill, O.L. (Eds.), *Amnesia* (pp. 109–133). London: Butterworths.

Murray, D.J. (1968). Articulation and acoustic confusability in short-term memory. *Journal of Experimental Psychology, 78,* 679–684.

Paivio, A. (1971). *Imagery and verbal processes.* New York: Holt Rinehart and Winston.

Peterson, L.R., & Peterson, M.J. (1959). Short-term retention of individual verbal items. *Journal of Experimental Psychology, 58,* 193–198.

Phillips, W.A., & Christie, D.F.M. (1977). Interference with visualization. *Quarterly Journal of Experimental Psychology, 29,* 637–650.

Salame, P., & Baddeley, A.D. (1982). Disruption of short-term memory by unattended speech: Implications for the structure of working memory. *Journal of Verbal Learning and Verbal Behavior, 21,* 150–164.

Shallice, T., & Warrington, E.K. (1970). Independent functioning of verbal memory stores: A neuropsychological study. *Quarterly Journal of Experimental Psychology, 22,* 261–273.

Tzeng, O.J.L. (1973). Positive recency effect in delayed free recall. *Journal of Verbal Learning and Verbal Behavior, 12,* 436–439.

Vallar, G., & Baddeley, A.D. (1984a) Fractionation of working memory: Neuropsychological evidence for a phonological short-term store. *Journal of Verbal Learning and Verbal Behavior, 23,* 151–161.

Vallar, G., & Baddeley, A.D. (1984b). Phonological short-term store, phonological processing and sentence comprehension: A neuropsychological case study. *Cognitive Neuropsychology, 1,* 121–141.

Wright, P., Holloway, C.M., & Aldrich, A.R. (1974). Attending to visual or auditory information while performing other concurrent tasks. *Quarterly Journal of Experimental Psychology, 26,* 454–463.

Part III Perspectives from Developmental Psychology

CHAPTER 7

Remembering: A Functional Developmental Perspective

Katherine Nelson

Remembering past events is a universally familiar experience. It is also a uniquely human one. As far as we know, members of no other species possess quite the same ability to experience again now, in a different situation and perhaps in a different form, happenings from the past, and know that the experience refers to an event that occurred in another time and in another place. Other members of the animal kingdom . . . cannot travel back into the past in their own minds. (Tulving, 1983, p.1).

With this provocative statement, Tulving opened his book on episodic—in contrast to semantic—memory. It is a position that has provoked a number of demurrers, and Tulving himself seems to have at least half backed away from it (Tulving, 1984). Nonetheless, I believe there is considerable truth to this position, although not all of the phenomena that Tulving attempted to include in the notion of episodic memory can be emcompassed within it. Rather I believe that a close study of the ontogeny of memory in infancy and early childhood can lead to an understanding of just which aspects of the human memory system are unique to our species and which are not. The question, then, is whether there is some sense in which Tulving's claim is true in ontogeny as well as phylogeny.

The position that I will be defending here is that the autobiographical memory system is the uniquely human capacity implicated in Tulving's claim, and further that this system is distinguishable as a separate subsystem within the general episodic memory system. Evidence that such a subsystem is established after the infancy period and is related to the development of language skills and engagement in socially shared memory talk supports the proposal that it is a species-specific capacity. This position necessarily implies that there are basic changes in memory after the close of the infancy period during early to mid childhood. An important part of the research effort, then, is to identify the existence of and the nature of such changes.

Memory Changes in Infancy and Early Childhood

Considerable research and theoretical analysis have established that there
are basic changes in memory and representation during the latter part of
the first year. For example, the work of Kagan, Kearsley, and Zelazo
(1978), of Mandler (1984), and of Schacter and Moscovitch (1984) posits
development of recall in addition to recognition memory, declarative as
well as procedural memory, and late as well as early memory, respectively. In each case, the later memory "system" is assumed to be an
addition to the earlier one, not a replacement of it. Schacter and
Moscovitch compared the development of memory with its dissolution in
amnesics, and they summarized the two systems as follows:

> The early system corresponds to the "unconscious" or "procedural" memory
> that is preserved in amnesics and . . . is available to the infant almost immedi-
> ately after birth. The late system corresponds to the "conscious" or "episodic"
> memory that is impaired in amnesics . . . [it] is not available to infants until the
> latter part of the first year. (p. 179)

This late memory is characterized further as "one that entails conscious
access to recently established representations of events and information"
(p. 178). Schacter and Moscovitch suggest that these two memory
systems constitute the basic mechanisms of the adult human memory;
that is, that no further basic developments take place in the system.
Changes in mnemonic abilities thereafter are attributed to "the emergence of crucial cognitive abilities, such as language and self-concept, and
with ongoing expansion of general knowledge and strategies" (p. 209).
This position is typical of students of memory development, who tend to
attribute changes in memory strategies to the ability to engage in
"metamemory" processes, that is, to reflect on one's own memory and
strategies for remembering.

But I will argue here that the late system that Schacter and Moscovitch postulated is not sufficient to account for all of the characteristics
that Tulving (1983) attributed to episodic memory, in particular to the
ability of humans to "travel back into the past in their own minds." I will
argue (and in citing parallels with the animal literature Schacter and
Moscovitch would appear to agree) that both the early and late systems
that they describe are established in other mammalian species, but that,
as Tulving claimed, there is something uniquely different about human
memory. Specifically, the establishment of autobiographical memory in
early to mid childhood is not accounted for in the Schacter and Moscovitch proposal.

It is striking that until very recently virtually no attention has been
given in memory development research to autobiographical memory and
to one of the most dramatic phenomenon of human memory, namely, the
phenomenon of childhood or infantile amnesia. Research with older

children and adults has established that autobiographical memories begin for most people sometime in early childhood (see Dudycha & Dudycha, 1941, for review). Rarely do they begin prior to 3 years of age, and the frequency of early memories increases slowly until 5 to 8 years. Various authors (Freud, '1963; Wetzler & Sweeney, 1986) date childhood amnesia as lasting until 5 to 6 years of age. There is no problem of retention of autobiographical memory over long periods of time after the age of 3 to 8 years. A 60-year-old can easily remember episodes from 20 or even 40 years earlier, whereas a 20-year-old cannot remember episodes from more than 15 years earlier. The existence of memories stretching back for decades into early childhood makes the barrier to memories before that cutoff point of considerable theoretical interest.

The timing of this development indicates that the study of memory during the preschool period may shed significant light on the meaning of this important transition. A basic question to be answered is whether there is a problem for the child in retaining memories before the age of 3 or 4. Most students of childhood amnesia (as distinct from infantile amnesia in animals) have looked at the phenomenon as Freud (1916) did, asking what happens to block early memories, implicitly assuming that such memories do exist. In contrast, I have taken the opposite approach, asking what happens during the early childhood years that makes enduring memories possible? The research that I report here is motivated at least in part by the goal of uncovering what developments in the memory system may take place during this period and thus ultimately understanding whether the onset of autobiographical memory represents a real discontinuity and thus a separate system.

Early childhood—the years roughly between 2 and 5—comprises a period of critical cognitive development. The boundaries of this period include the most dramatic transitions in all of child development, the first from prelinguistic infancy to language-using childhood. The second transition is harder to characterize concisely, and indeed there is considerable controversy as to whether there is a necessary dramatic shift in functioning or whether observed changes between the ages of 5 and 8 are artifacts of the onset of schooling in literate cultures. Without entering into this discussion (which is irrelevant to the present purpose) it can be said with confidence that the period of early childhood itself consists of important transitions that set the stage for the cognitive achievements of the school years. One might well expect to find, then, important changes in the memory system during this period.

Before we move to consider in some detail memory in early childhood, it is important to be clear about how memory is defined for the present purposes. Roughly speaking there are two approaches to this question. One possibility is to embrace the broadest possible definition of memory, an approach exemplified by Oakley (1983). This enables the theorist to set memory into a broad evolutionary scheme and to make distinctions among different types of memory, or perhaps more appropriately, among types of information storage. This approach has some merit, and I will elaborate on it later.

On the other hand, one may insist on the narrowest definition of memory, restricting memory only to that which provides the rememberer with a valid conscious awareness of having experienced something at a definite point in the past. This is the approach taken by Lockhart (1984)[1] and is roughly what Tulving seems to have intended by the concept of episodic memory; again, it has merit. It excludes from memory all evidence of learning or knowledge that is not accompanied by an awareness on the part of the learner that this bit of knowledge or belief was established on the basis of an experience on a *particular* occasion in the past. This view of memory necessarily excludes virtually all nonhuman memory studies, as well as infant memory research, on the grounds that without language the organism cannot indicate an awareness of pastness (Tulving, 1984, contra Olton, 1984). This view also exludes what is usually referred to as *semantic memory,* as well as other general knowledge representations that may not fit neatly under the semantic memory notion (e.g., Hirst, 1984). Moreover, this view seems to define autobiographical memory as the only valid memory.

To make sense of memory *development* it is necessary both to view memory within a broad evolutionary perspective and to distinguish between different types of memory and of episodic memory in particular, recognizing that some types of episodic memory exist that have an uncertain tie to specific temporal-spatial markers, whereas others are definitely marked in such a way that it is natural to say "I remember we did X on Y occasion." Autobiographical memory in this perspective, then, is viewed as a subtype of episodic memory.

Autobiographical memory, however, seems to have characteristics of both early and late memory systems (Schacter & Mocovitch, 1984), and both semantic and episodic memory (Tulving, 1984). Like episodic memory and late memory, it is based on a specific episode and represents a conscious awareness of an experience in the past; like semantic and early memory it is often invulnerable to loss—it may endure over long periods of time without conscious rehearsal. As noted previously, an important distinctive characteristic of autobiographical memory is that it is not present in infancy but tends to be established in early childhood, usually between 3 and 8 years of age. The study of episodic memory before and after this point should thus be revealing with regard to whether there are special characteristics of the young child's memory that can be identified with the establishment of this system. Thus important questions include: Do very young children have episodic memories or only generic

---

[1] This is also what was meant by Piaget and Inhelder (1969), who distinguished memory in the strict sense in contrast to memory in the broad sense.

(semantic) memories? Are episodic memories of very young children vulnerable or long-lasting?

Another characteristic of autobiographical memory is its organized character. Research suggests that people tend to remember (or to reconstruct) whole episodes in narrative form, reflecting temporal-causal coherence, motivations, intentions, affect, and the interactions between people. Fragments of memory—faces from the past, physical locations such as buildings visited on a trip, songs learned in childhood—may exist within autobiographical memory, but the unique character of this system is reflected in the narrativized episodes that seem to be a part of it.

A final important characteristic of autobiographical memory is that to a large extent it does not seem to be pragmatically motivated, but rather is memory valued for its own sake. This makes it a good candidate for a specifically human characteristic. Autobiographical memory can be enjoyed (or contrastively can serve to embarrass or annoy) and can be shared with others. It might be suggested that the critical differences between autobiographical memory and other types of episodic memory that makes it invulnerable to decay or interference is the fact that it is not utilitarian. It is neither entered into the general knowledge system where it can be used at will, nor forgotten once its utility in a specific situation is past. Rather, it is retained as a kind of personal and social treasure, a continuing reservoir of knowledge about self and others.

To claim that this type of memory is the only legitimate memory as distinct from all other types of learning and knowledge, as Lockhart's discussion seems to do, is to lose the possibility of distinguishing similarities and differences among them and to discern what might be involved in the evolution and development of what we may call "remembering." In particular, there may be kinds of episodic memory that do not include a specific sense of pastness and that thus provide an evolutionary bridge to what may well be a specifically human ability. Moreover, there may be "strict" episodic memories, tied to a specific space-time framework, that do not become part of the autobiographical system.[2]

In considering how these putative types may be related developmentally, it is helpful to note first the characteristics of early childhood memory (in the broad sense) that distinguish it from the earlier and later periods. First, like memory in infancy, memory in early childhood is rarely deliberate. Young children are exposed to a variety of experiences, they are talked to, read to, sung to, sometimes they are even exhorted to remember. But for the most part, they are not expected to use deliberate strategies or to intentionally commit facts to memory, and they do not. Memory is a by-product of everyday life; what children remember is an indicator of interest, salience, importance, or affective intensity.

Second, like memory in infancy, memory in early childhood is pri-

---

[2] Most laboratory experiments no doubt fall into this category.

marily memory of directly experienced events rather than information mediated through instruction or verbal presentations. This characteristic is one that is subject to change over the period. At the onset, when the child is just beginning to learn language, virtually everything known is known through direct experience. By the beginning of the school years, children in our culture have been exposed to considerable mediated knowledge, through stories, TV, and the efforts of adults to enculturate them in the categories considered basic and important, such as colors, shapes, letters, numbers, days of the week, months of the year, and so on. Nonetheless, throughout this period a great portion of the child's daily life is directly experienced. Of course, once language is attained adults may impart to that experience their own interpretation of its structure and meaning. Thus increasingly the child's representation of experience may be expected to take on a form that matches that of the adult. This shift from direct to mediated experience may have an important influence on cognitive development during this period, including development of the memory system.

Third, again like memory in infancy, most of the content of the young child's memory is inaccessible to retrieval later in life, as already discussed.

Fourth, unlike memory in infancy, and like later childhood memory, memory in early childhood can be manifested in a variety of intentional behaviors, including verbal reports. This is a critical difference between the study of memory in infancy and in early childhood in that evidence may be obtainable to indicate not only that information is stored (i.e., that previously presented stimuli are recognized as old), but that the child is aware of having experienced something before and intends to retrieve it. To be sure, Mandler (1984) has presented evidence supporting the claim that infants have established declarative memory enabling them to engage in recall as well as recognition memory prior to the age of 1 year; and Moscovitch and Schacter (1984) have shown that the awareness associated with what they call "late memory" is evidenced by the end of the first year. Still, an awareness of "something happened" is not the same as the awareness that something happened at X time and in Y place. The possibility of a verbal report provides unassailable evidence of intentionality and awareness of a specific experience that eliminates ambiguity on this point. Of course there is still the problem of negative evidence: The child may remember more than he or she can tell. Nonetheless, positive evidence of remembering is of signal importance.

Originally the research questions that were addressed in the study of memory in early childhood were the same as those posed for older children, and the question of interest was, at least in part, how different younger children were from older on memory tasks. Differences could then be used to suggest a course of development. In this mode the younger child was understandably generally seen as quite deficient, and a variety of problems that needed to be overcome was suggested.

A different set of questions has emerged from the concerns of researchers who view memory not as an end in itself, but rather as a function within the general cognitive system. From this view, the younger child's nondeliberate memory could be seen as directed by the needs and goals of current activity. Soviet researchers working within the activity theory originally developed by Vygotsky (1978; see Wertsch, 1985) were pioneers in exploring this approach. Within this general approach, the question is not, how do preschool children differ from older children, but rather what are the characteristics of their memory system as it is displayed in everyday activities? Basic research questions have not disappeared; it is still of interest to know how accurate and long-lasting memory is during this age period. Moreover, of particular interest are such questions as what is remembered (since the preschool child's activities and goals may differ from those of older children and adults, we might expect different aspects of a situation to be encoded and retained), and how is it organized (it might be organized in terms of everyday activities, in contrast to abstract categories, for example). Are there changes in these dimensions during the period in question? Of central interest are any indications that changes in the way episodic memories are organized, stored, and retrieved take place over this age period.

In the next section I review some findings relevant to these questions that have emerged from research carried out by my research group. On the basis of considerations just outlined, our approach employed the strategy of studying nondeliberate memory for naturally occurring events by children aged 2 to 5 years.

Episodic Memory in Early Childhood

A major focus of our research was the investigation of the relation between specific memory and the child's general knowledge system, which we viewed as in large part organized in terms of event representations. The relation between a specific episodic memory and the representation of a general schema for episodes of that class of events is an intricate one that has received limited attention in the general memory literature (e.g., Linton, 1975, 1982). Our interest was developmental: How are event schemas built up from specific experiences, and how might the availability of a general schema affect the memory for a specific instance of that event? This relation in turn seemed to have implications for understanding the development of autobiographical memory.

Diary Studies

One method adopted by several researchers to investigate memory in very young children (Ashmead & Perlmutter, 1980; Wellman & Somerville, 1980) relies on diaries kept by mothers. This method has an ancient history in the field: Developmental psychology originally relied extensively on parental diaries for basic descriptions of the sequence of motor, perceptual, and language development. Later this methodology was largely abandoned in favor of more direct observational and experimental methods, but in the study of language development in particular it still plays a significant role and has made important contributions to our understanding in that field. Diaries are useful in areas where the phenomena under study cannot be experimentally elicited, are spontaneous, and are sporadically and infrequently observed. These conditions hold for the use of words early in language acquisition, as well as for evidence of sponaneous remembering in infants and young children.

To address the first research question, do children have episodic memories prior to 3 years of age, Gail Ross and I (Nelson & Ross, 1980) asked mothers of toddlers (21, 24, and 27 months of age) to keep diary records of their children's memories over a 3-month period. Mothers were provided with a notebook with instructions as to what aspects of each memory episode they were to record, including what cued the memory, how long in the past the remembered episode had occurred, whether it was a frequent or infrequent event, and a basic description of the child's behavior that revealed evidence of a memory. Our aim was to discover whether children of this age could be said to remember specific episodes (memory in the strict sense) as contrasted to general knowledge such as where objects are usually kept. As has been noted before and will be discussed again later, evidence for specific memory is elusive. Even though an episode may have happened only once in the child's life, it is difficult to say with certainty that a memory for that episode has a unique place in the past for the child without some corroborative evidence such as that provided verbally. When the child can state something like "when I went to Grandma's last time we played cards" we can be sure that there is an episodic memory (whether accurate or not). But when the only evidence we have is the child going to the drawer where the cards were kept, we do not know that she is remembering a specific episode or has simply entered "cards are in that drawer at Grandma's house" into a general knowledge system.

Among the findings from this study, based on 19 children and 114 recorded memories, were the following: The most common memory among the youngest children was the location of an object such as the cards in the example just given. This finding accords with DeLoache's (1980) systematic investigation of highly accurate long-term memory for locations of objects by 2-year-olds. An increasing number of episodes among the oldest (27-month) group (53%) involved the recall of some aspect of an event. For example, one child looking at pictures of his birthday party 3 months earlier recalled that a guest had broken a toy bus, one of the gifts. This type of memory appears to be evidence of the specific past in that a reminder of one novel event (the birthday party) elicited the memory for a specific happening within that event. The coordination of one event with another is a necessary condition for concluding that such specific episodic memory exists. While verbal evidence is not necessary, it is generally the best evidence, and all but a handful of memories reported in this study were evidenced verbally. Unfortunately, it is also true that positive evidence of the sort presented here is not conclusive, but only suggestive. The child could have only a general representation of birthday parties that was triggered by the photograph of the specific party in question. Considerable verbal ability on the part of the child is necessary to disambiguate such evidence.

These reports suggested that strict episodic memory was emerging or had emerged by 2 to 2 1/2 years of age. It is of considerable interest that some memories that were expressed verbally were based on events that had happened before the child could talk; 21% of the memories were of events that had happened more than 3 months previously. While about half the reported memories were of novel rather than recurrent events, novelty in itself is not evidence for the specificity of memory. In summary, this study provided clear evidence that 2-year-olds remember experiences over relatively long periods of time—up to 1 year in some cases—and they remember things that happened only once as well as things that happened often. Whereas some evidence was provided that children in the 2-year-old age range had specific episodic recall, the onset or development of such memory was not clarified. Of particular interest was the ambiguity of the possible relation between such specific memories for episodes in the life of the young child and the establishment of an autobiographical memory system. If the 2-year-old has memories as vivid and long-lasting as our evidence seemed to suggest, why did at least some of these memories not enter into an enduring autobiographical system?[3]

Interview Studies

In an effort to determine what and in what form young children might represent properties of events to themselves, my colleagues and I had carried out a series of studies in which we interviewed children about familiar events such as having lunch, and used the results of these interviews to construct the child's script for that event. We determined that children as young as 3 years had very good general representations of recurrent events (Nelson, 1986; Nelson & Gruendel, 1981). One revealing characteristic of their script reports was the framing of the report in the simple present (or timeless) form of the verb, such as "you get your food and then you eat it." This use is standard in adult speech for the reporting

---

[3] While we did not follow our subjects to adulthood or even later childhood, evidence from other studies is quite convincing that memories in the 2-year old do not last a lifetime, while some memories at ages 4, 5, and later years often do.

of norms or usual expectations (Gerhardt & Savasir, 1986; Quirk, Greenbaum, Leech, & Svartik, 1972).

In a study carried out with Judith Hudson (Hudson & Nelson, 1986), we constrasted these general reports with a specific report of one occasion of the event. Specifically, working with 3- and 5-year-olds we contrasted the question, "What happened when you had snack at school (or dinner at home) one time" with the general question, "what happens when you have snack at school (dinner at home)?" Two findings stand out from this study: The reports on the specific episode were significantly shorter and included less information than those on the general event, and relatedly, while children used the simple present—and not the past—tense appropriately for the general report, they frequently slipped from past to present tense in their specific one-time reports. These findings seemed to indicate that preschoolers' memories for familiar recurrent events are entered into a standard event schema or script, making it difficult for them to retrieve a specific instance of that event.

Although adults too may have difficulty retrieving a specific happening of a recurrent event (Linton, 1982), they are usually able to reconstruct an account of a specific episode that has taken place within a reasonably short period of time (days or weeks). Preschoolers, on our present evidence, have difficulty retrieving and reconstructing an account of a specific episode of a familiar event even from the immediate past. In this respect, specific memories seem to be lost in the general representational system. It appears on this evidence that general memory not only directs but even interferes with specific memories for young children.

But what then of the evidence from our diary study that 2-year-olds retain specific memories for long periods of time? Another part of the first Hudson and Nelson study asked children to report on something special that had happened to them one time. Unlike the familiar (and perhaps uninteresting) event reports, these reports were relatively long and full of detail. They concerned such episodes as going to the zoo, taking trips, going to museums, and so on. These data accord with that from other studies of memory for interesting events (Todd & Perlmutter, 1980; Fivush, Gray, Hamond& Fromhoff 1986; Ratner, 1980,1984). Thus again there is clear evidence that preschool children remember specific novel happenings for up to a year and possibly longer.

A follow-up study to the original study of specific and general reports (Hudson & Nelson, 1986) systematically varied the degree of familiarity of the event to be reported. Mothers were asked to provide information on experiences that their children had had only once, two to five times, or more than five times, and 3-, 5-, and 7-year-old children were queried about these events in either a script ("What happens when you go to the beach?") or an episodic ("What happened when you went to the beach last year?") condition. Although there were no differences in the length of reports in the two conditions, familiarity of the experience had a strong effect on both types of reports. Events that had been experienced more than five times were reported with significantly fewer episodic details and significantly less use of the past tense in both reporting conditions. Thus, for both the general and specific reports, greater experience led to more general and less episodic memory reports. Older children generally gave longer accounts, but there were no differences with respect to the degree of generalization. The youngest children (3 years old), however, often gave simple script reports rather than specific memories when they were asked to recall an episode of a very familiar event, similar to the findings from the first study.

Experience-Test Studies

The studies described thus far have been based on diaries or interviews that could not control adequately for the frequency of an event, its recency, rehearsal by the child of memory for it, cues for recall, or its particular characteristics. Several studies have since been carried out in the effort to overcome these deficiencies. In one study (Fivush, Hudson, & Nelson, 1984) kindergarten children were interviewed about their experience of going to a novel museum. Although all of the children had been to museums before, this visit was unique because they were allowed to handle archeologists' tools, they pretended to dig for artifacts, and they made clay models of artifacts. The experimenters accompanied the children to the museum and took pictures of salient experiences there. Some of the children were interviewed immediately after the trip and others only 6 weeks later; all of the children were reinterviewed 1 year later. After 6 weeks, children's memory for the episode was as accurate and detailed as their immediate recall. After 1 year, children's recall was equally accurate, but they required more specific cues to recall the same information that was easily accessed before. Immediate rehearsal had no apparent effect on subsequent memory. The child's general museum script did not appear to influence this memory, nor did the experience affect the general museum script; that is, elements of this experience did not get entered into the general representation. Even though from the adults' point of view it was an instance of "museum trips," from the child's point of view it appeared to be novel and memorable.

A study by Hudson (1984) examined preschool children's recall of specific episodes when familiarity, time delay, rehearsal, and cueing were all controlled. Nursery school and kindergarten children participated in either a single creative movement workshop (the episodic condition) or a series of workshops once a week for 4 weeks (the script condition). Four weeks after the first and last workshops in the series, children in the script condition were asked to recall those specific episodes. In the episodic conditions, children experienced a workshop identical to either the first or the last workshop that children in the script condition experienced; they also recalled the workshop 4 weeks later. In addition, half of the children in each age group and condition were asked to recall the workshop on the same day it was experienced, which gave the children additional verbal rehearsal of the experience. Children were not told, however, that their memory for the workshop(s) would be tested later.

Age, repetition, and rehearsal all produced significant effects on the amount remembered, but there were no interactions among these variables. Although children in the script condition remembered more details, they also produced more intrusion in recall, as they had difficulty distinguishing between particular workshops. The younger children in this study tended to rely more heavily on specific cues in recall, suggesting that they were less efficient at directing their own memory search or at reconstructing a memory.

Thus the results from these studies support the findings from the interview studies in showing that, whereas a novel experience may result in a memory that lasts for as long as a year, repeated experiences of the same type of event or even the expectation of a repeated event tend to make accurate retrieval of a particular occasion of that event difficult even if it is verbally recounted immediately after the event. Moreover, these effects seem to be especially strong for younger children— 3- and 4-year-olds—who have difficulty retrieving specific episodes of repeated experiences at all without the help of specific cues.

As this point then, we know that preschool children are good at constructing a general representation of repeated events (what we may call general memory) and are equally good at forming and retaining a specific memory of a novel experience over a long period of time (i.e., strict episodic memory). However, the general representation, rather than facilitating the episodic memory, actually appears to interfere with it. Thus the two do not seem to be separate but rather interacting systems. When a novel experience is repeated, it enters into a general representation and displays the interference effects noted for such experiences.

Memory Revealed in Crib Monologues

Data collected from a single subject between the ages of 21 months and 3 years suggest changes in the way that memories are organized and spontaneously recalled during early childhood. In this study monologues of the child Emily talking to herself in her crib before sleep were tape recorded at intervals over the 16-month period. These monologues were transcribed, were annotated by her mother to clarify references to happenings, and have been analyzed to reveal the content and form of her prebed narratives with particular attention to aspects of memory (Nelson, 1984, in press). Spontaneous reference to a happening in talk for oneself provides a unique view of what is remembered and how by the young child. While no control over the material to be remembered is possible, knowledge of the frequency and timing of the events that were the basis for the memories and the accuracy of the account is provided by the mother's comments in most cases.

To address the issues under examination here in terms of memory for different types of events, the findings can be summarized as follows. Evidence of memory for specific episodes is present from the first recordings made at 21 months. In one such "narrative" Emily talks about one of the family cars being broken, a happening from 2 months prior to this account. For Emily this was a novel happening; it recurred as a memory topic several times during the next 4 months. However, the earliest monologues do not place the episode in a specific time-space framework, and they tend to chain together bits of seemingly unrelated episodes rather than narrating a coherent account of a single episode.

On the whole, the novel topics that showed up in Emily's monologues were not ones that were likely to seem especially memorable or important to adults—a trip to the library on the bus, watching a tow truck tow a car, getting a TV set, Daddy making cornbread. Adults would be likely to rate such events as Christmas, the birth of a baby brother, plane trips to visit relatives in distant states as more novel, salient, important, and memorable, but these events did not show up as memory topics in Emily's monologues. It may be speculated on the basis of this evidence that some of the differences between the nondeliberate memory of young children and older children may reside in what is considered memorable by the child's general cognitive system. I hypothesize that the very novel events were unassimilable to the child's current representations of reality and thus were not retained, whereas the moderately novel stood out and served as material for further thought, possibly in the service of becoming assimilated into the general representational system. Most of the memories recorded in the monologues were even less novel, being variations on daily events, such as sleeping in mommy and daddy's bed, being picked up by mommy at the babysitter's, incidents of fighting by other children. Of course we could not ask Emily to rate these incidents for importance or novelty, but the impression is strong that these variations on familiar events were ruminated upon and then forgotten. No memory from the first 6 months of the study was repeated in a recorded monologue during the last 6 months, and the longest lasting memory (by mother's report) was about 6 months.

The observation that most memories in the monologues were of repeated events seems in conflict with the findings from our other studies. It must be remembered though that these data come from a child talking to herself, a situation that may be viewed as revealing the workings of the cognitive system. That is, what we may have recorded are efforts of that system to reconcile new data with already known material. Such self-directed efforts are qualitatively different from requests by another person to recall and report a particular episode at a later time. They may be better viewed as direct views of the child's processing system rather than as memories per se.

A question relevant to our concerns is whether Emily's memories are organized in terms of the specific past in contrast to simply a concept of temporal displacement or "not nowness." For example, when Emily talked about the broken car, did she mentally place it at a specific point in time in relation to other events that took place before and after it? In a previous report on these data (Nelson, 1984) I suggested that the evidence indicated that Emily moved from a state of the undifferentiated non-present to a specific representation of past and future. The basis for this conclusion was primarily the development of her use of language forms, both verb tense and temporal adverbials such as "not now," "tomorrow," "yesterday," and "usually." These forms appeared in a systematic order, representing first future, then past, and finally the general case. While this argument may appear to be tautological, given that (as noted earlier) evidence for a sense of pastness is difficult to come by without the use of appropriate language forms, it is supported by the contemporaneous development of the organization of her memories into coherent narratives about specific past episodes, in contrast to the earlier ruminations on seemingly randomly associated elements from different points in her past experience.

It was also after this point in development (at 23–24 months) that she began to explicitly formulate rules for the general case, (e.g., "You can't go down the basement with jamas on") and distinguish the usual from the sometimes ("when Emily go mormor in the daytime . . . that's what Emmy do sometime"). She also began speculating on what might happen on the basis of general knowledge and past experiences (e.g., "Maybe the doctor take my jamas off." "I don't know who gonna bring book to Tanta's."). All of these developments, which emerged during her 24th and 25th months, seem to indicate that she had acquired a sense of the specific past, the anticipated future, and the general norm (or script). It is not just the emergence of the appropriate tense forms and adverbials that leads to this conclusion, but also the related developments in the substance of her accounts and how she organized her talk about past episodes and future events (see Nelson, 1988, for further discussion of this point.)

More could be said about what Emily found to be memorable and its relation to her life experience and to her anticipation of coming events (Nelson, in press). For the present purpose it is sufficient to note that these data provide unique suggestive evidence for the emergence of the organization of strict episodic memory tied to a specific time and its differentiation from a general representation of how things are. This emergence is placed for Emily at approximately 2 years of age. Whether this age is significant for other children and whether it is related to their acquisition of language forms to express the past remains to be seen.

To summarize thus far: There is good evidence that young children remember specific episodes for fairly long periods of time and that at least some of them formulate these memories in well-organized narratives by 3 years of age. But the autobiographical memory system, it will be recalled, is not well established for the vast majority of children until somewhere around 5 or 6 years of age. What then delays its development? What precipitates its onset?

Mother-Child Interaction Studies

Whereas talk for self reveals some of the characteristics of spontaneous memory for past events, talk between parents and young children may be revealing of how verbal input influences the child's ability to recall an event, as well as how the memory for that event is organized. Several studies have specifically addressed this issue, examining how adults talk about the past with their young children (DeLoache, 1984; Eisenberg, 1985; Engel, 1986; Hudson, 1986; Lucariello & Nelson, 1987; Sachs, 1983). These studies all indicate that young children are quite explicitly taught how to talk about the past.[4] As Eisenberg noted, children seem to have to learn the point of talking about the past. Sachs (1983) did not find evidence of memory sharing until 3 years of age in her study of a single child, but Engel, Hudson, and Lucariello and Nelson all reported such shared talk by 2 years. Ratner (1980,1984) studied the memory demands made by mothers in naturalistic home situations and related these to the memory performance of children on standard tasks. She found a significant relationship for 3-year-olds on both cotemporaneous tests and tests carried out 2 years later. Several other studies suggest that the social-linguistic input to the child is important in establishing *what* is to be remembered and also that *memory* is important in its own right.

Two studies from our group have looked at mother-child memory talk from the perspective of considering memory as a socially constructed skill.[5] Susan Engel (1986) studied spontaneous memory talk between mothers and their children when the children were between 19 and 24 months of age. An important finding of her study was the distinction between two types of memory talk engaged in by mothers.[6] In one type of talk, termed "reminiscing" by Engel, mothers engaged in narratives about past experiences shared with the child (e.g., "Remember when we

---

[4] As always, such a statement needs to be qualified by the cautionary "in our culture."

[5] This perspective draws on the Vygotskian theory of development, which views cognitive achievements as being first carried out interpersonally, as a transaction between adult and child, before being accomplished intrapersonally, as an individual achievement of the child.

[6] A similar distinction has been verified in other studies since by Hudson (1986) and by Fivush et al (1986).

went to Vermont and saw Cousin Bill?''). In the other type, termed "practical remembering" by Engel, mothers referenced memory for a specific purpose; the reference was not embedded in the recall of an episode but rather asked the child to use memory to solve a problem or to remember a particular fact (e.g., working on a puzzle: "Where does this piece go? You remember we did that one yesterday.")

By a number of measures Engel demonstrated that the children of mothers in her longitudinal study who primarily engaged in reminiscing were able to enter into memory talk with their mothers more extensively and to make more spontaneous substantive contributions to the talk. These findings were replicated in a cross-sectional study that focused specifically on mothers' attempts to elicit memories. Thus it appears that, consistent with Ratner's findings, a certain type of mother-child interaction may facilitate the development of the child's memory. This possibility has received support as well from a study by Hudson (1986) as well as by the following study.

Minda Tessler (1986) studied 10 3-year-old children and their mothers. Her intent was to focus on how mothers might influence children's encoding of an event (in contrast to its subsequent recall) through framing it, that is, describing aspects of it and asking questions about it, as the child experienced it. In this study the experimenter took the mother-child dyad to a natural history museum and tape recorded their conversations as they proceeded through the museum. Half of the mothers were told to interact naturally with their child, while half were asked not to initiate discussions but to respond to any comments the child might make. A week later the experimenter returned to interview mother and child separately. Each member of the dyad was asked for free recall and was also given a set of 30 questions about particular objects that had been viewed the week before. These questions included (for the freely interacting group) some that the dyad had talked about together, others that only the mother or only the child had mentioned, and some that neither mother nor child had mentioned. The striking result here was that only those objects that were discussed by mother and child together were remembered by the children. None of the questions referring to objects mentioned by mother alone, child alone, or neither one were answered correctly by any child. This appears to be good evidence for the claim that there is a strong influence of social interaction on child memory for an event.

It was also the case that the children in the freely interacting group gave more correct responses than the others. An analysis of mothers' interaction styles, similar to that carried out by Engel, provided evidence that interaction had a powerful influence on what was remembered. Tessler identified four mothers as employing a narrative style[7] (similar to Engel's

---

[7] Following Bruner's (1985) discussion of types of thinking.

reminiscers), all but one of whom was included in the freely interacting group. The other six mothers were characterized as using a paradigmatic style (similar to Engel's practical rememberers). When the responses of the children of the mothers using different styles were compared, the narrative group gave an average of 13 (out of 30) correct responses to questions, while the paradigmatic group gave only 4.7 ($P <.001$ by the Mann-Whitney U test).

Thus it appears that the way in which an experience is framed through talk has an important impact on what is remembered of that experience a week later. On reflection, this may not be very surprising, but it highlights a neglected variable in discussions of memory development, and it has an important bearing on how we think about the development of children's memory. Together with the findings from Engel's and Ratner's studies that the way mothers engage in remembering with their children affects the children's skill at remembering, it suggests an important social influence on the development of memory. Mothers appear to differ in the way they characteristically talk about events, both ongoing and past, with their young children, and children apparently are better able to make use of the narrative or reminiscing style in encoding and retrieving information.

Summary of Research Results

The studies reviewed here have been concerned with nondeliberate memory for naturally occurring events by children between 2 and 5 years of age. What these studies have revealed is that, in the course of their natural real-life experiences, children take in, store, and may retrieve when asked to do so a great deal of information about those experiences. This information is not randomly stored, but is organized in terms of sequentially arranged schemas, scripts, or general event representations (the particular terminology employed does not seem crucial to the present account). When an experience is repeated, the specific details of the episode tend to become confused with others, and younger children may not be able to retrieve an episode of a familiar experience at all. What is remembered may be very skeletal at first and incorporates those things that seem most important to the young child (not necessarily to the adult), probably including elements that need to be assimilated to the child's current model of the world. Unusual experiences may be remembered in some detail for a year or more. Such persistent memories appear to be in some way novel, but not too novel. The evidence from Emily indicates that episodic memories are not at first well organized in sequential narrative form and are not located in a specific spatiotemporal context, but the later transcripts from that study and the reports of novel episodes from older preschool children indicate that by 3 years of age children do report episodes from as long ago as a year in well-organized form and relate them to a specific spatiotemporal context. Thus these two characteristics of the autobiographical system appear to be present—at least in some children—by that critical age. However, the last studies reported here indicate that children *learn* to talk about their memories of past experiences in an organized form through the examples and framing presented by their parents. Listening to stories may also influence their organization in narrative form. Further, such talk has been shown to influence what aspects of their ongoing experience children remember. The way that adults frame experiences for the child and talk about them after they have happened influences both what is remembered and how it is remembered. What remains to be discussed is what implications these findings have for understanding the establishment of autobiographical memory.

A Functional Perspective on Memory Development

This section introduces a framework for thinking about the natural history of memory, particularly the ontogeny of different types of memory, with possible reference to phylogeny as well. It is striking how little discussion of evolutionary and functional issues there is in the field of memory (cf. Bruce, 1985; Oakley, 1983). But when the topic is memory development, the question naturally arises, why remember? What purposes does memory serve? Does one type of memory serve a different function than another? In the present context, what function does autobiographical memory serve, if any?

The answer to the general question seems obvious: Remembering the past has value insofar as it serves action in the present or future. Thus what is remembered should be that that enables the individual to carry out activities, to predict, and to plan. How does the organism know which bits of information to remember from an experience, that is, which will be useful to future activity? A nonverbal organism—including the human infant and young child who has not yet attained mastery of language and whose experience is thus unmediated by language—is guided by innate selection mechanisms including such factors as salience, novelty, and importance to goals. Regardless of the fact that these constructs are difficult to define, they seem to play a role in anyone's theory of functional significance (e.g., Brown & Kulick, 1977, on flashbulb memory).

Oakley (1983) laid out an interesting taxonomy of varieties of memory in phylogeny which incorporates different mechanisms of functionally significant information storage by organisms at different levels of complexity, including genetic storage, specialized individual learning and memory systems, and culturally stored and transmitted information. This taxonomy seems to be a useful way of thinking about the ontogenetic development of memory as well as the phylogenetic. Although Oakley pointed out that culturally transmitted information (what he called level 4) occurs in many species through imitation and observational learning, the nonverbal animal (again including the human infant and young child) primarily relies on individual memory (what Oakley referred to as level 3). The point to be emphasized here, without going into the details of Oakley's taxonomy, is that the memory systems of the young child (and I use "systems" here informally without claiming hard and fast distinctions among them) may be thought of as on a continuum, sharing much in common with the memory systems of other mammals including other primates, and with little impact from the culturally transmitted level 4 systems.

Within this general framework, the following developmental course is hypothesized, based on the information presently available. With regard to the question of what shall be remembered by the young organism, our studies have indicated that what is significant to the child may not be significant for the adult. But what is of more fundamental interest is that specific episodes may not be initially identified as such, but rather that in development there may exist a state of undifferentiated event memory. In this state, recurrent events are recognized as "the same" when some critical features or patterns are identified, and thereafter the general memory for the event serves the purpose of organizing action and predicting what will be encountered next. The fact that a novel episode may be retained intact for a considerable period of time may be significant only in that the event has not yet been repeated, that is, the system does not recognize critical similarities between it and other episodes, and thus is has not yet been assimilated into a general scheme. The general representation of an event (i.e., a script) is not then distinguished from memory per se but rather differs from it only in being more schematized, with specific details that are irrelevant to taking action or that are too variable to be of predictive use dropping out or being randomly stored.

From this undifferentiated memory system, several subsystems appear to emerge. First there emerges a representation of an expected event, based on experience with similar events in the past. Next there emerges a representation of a specific past happening, specifically indexed as such. Next comes an organized conception of events, a general event representation from which rules and principles and abstract systems can be extracted (see Nelson, 1986; Nelson & Gruendel, 1981; also Oakley, 1983). All of these developments appear to take place in very early childhood and are no doubt facilitated by the acquisition and employment of language, although whether language is necessary to their initial development seems unlikely.

Still, Tulving's (1984) claim with respect to the uniqueness of human memory does not apply to any of the developments described thus far, which may all be shared with other phylogenetically closely related species. Rather, this claim must be restricted to the one discontinuity of childhood memory, the emergence of an autobiographical memory system, which is not entailed by these prior developments.

Most of the usual explanations for the discontinuity represented by this development cannot stand up to examination. Memories do exist in early childhood, and so far as we have been able to tell they do not differ in organization in any major way from later memories. Nor are they too short-lasting to be retained: We have found evidence for memories lasting at least a year, and there is no reason to believe that 1 year is a final limit (Fivush, 1988). Freud's repression theory has been found to conflict with both clinical data (see White & Pillemer, 1979) and our own studies, which have not found memories in early childhood to be primarily emotionally laden. That is, if some memories are repressed or replaced with screen memories, this explanation does not apply to the majority of very young children's memories. The hypothesis that memories are coded and stored differently in early childhood and thus cannot be retrieved using cues available later (e.g., Neisser, 1962; Schachtel, 1947; White & Pillemer, 1979) does not seem supportable for two reasons. First, although young children seem to need more cues to access their memories (Hudson, 1984), these are not different from the cues used by older children. Second, there does not seem to be any one point in childhood when the organization of the cognitive system undergoes a discontinuous shift such that previously used cues would no longer be useful in encoding or subsequent ones no longer useful for retrieval. For example, the difference between the child's cognitive structures at 4 and 7 years of age seems no greater that that between 7 and 16 years of age, yet the former discrepancy is held by these theorists to explain the irretrievability of memories, while the latter does not interfere. Why one restructuring should pose a barrier to the retrieval of prior memories and the other not is not obvious.

The crucial question to be addressed is not what happens to block early memories, but what happens in the preschool period to enable an autobiographical memory system to become established? The present state of research suggests that the critical development is that through language the child enters into and begins to participate in Oakley's level 4, culturally stored and transmitted information. On a very trivial but potentially portentous level, the young child begins to listen to and learn stories, poems, and songs and at the same time begins to listen to and exchange information about previous experience with adults. As shown in the last series of studies reported here, adults typically frame events for the child in such a way that certain things are made salient and are organized in a conventional way. Adults also talk to the child about what has happened in the past, and do so in distinctive manners. Thus what the child remembers, or how the child learns to reconstruct the past, is influenced by how the adult frames the past experience both at the time of its occurrence and later when it is recalled. In the course of this kind of talk about the past, the child come to value the past for its own sake, or rather for the culturally significant activity of sharing and exchanging stories about it. Equally and perhaps more important, the child comes to view her or his own experience as an objective socially shareable fact, having a status similar to stories and other culturally valued semiotic objects.[8] As Engel, Hudson, Lucariello and Nelson, Tessler, and others have shown, parents provide models for what should be remembered from an experience through questioning about particular aspects of the event, thus conventionalizing the subjective account (cf. Neisser, 1962, and Schactel, 1947, on the socialization of memory). It is thus the conventional and "objective" memory that survives, replete with interpretations of affect, beliefs, and desires, whether or not a specific memory has been discussed with others.

It is clear that autobiographical memory develops during and in conjunction with the period that the child is gaining control over language and the ability to communicate thoughts, feelings, and experiences with others. Since these abilities are also specifically human and dependent upon language, it is not unreasonable to claim that just so is autobiographical memory. But does that indicate that its development is external to the memory system, simply an adjustment of basic processes, as Schacter and Moscovitch (1984) implied? I suggest rather that autobiographical memory is as representative of human functioning as language itself, and that it is reflected in and forms the basis for song, story, epic, and myth in all human cultures. Any complete account of human memory, and the development of human memory, must include it as a specific and distinct type of memory. However, this claim does not necessarily mean that it is an independent memory system. Indeed, we have seen its beginnings in the episodic system emerging from infancy. There must be connections among general memory, episodic memory, and autobiographical memory, as well as various abstract knowledge stores derived therefrom.

In summary, on the basis of the developmental evidence presented here, there appear to be three important developments. First the episodic system is developed, as Schacter and Moscovitch (1984) have outlined. Next, episodes are identified as belonging to a specific point in the past. This move is facilitated by but may not be dependent upon acquisition of language forms. Finally, episodes are reconstructed and organized, are repeated to self and others as communicative and narrative skills develop,[9] and are entered into a separate autobiographical memory system,

---

[8] This objective character may be related to the confusions in memory as to whether something is a "real" memory or a story told by someone else. Since this characteristic of early memory is part of what is to be explained, the veridicality of such memories is not in question here.

[9] The fact that reconstruction of an event and organization of a narrative are language-dependent skills which may be improved with communicative practice suggests also an explanation for the wide variation in age of early memories among individuals, variation which has sometimes been found to be correlated with language development.

which serves as a self-history defined in collaboration with the important others who exchange and redefine experiences from the past.

References

Ashmead, D.H., & Perlmutter, M. (1980). Infant memory in everyday life. In M. Perlmutter (Ed.), *Children's memory: New directions for child development* (No. 10, pp 1–16). San Francisco: Jossey-Bass.

Brown, R., & Kulik, J. (1977). Flashbulb memories. *Cognition, 5,* 73–99.

Bruce, D. (1985). The how and why of ecological memory. *Journal of Experimental Psychology: General, 114,* 78–90.

Bruner, J. (1986) *Actual Minds, Possible Worlds.* Cambridge MA: Harvard University Press.

DeLoache, J.S. (1980). Naturalistic studies in memory for object location in very young children. In Perlummter, M. (Ed.), *Children's memory: New directions for child development* (No. 10, pp 87–101). San Francisco: Jossey-Bass.

DeLoache, J.S. (1984, October). What's this? Maternal questions in joint picture book reading with toddlers. *The Quarterly Newsletter of the Laboratory of Comparative Human Congition, 6*(4), 87–95.

Dudycha, G.J., & Dudycha, M.M. (1941). Childhood memories: A review of the literature. *Psychological Bulletin, 38,* 668–682.

Eisenberg, A.R. (1985). Learning to describe past experiences in conversation. *Discourse Processes, 8,* 177–204.

Engel, S. (1986). *Learning to reminisce: A developmental study of how young children talk about the past.* Unpublished doctoral dissertation, City University of New York, New York.

Engel, S., Kyratzis, A., & Lucariello, J. (1984, April). Early past and future talk in a social interactive context. Paper presented at the symposium on *Memory development and the development of "memory talk,"* International Conference on Infant Studies, New York City.

Fivush, R. (1984). Learning about school: The development of kindergarteners' school scripts. *Child Development, 55,* 1697–1709.

Fivush, R. (1988). The functions of event memory: Some comments on Nelson and Barsalou. In U. Neisser (Ed.), *Real events remembered.* New York: Cambridge University Press.

Fivush, R., Gray, J.T., Hamond, N.R., & Fromhoff, F.A. (1986). Two studies of early autobiographical memory (Report No. 11, Emory Cognition Project). Atlanta: Department of Psychology, Emory University.

Fivush, R., Hudson, J., & Nelson, K. (1984). Children's long term memory for a novel event: An exploratory study. *Merrill-Palmer Quarterly, 30,* 303–316.

Freud, S. (1963). Three essays on the theory of sexuality. In Strachey, J. (Ed.), *The standard edition of the complete works of Freud* (Vol. 7). London: Hogarth Press. (Original work published 1905).

Gerhardt, J., & Savasir, I. (1986). The use of the simple present in the speech of two three year olds: Normativity not subjectivity. *Language in Society, 15,* 501–536.

Hirst, W. (1984). Factual memory? *The Behavioral and Brain Sciences, 7,* 241–242.

Hudson, J.A. (1984). Recollection and reconstruction in children's autobiographical memory. Unpublished doctoral dissertation, City University of New York, New York.

Hudson, J.A. (1986, April). *Effects of repetition on children's autobiographic memory*. Paper presented at the Conference on Human Development, Nashville, TN.

Hudson, J., & Nelson, K. (1986). Repeated encounters of a similar kind: Effects of familiarity on children's autobiographic memory. *Cognitive Development, 1,* 253–271.

Kagan, J., Kearsley, R.B. & Zelazo, P.R. (1978). *Infancy: Its place in human development*. Cambridge MA: Harvard University Press.

Linton, M. (1975). Memory for real-world events. In Norman, D.A., & Rumelhart, D.E. (Eds.), *Explorations in cognition*. San Francisco: W.H. Freeman.

Linton, M. (1982). Transformations of memory in everyday life. In Neisser, U. (Ed.), *Memory observed* (pp. 77–91). San Francisco: W.H. Freeman.

Lockhart, R.S. (1984). What do infants remember? in Moscovitch, M. (Ed.), *Infant memory* (pp. 131–144). New York: Plenum Press.

Lucariello, J., & Nelson, K. (1987). Remembering and planning talk between mothers and children. *Discourse Processes, 10,* 219–235.

Mandler, J.M. (1984). Representation and recall in infancy. In Moscovitch, M. (Ed.), *Infant memory* (pp. 75–102). New York: Plenum Press.

Neisser, U. (1962). Cultural and cognition discontinuity. In Gladwin, T.E., & Sturtevant, W. (Eds.), *Anthropology and human behavior* (pp. 54–71). Washington, DC: Anthropological Society of Washington.

Nelson, K. (1984). The transition from infant to child memory. In Moscovitch, M. (Ed.), *Infant memory. Vol. 10. Advances in the study of communication and affect* (pp. 103–130). New York: Plenum Press.

Nelson, K. (1986). *Event knowledge: Structure and function in development*. Hillsdale, NJ: Lawrence Erlbaum Associates.

Nelson, K. (1988). The ontogeny of memory for real events. In Neiser, U. (Ed.), *Real events remembered*. New York. Cambridge University Press.

Nelson, K. (Ed.) (in press). *Narratives from the crib*. Cambridge MA: Harvard University Press.

Nelson, K., & Gruendel, J. (1981). Generalized event representations: Basic building blocks of cognitive development. In Lamb, M., & Brown, A. (Eds.), *Advances in developmental psychology* (Vol. 1, pp 131–158). Hillsdale, NJ: Lawrence Erlbaum Associates.

Nelson, K., & Ross, G. (1980). The generalities and specifics of long term memory in infants and young children. In Perlmutter, M. (Ed.), *Children's memory: New directions for child development* (no. 10, pp. 87–101). San Francisco: Jossey-Bass.

Oakley, D.A. (1983). The varieties of memory: A phylogenetic approach. In Mayes, A. (Ed.), *Memory in animals and humans*. Workingham, England: Van Nostrand Reinhold.

Olton, D.B. (1984). Comparative analysis of episodic memory. *Behavioral and Brain Sciences, 7,* 250–251.

Quirk, R., Greenbaum, S., Leech, G., & Svartik, J. (1972). *A grammar of contemporary English*. London: Longman.

Ratner, H.H. (1980). The role of social context in memory development. In

Perlmutter, M. (Ed.), *Children's memory: New directions for child development* (No. 10, pp. 49–68). San Francisco: Jossey-Bass.

Ratner, H.H. (1984). Memory demands and the development of young children's memory. *Child Development, 55,* 2173–2191.

Sachs, J. (1983). Talking about the there and then: The emergence of displaced reference in parent-child discourse. In Nelson, K.E. (Ed.), *Children's language* (Vol. 4, pp 1–28). New York: Gardner Press.

Schachtel, E. (1947). On childhood amnesia. *Psychiatry, 10,* 1–26.

Schacter, D.L., & Moscovitch, M. (1984). Infants, amnesics and dissociable memory systems. In moscovitch, M. (Ed.), *Infant memory* (pp. 173–216). New York: Plenum Press.

Tessler, M. (1986). *Mother-child talk in a museum: The socialization of a memory.* Unpublished manuscript, City University of New York, New York.

Todd, C.M., & Perlmutter, M. (1980). Reality recalled by preschool children. In Perlmutter, M. (Ed.), *Children's memory: New directions for child development.* (No. 10). San Francisco: Jossey-Bass.

Tulving, E. (983). *Elements of episodic memory.* Oxford, England: Oxford University Press.

Tulving, E. (1984). Author's response. *Behavioral and Brain Sciences, 7,* 257–268.

Vygotsky, L.S. (1978). *Mind in society.* Cambridge: MA: Harvard University Press.

Wellman, H.M., & Somerville, S.C. (1980). Quasi-naturalistic tasks in the study of cognition: The memory related skills of toddlers. In Perlmutter, M. (Ed.), *Children's memory: New directions for child development* (pp. 33–48). San Francisco: Jossey-Bass.

Wertsch, J.V. (ed.) (1985). *Culture, communication and cognition: Vygotskian perspectives.* New York: Cambridge University Press.

Wetzler, S.E., & Sweeney, J.A. (1986). Childhood amnesia: An empirical demonstration. In Rubin, D.C. (Ed.), *Autobiographical memory* (pp. 191–201). New York: Cambridge University Press.

White, S.H., & Pillemer, D.B. (1979). Childhood amnesia and the development of a socially accessible memory system. In Kihlstrom, J.F., & Evans, F.J. (Eds.), *Functional disorders of memory* (pp. 29–74). Hillsdale, NJ: Lawrence Erlbaum Associates.

CHAPTER 8

The Joy of Kicking: Memories, Motives, and Mobiles

Carolyn Rovee-Collier

A central question in developmental psychology is whether young infants can profit from experience, and if so, how. The answer is critical not only for our practical understanding of the effects of early experience on later behavior but also for theories of development, most of which include strong assumptions regarding the mechanisms underlying early behavioral transitions. Given the importance of this problem, it is surprising that the study of memory early in infancy has been and continues to be a neglected research topic. This neglect has arisen both from the methodological difficulties associated with questioning prelinguistic infants about their memories and from philosophical differences regarding the representational abilities of nonverbal organisms and the role of consciousness in memory processing (see chaps. 4 and 6 in this volume; J. Mandler, 1984; Strauss & Carter, 1984; Tulving, 1985). As a result, today there is a general consensus among authorities of human memory and human development that the capacity for long-term memory does not emerge until sometimes after the first 8 or 9 months of life (chap. 6 in this volume; Kagan, 1984; Nadel & Zola-Morgan, 1984; Olson & Strauss, 1984; Schacter & Moscovitch, 1984).

Animal researchers, who also encounter the problem of asking a nonverbal organism its past experiences, have traditionally studied memory in a learning context (see Bolles, 1976). For an animal to learn the predictive relation between two events, for example, it must remember the first event in some fashion until the second event occurs. In addition, the characteristic learning curve describing the cumulative effects of experience within a session reflects not only retention from one event to the next but also from one trial to the next. This relatively short-term retention of prior experience has been described as "associative memory" (Revusky, 1971) or "memory *in* learning" (Watson, 1984) and has been documented for even the youngest of human infants (for review, see Rovee-Collier, 1987). A long-term memory capacity is clearly required, however, to account for the cumulative effects of experience from one session to the next (or from a training session to a test session), particularly if sessions are separated by 24 hours or more. This long-term effect of prior experience has been described as "retentive memory" (Revusky, 1971) or "memory *of* learning" (Watson, 1984). Over the past decade, evidence of retention after intervals of days and even weeks has been obtained during the first few months of life in studies of prenatal exposure learning (DeCasper & Fifer, 1980), classical conditioning (Little, Lipsitt, & Rovee-Collier, 1984), and operant conditioning (Rovee & Fagen, 1976; Sullivan, Rovee-Collier, & Tynes, 1979).

More recently, inspired by findings from animal research on the effects of reminders on long-term retention (Campbell & Jaynes, 1966; Campbell & Spear, 1972; Spear, 1973; Spear & Parsons, 1976), my colleagues, students, and I have found that a reminder procedure can extend the influence of prior experience for even longer time periods (for review, see Rovee-Collier & Hayne, 1987).

In this chapter I review briefly the different procedures that have been used to study memory in very young infants, including the simple forgetting and reminder paradigms that we have developed, and the characteristic findings that these procedures have yielded. In addition, I describe some of our recent findings on the specificity of infant memory, the role of contextual information in retention, the time-dependent course of retrieval for different types of memory attributes, and the malleability of memories. Finally, I attempt to place our research within the general framework of animal and adult-human memory processing.

Visual Recognition Memory Paradigms

Paired-Comparison Paradigm

Until recently, most of what was known about early memorial abilities came from studies of infant looking patterns. Fantz (1956), using a paired-comparison procedure, made the original observation that infants' looking was not randomly distributed with respect to members of a pair of stimuli; rather, some visual patterns were fixated reliably longer than others. The paired-comparison paradigm was subsequently modified to study the effect of a brief preexposure to one member of the test pair (the sample) on the infant's subsequent distribution of looking when the sample was then presented concurrently with a novel distractor. In general, it was typically found that infants younger than 8 to 10 weeks of age looked reliably longer at the preexposed sample than at the novel member of the test pair, whereas infants older than 8 to 10 weeks of age looked reliably longer at the novel member of the test pair than at the preexposed sample (for review, see Fagan, 1984). Fagan (1970) introduced a delay between exposure to the sample and the paired-comparison test and asked after what interval preexposure to the sample no longer yielded the novelty response. He described this as a *delayed recognition-*

memory procedure. The maximum delay between the sample and the test that yielded nonrandom looking behavior was considered to index the limit of the infant's "recognition memory."

The paired-comparison paradigm is procedurally and conceptually identical to the delayed matching-to-sample paradigm—the traditional paradigm used to study short-term memory and attention in pigeons (Roberts & Grant, 1978) and in monkeys (D'Amato & Cox, 1976). From this perspective, it is not surprising that paired-comparison studies of infant recognition memory have yielded evidence of forgetting after the same brief delays that characterize forgetting in delayed matching-to-sample studies with animals, older infants (Brody, 1981), and preschoolers (Timmons, Lapinski, & Worobey, 1986).

Habituation Paradigm

Other investigators, inspired by Sokolov's neuronal model of the habituation of the orienting reflex (Sokolov, 1963), developed a similar assessment of infant recognition memory (Caron, 1967; Cohen, 1973; Cornell, 1974; McCall, 1971). Sokolov's model assumes that the subject constructs an internal representation or template of each attended stimulus ("engram"). Attention to a given stimulus on each subsequent occasion is determined by the magnitude of the discrepancy between the physical stimulus and its internal representation. When the engram matches the physical stimulus (zero discrepancy), the subject no longer attends to it. The decline in attention to a previously encountered stimulus, therefore, reflects the reduction of the effective stimulus, that is, the discrepancy. As time passes, however, the representation decays, and the discrepancy between the template and the physical stimulus correspondingly increases. When there is no longer any trace of the template, the discrepancy is again at a maximum. By this account, when the habituated stimulus is again attended as fully as a completely novel stimulus, forgetting is assumed to be complete. A similar account based on the discrepancy between the external stimulus and its internal representation has been applied to changes in looking time in the paired-comparison paradigm.

In habituation studies of infant recognition memory, trials are presented in rapid succession until a criterion of response decrement (typically, a percentage of the initial response magnitude) is attained, at which point different groups of infants are tested for retention after different delays with either the habituation stimulus or a novel stimulus. When testing immediately follows the final habituation trial, responding to the habituation stimulus remains low, and habituation generalizes to novel test stimuli as a function of their similarity to the habituation stimulus. When a delay is introduced between the habituation series and the posthabituation test trial, spontaneous recovery to the original habituation stimulus is a function of the delay interval, and infants may ultimately fixate the test stimulus for as long as they did on their original encounter with it. The maximum delay that can be tolerated before spontaneous recovery is complete indexes the limit of the infant's memory span. In general, studies of visual recognition memory, irrespective of paradigm or infant age, have indicated that forgetting is complete (i.e., spontaneous recovery to the original level) after only a few seconds or minutes (for review, see Cohen & Gelber, 1975; Olsen & Sherman, 1983; Werner & Perlmutter, 1979).

Distinctions Between Short- and Long-Term Memory

Both the specificity of the response decrement to the preexposed stimulus and the spontaneous recovery of responding to that stimulus after a delay are basic characteristics of habituation (Thompson & Spencer, 1966) that have been repeatedly documented in many species, invertebrate (Wyers, Peeke, & Herz, 1973) as well as vertebrate (Groves & Thompson, 1970; Thompson & Glanzman, 1976; Thompson & Spencer, 1966). However, evidence that either longer interstimulus intervals or a greater number of trials can maintain habituation over a longer time period (Kandel, 1979; Leaton, 1976; Wagner, 1976) has led to a distinction between short-term and long-term habituation that resembles the distinction between short-term and long-term memory.

Bashinski, Werner, and Rudy (1985) explored the possibility that the young infant's visual habituation curve may be the sum of two independent processes—a sensitization process and an habituation process (Groves & Thompson, 1970). When they increased the interval between trials to 30 seconds—an interval exceeding the memory span previously reported for 4-month-olds (Stinson, 1971), habituation was established even more rapidly, presumably because longer interstimulus intervals allowed the sensitization induced by each stimulus presentation to dissipate between trials. These data suggest that young infants may be capable of relatively long-term habituation, but thus far this possibility has not been tested. To date, all habituation studies of infant recognition memory have been of the short-term variety.

The Function of Memory

Bruner (1964) has argued that what is important about memory is not that an organism possesses it but that it can be retrieved and used to guide behavior. The central assumption of paired-comparison and short-term habituation studies—that is, that what the infant remembers can be inferred from the extent to which a preexposed stimulus is subsequently *not* fixated—is inconsistent with this function. Moreover, if only aspects of a prior event that are represented in the memory of that event can cue its retrieval, as most authorities on memory agree (for review, see Tulving, 1983), then, by definition, novel stimuli cannot serve as retrieval cues for the memory of an event. Moreover, to the extent that novel stimuli compete with effective retrieval cues for the allocation of attention, they actually impede memory processing: Unless the preexposed stimulus is attended at the time of testing, the requisite retrieval cues cannot be sampled, and retrieval cannot be initiated.

It seems highly unlikely that all sensory information that is encountered is encoded. Rather, there must be a means by which attention is directed to potentially significant events in the immediate environment. This *attention-gating* (Reeves & Sperling, 1986) or *perceptual processing* (Jeffrey, 1976) function is what studies of short-term memory assess. Attention-gating (or perceptual processing) is a precursor of memory processing but is not synonymous with it. Insofar as attention-gating involves no encoding, "short-term memory" is a misnomer. The infant's novelty-detection response, analogous to Pavlov's "what is it" reflex, reflects the momentary *vigilance function* of this attentional-perceptual mechanism (Rovee-Collier & Hayne, 1987). Although vigilance has obvious biological relevance, it has little to do with the adaptive function of memory to which Bruner referred. If the events to which the organism attends are *informative,* however, then they may be encoded and remembered; these are the memories that can guide behavior.

Memory Research with Motivated Infants

A decade ago, after reviewing the status of knowledge of memory development, Campbell and Coulter (1976) concluded:

Child development psychologists have not yet studied memory over long time intervals. Our best estimates come from retrospective studies of early childhood memories. . . . We cannot overemphasize the differences between these indices of long-term memory in man and those used to study memory in the developing rat. The human is asked to recall events of early childhood in the absence of any stimuli associated with that era. The rat, on the other hand, is returned to a highly distinctive setting and asked to reproduce a specific response. If these same procedures were used with man, it seems quite likely that evidence for long-term memory would appear much earlier. . . ." (pp. 144–145)

Our studies of retention in human infants have followed this advice, exploiting the logical relation between learning and memory. We introduce motivated infants to a novel task that requires the learning of a unique response. After a delay, we reinstate the original experimental context and record whether the infants produce the learned response. Our procedure differs from recognition memory procedures in that we are not recording a continuously distributed variable (visual attention) but the extent to which a unique and distinctive response is produced during a retention test. We do not have to *infer* retention. Although recognition of familiar cues in the experimental context is prerequisite to producing the correct response, recognition alone is insufficient to ensure that the correct response will be exhibited. In addition to recognizing the context, infants must also remember what to do in that context. This is analogous to cued-recall tasks used with animals and older humans (Spear, 1978) in which a cue is presented and, in the absence of other information, the response appropriate to that cue must be generated. As in those tasks, the infant's operant response is emitted, not elicited—as has been mistakenly concluded (Moscovitch, 1984). Also, because retention is assessed during a "baseline" condition and not during reacquisition, test performance is the exclusive product of a memory component rather than a result of new learning at the time of testing (Spear, 1978).

Finally, our retention paradigm differs from recognition-memory paradigms in that it involves the study of motivated infants. We have found that when young human infants have a *reason* to remember an event—that is, when they are motivated—their long-term retention is quite remarkable.

The Mobile Conjugate-Reinforcement Retention Paradigm

In most of our studies, 2- to 3-month-olds learn to kick one foot to move an overhead crib mobile. After periods ranging from a few hours to several weeks, we reintroduce them to the mobile to see if they will still perform the previously acquired response. In our standard procedure, infants are trained for two 15-minute sessions that are 24 hours apart. The training phase consists of a 9-minute reinforcement period when an ankle ribbon is attached from the infant's ankle to an overhead hook from which a mobile is suspended (see Fig. 8.1, left). When this arrangement is in effect, the infant's kicks activate the mobile with an intensity proportional to the rate and vigor of kicking. Preceding and following each training phase is a 3-minute nonreinforcement phase during which the mobile is suspended overhead as before, but the ribbon is shifted to a second, "empty" mobile hook. When this arrangement is in effect, the infant can see the mobile but cannot move it by kicking. It is emphasized that the reinforcement is the conjugate movement of the mobile—not the visual presence of the nonmoving mobile.

The initial 3-minute nonreinforcement period of session 1 is a *baseline phase* during which the response rate of the leg with the ankle ribbon is measured (i.e., operant level). Responding during the final 3-minute nonreinforcement period of session 2 provides a measure of the infant's final level of acquisition. Because responding during this period is based on the infant's memory of prior training after "zero" delay, this period also serves as an *immediate retention test* phase. Performance during the immediate retention test is expected to be better than at any later time and

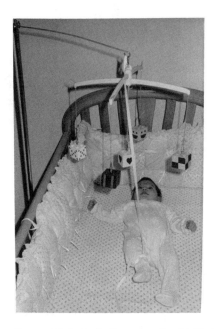 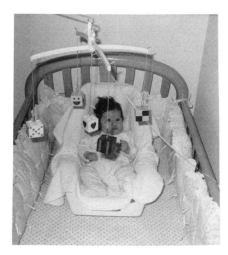

FIGURE 8.1. *Left:* Two-month-old Christina during a training phase in the mobile conjugate reinforcement paradigm. During baseline and all retention tests, the ankle ribbon is shifted from the hook suspending the mobile to a second stand (not shown) so that kicking cannot activate the mobile. *Right:* The experimental arrangement during a brief reactivation treatment. The arrangement of the mobile stands is identical to that of training, but the mobile will be moved by an experimenter drawing and releasing the ribbon. The infant seat minimizes random kicking during the procedure. (Photographs courtesy of M. Capatides.)

therefore is used as the standard of comparison for performance during the *long-term retention test*—a procedurally identical, 3-minute nonreinforcement phase at the end of the delay interval (i.e., at the outset of session 3).

The retention paradigm is illustrated in Figure 8.2. A reacquisition phase is introduced after the long-term retention test to confirm that infants who did not respond during the long-term retention test are still interested in the game and are physically able to respond at their previous rate on the test day.

Measures of Retention

Forgetting and retention are operationally defined in terms of the infant's kick rate during the long-term retention test relative to the same infant's kick rate at the end of training (during the immediate retention test) and before training was ever instituted (during the baseline phase), respectively. Thus, if an infant responds at the same rate during the long-term

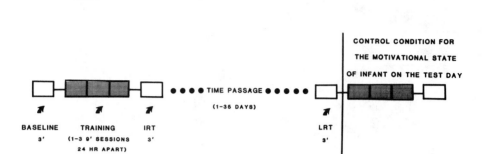

FIGURE 8.2. The standard retention paradigm, showing the immediate retention test (IRT) at the end of training and the long-term retention test (LRT) at the end of the retention interval.

retention test (*B*) at the end of the retention interval that he or she did during the immediate retention test (*A*) at the beginning of the retention interval, then that infant will have shown no forgetting: The infant's *retention ratio* (*B/A*) will equal 1.00. The greater the forgetting over the retention interval, the less the infant will kick during the long-term retention test, and the lower will be the retention ratio. A mean retention ratio significantly less than 1.00 confirms that forgetting has taken place.

Even though infants' test performance may be indicative of some forgetting, it may not be complete. If infants still remember something of their original training experience, then their retention test performance should be better than their pretraining response rate. To measure the extent of retention, we determine the extent to which performance during the long-term retention test exceeds an infant's operant level. A *baseline ratio* (*B/P*) is obtained by dividing an infant's kick rate during the long-term retention test (*B*) by that infant's kick rate during the pretraining baseline phase (*P*). If performance during the long-term retention test reflects a memory component, the mean baseline ratio will be significantly greater than 1.00. Forgetting is said to be complete when responding during the long-term retention test has returned to operant level (i.e., a mean baseline ratio not significantly different from 1.00).

Evidence of Long-Term Retention

The simple forgetting functions that are obtained from independent groups of 2- and 3-month-olds, trained for two sessions and tested in the mobile conjugate reinforcement paradigm, are presented in Figure 8.3. Note that the X-axis on this figure is in units of days. This stands in sharp contrast to data from visual recognition-memory studies, which typically

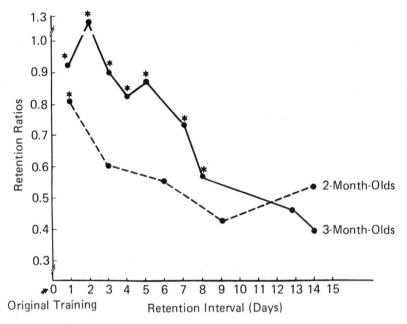

FIGURE 8.3. Retention ratios of independent groups of 2- and 3-month-olds who were trained for two sessions and tested after delays of 1 to 14 days in the standard retention paradigm (Fig. 8.2). Stars indicate performance above operant level (mean baseline ratio > 1.00). (From Greco, Rovee-Collier, Hayne, Griesler, & Earley, 1986).

characterize infant retention during the first year of life in terms of only seconds (e.g., Stinson, 1971; Werner & Perlmutter, 1979). Three-month-olds display virtually no forgetting after a 3-day delay, and even after 8 days, their performance is still above operant level. After a 13-day delay, however, forgetting is complete; response rates during the 13- and 14-day long-term retention test are at operant level. Although 2-month-olds, as a group, forget more rapidly following identical training, their test performance is highly variable. When the same amount of training (18 minutes) is distributed into three sessions, 2- and 3-month-olds exhibit excellent and equivalent retention after 2 weeks (Enright, Rovee-Collier, Fagen, & Caniglia, 1983; Vander Linde, Morrongiello, & Rovee-Collier, 1985).

Not only do very young infants remember for many days, but their memories are very precise. If different numbers of novel mobile objects are substituted for familiar ones during a retention test 1 day after training, such that some infants are tested with a mobile containing four original objects and one new object, others are tested with a mobile containing three original and two new objects, and so on, infants' responding during the retention test is reduced (Fagen, Rovee, & Kaplan, 1976), indicating that they discriminate the change in the original training mobile even though they last saw it on the preceding day. In fact, their memory of the details of the training mobile is so keen that if more than a single object is changed on the test mobile, their 24-hour test performance plunges to operant level. Two-month-olds are equally competent in performing this highly precise discrimination after a 24-hour delay (Hayne, Greco, Earley, Griesler, & Rovee-Collier, 1986). Thus, even for the youngest infants tested, effective retrieval cues are highly specific to the original training context; generalized stimuli cannot cue retrieval.

These data are clearly at odds with conclusions that the memories of infants less than 8 months of age are generalized and undifferentiated (chap. 6 in this volume; Olson & Strauss, 1984). In addition, they challenge Kagan's (1979, 1984) conclusion that, prior to the eighth month, infants are incapable of maintaining a representation "on the stage of memory" for more than a few seconds. Presumably, for the first time at 8 months, infants are able to maintain a memory representation of their mother, who left the room seconds or minutes earlier, long enough to compare it with the characteristics of a stranger who is physically present. The resulting discrepancy, according to Kagan, results in crying. The fact that infants first show stranger distress between 8 and 9 months of age is taken by Kagan as evidence that an "enhanced memory" capacity first emerges at that age. The difference between previous conclusions regarding early memory capacities and our data are particularly striking when one considers that the 2- and 3-month-olds in our studies were exposed to their training mobile for only 15 minutes on each of three successive days and were then tested after a delay of 24 hours. Kagan's analysis, which assumes a failure to remember, after delays of just a few seconds, the details of an individual to whom infants three to four times older have been exposed daily for almost 8 months, appears untenable.

Reactivation of Infant Memories

When we asked motivated infants what, how much, and for how long they remember a distinctive task in a particular setting, we obtained quite a different picture of long-term memory abilities, as Campbell and Coulter (1976) originally anticipated. Even so, however, were events that are significant to the infant remembered for only slightly more than a week, this would hardly advance our understanding of infantile amnesia or provide insights into how prior experience might influence behavior over the long term. Our recent studies of reminder effects and the conditions under which such effects are obtained has led us to hypothesize that *memory reactivation*, that is, the presentation of a context-specific retrieval cue prior to the time that its efficacy is formally assessed, is the mechanism by which infants accumulate information over long periods of development (Hayne, 1988; Rovee-Collier & Hayne, 1987). We believe that memory reactivation is the fundamental process underlying long-term retention over both ontogeny and phylogeny (Campbell & Jaynes, 1966; Campbell & Spear, 1972; Spear, 1973, 1978).

In 1966, Campbell and Jaynes discovered that baby rat pups could remember a fear response over a period of 4 weeks if, each week, the pups were exposed briefly to the original training conditions. The exposure consisted of partial training trials that were too brief for new learning to take place. Pups who received only the interpolated partial training trials without the original training experience showed no fear at the end of the 4-week period. Also, pups who were trained but who received no intervening reminders exhibited complete forgetting after the 4-week delay. Campbell and Jaynes termed this phenomenon "reinstatement," referring to the reinstatement of a portion of the original training context as the condition for perpetuating the original memory. Subsequently, it was demonstrated that reinstatement-like facilitation of retrieval could occur even when the subject did not receive a complete training trial (e.g., a conditioned stimulus [CS]-unconditioned stimulus [US] pairing) but was exposed to only a fractional component of the original training context (e.g., the CS, US, or original training apparatus) during the retention interval (Riccio & Haroutunian, 1979; Spear & Parsons, 1976). Spear (1973) described this prior-cuing procedure as a "reactivation treatment" and its facilitating effects on retention as "reactivation." He hypothesized that the reminder or reactivation stimulus primed or recycled the dormant memory, making it more accessible during the actual retention test. Spear distinguished four classes of reactivation treatments: (a) *warm-up,* which involves exposure to contextual attributes (motoric, environmental) either immediately preceding a retention test or during the first few test trials; (b) *reinstatement,* or the interspersed presentation of multiple reactivation treatments throughout the retention interval; (c) *direct reactivation,* in which a single reactivation treatment is presented in the retention interval, and (d) *implicit reactivation,* in which a single reactivation treatment is immediately followed by a second procedure designed to disrupt the active memory aroused by the reactivation treatment. Considerable research has been reported on reactivation effects in both mature and immature animals and with both internal (pharmacological state, illness) and external contextual cues (for reviews, see Gordon, 1979, 1981; Riccio & Haroutunian, 1979; Riccio, Richardson, & Ebner, 1984; Spear, 1978).

The direct-reactivation phenomenon is of major theoretical significance in that it demonstrates a distinction between the *accessibility* and the *availability* of memories that has also been made in adult verbal learning and memory research (Tulving, 1972, 1983; Tulving & Thompson, 1973). A memory that is not expressed in the presence of a previously effective retrieval cue may not have decayed or become permanently "lost" (i.e., "unavailable"); rather, it may only be temporarily "inaccessible." This analysis shifts the focus of blame for poorer retention early in human development from encoding deficits to retrieval deficits (for reviews, see Ackerman, 1985; Perlmutter, 1984). In short, because overt behavior is ultimately required as a demonstration of retention in nonverbal organisms and retention requires a retrieval process, there is always the possibility that poor performance is a result of a retrieval failure. Evidence that retention can be improved by manipulating retrieval cues not only subsequent to the original encoding opportunity but even after forgetting is complete unequivocally supports this conclusion (Spear, 1973, 1976, 1978).

Spear and Parsons (1976) exposed infant rat pups to a single presentation of the US (shock) 27 days following the conclusion of training, when forgetting was complete. During the long-term retention test 24 hours later, these pups displayed excellent performance relative to that of pups who received no interpolated reminder in the interval and to that of pups who received the reminder without prior training. To study the possibility of memory reactivation in human infants, we adapted Spear and Parsons' reactivation treatment and testing procedure to our paradigm. If a memory acquired early in life can still be retrieved even after it has, by definition, been forgotten, then it is conceivable that forgotten memories could influence an infant's behavior after even more substantial periods.

In the mobile task, forgetting by 3-month-olds was complete 13 days after two training sessions (see Fig. 8.3). Therefore, we attempted to prime the forgotten memory by introducing a reminder at this point, testing the effectiveness of the reactivation procedure 1 day later, 14 days after the conclusion of training, in the standard long-term retention test (see Fig. 8.4).

As a reactivation treatment, we briefly (for 3 minutes) exposed the

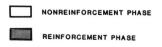

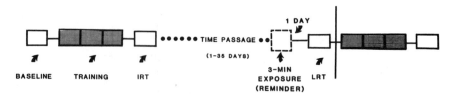

FIGURE 8.4. Timing of the 3-minute reactivation treatment relative to training and testing. The reminder is inserted into the standard retention paradigm (Fig. 8.2) when forgetting is complete and at some point (usually 1 day) prior to the long-term retention (LRT) test. IRT, immediate retention test.

infants to some salient aspect of their training context that was likely to have been noticed at the time of the original event (i.e., encoded as part of the memory of that event). In most of our studies, we have used noncontingent exposure to the reinforcer (the moving mobile) as a reminder (see Fig. 8.1, right). However, we have also used a distinctive crib bumper that lined the sides of the crib during training either as the sole reminder (Rovee-Collier, Griesler, & Earley, 1985) or in combination with the noncontingent exposure to the moving mobile (Borovsky, 1987; Butler, 1986; Hayne, Rovee-Collier, & Butler, 1986; Hill, Borovsky, & Rovee-Collier, 1988).

In all instances, infants who received a reminder responded during the 14-day long-term retention test at the same high rates that they had during the immediate retention test at the conclusion of training. In contrast, infants who saw no reminder and infants who saw a reminder without prior training responded at operant level during the long-term retention test (Sullivan, 1982). Figure 8.5 shows the forgetting function of the original memory following training as well as the reforgetting function of other groups of infants tested at comparable intervals following a reactivation treatment ("priming") administered 13 days following the conclusion of training (Rovee-Collier, Sullivan, Enright, Lucas, & Fagen, 1980).

Also shown in this figure is the effect of reminder treatments that were

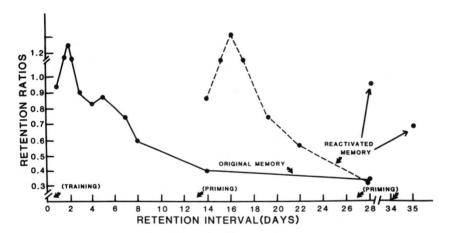

FIGURE 8.5. The original forgetting function of independent groups of 3-month-olds who were trained for 2 days and tested after delays ranging from 1 to 28 days in the standard retention paradigm. Retention ratios of groups receiving a single reactivation treatment ("priming") on days 13, 27, or 34 and results of tests at different delays following priming are also shown. The forgetting function of the reactivated memory of independent groups reminded on day 13 is indistinguishable from the original forgetting function. (Redrawn from Rovee-Collier et al., 1980).

first administered either 27 or 34 days after the end of training. The 3-month-olds' memory was restored to its final training level after a retention interval as long as a month. Even after a retention interval of 5 weeks, a reminder alleviated forgetting for almost half of the infants (Greco, Rovee-Collier, Hayne, Griesler, & Earley, 1986). Finally, this figure reveals that once an infant's memory of an earlier event has been reactivated, the memory is not transient but remains accessible as a potential influence on behavior for several days, after which time it is gradually reforgotten. The original forgetting function and the reforgetting function of a once-reactivated memory are virtually identical (Rovee-Collier, Enright, Lucas, Fagen, & Gekoski, 1981). These findings lead us to hypothesize that if a memory is repeatedly reactivated, the slope of the forgetting function may become progressively flatter and/or the intercept may become higher until, at some point, the memory attributes have become so accessible that the memory is not forgotten. At this point, the memory contents would be "general knowledge" or "semantic memory." In effect, we propose that general knowledge is simply the end point of a series of retrievals of specific-item information rather than the product of an altogether different memory system, as has been envisioned by many theorists (Schacter & Moscovitch, 1984; Squire, 1986; Tulving, 1983, 1985).

Time-Dependent Processes in Memory Retrieval

In spite of similarities, there are important differences between original and reactivated memories (see also Mactutus, Riccio, & Ferek, 1979). We reported previously, for example, that infants initially discriminated very minute changes in the training mobile during a retention test administered after a 1-day delay (Fagen et al., 1976; Hayne, Rovee-Collier, & Butler, 1986). In addition, we had found that responding to novel mobiles increasingly generalized over the days following training; during retention tests after delays of 3 to 4 days, infants responded as vigorously to completely novel test mobiles as to their original training mobiles (Rovee-Collier & Sullivan, 1980). This suggested that memory attributes corresponding to the specific details of the training mobile were forgotten more rapidly than those corresponding to its more general features, Similar findings have been reported in studies with animals (e.g., Riccio et al., 1984) as well as with adult humans tested in verbal-learning paradigms (e.g., Hasher & Griffin, 1978). As shown in Figure 8.6, this generalization function is reversed following a reminder treatment. Twenty-four hours after a reminder, infants generalize responding to completely novel test mobiles (Enright, 1981; Hayne, Rovee-Collier, & Butler, 1986); 72 hours later, however, infants once again discriminate the novel test mobile (Hayne, Rovee-Collier, & Butler 1986).

This finding suggests that different types of memory attributes are not only forgotten at different rates but also are retrieved at different rates.

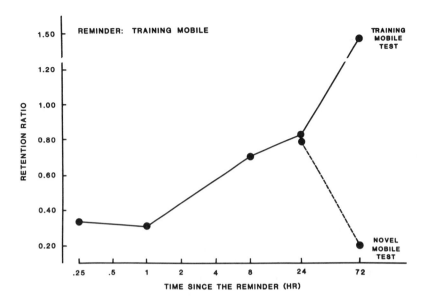

FIGURE 8.6. Retention ratios of independent groups of infants receiving a reactivation treatment with their training mobile 13 days following the conclusion of training and tested with the same mobile after delays ranging from 15 minutes to 3 days (solid line). Performance after the two shortest delays is at operant level. (Redrawn from Fagen & Rovee-Collier, 1983.) The dashed line depicts retention of independent groups who were trained and reminded with one mobile and tested with a different one after 1 or 3 days. Infants generalized to the novel test mobile 1 day after the reminder but discriminated it 3 days afterward.

Moreover, it appears that those memory attributes that were initially the last to be forgotten (e.g., memory attributes representing general information as opposed to attributes representing specific details) are the first to become accessible again following a reminder treatment. This offers strong evidence that retrieval is a time-dependent process (see also chap. 2 in this volume).

The finding of a time-dependent memory retrieval process for different types of memory attributes was surprising. However, this was not the first time-locked retrieval process we have observed. Figure 8.6 also displays the retention exhibited by independent groups of infants tested only once at different points in time following exposure to a reminder 13 days after the last training session (solid line). These data illustrate that the priming process, that is, the accessing of an inactive memory, takes time (Fagen & Rovee-Collier, 1983). Fifteen minutes and even an hour after the reactivation treatment, 3-month-olds showed no evidence of remembering the task. Eight hours afterward, some of the infants remembered a little better, and 24 hours afterward, retention was completely restored to the final training level. Moreover, retention continued to improve for 72 hours following the reminder—a hypermnesic effect virtually identical to that seen following original training. The longer infants in the 8-hour test group ($n=8$) napped between the reminder treatment and the long-term retention test, the higher were their retention ratios (correlation = .75). More recently, we have obtained data that suggest that memories which have been forgotten for longer periods take longer to be retrieved (Greco, Rovee-Collier, Hayne, Griesler, & Earley, 1986; Hayne, Greco, Earley, Griesler, & Rovee-Collier, 1986).

It is difficult to conceptualize physiological processes, other than endocrine actions, that endure for periods of several days and could mediate such a protracted phenomenon. The fact that similar time-dependence in memory retrieval has rarely been reported in studies of memory with older organisms except in cases of anterograde or retrograde amnesia (or in the tip-of-the-tongue phenomenon) suggests that infants may be model subjects for understanding the basic mechanisms that underlie adult memory retrieval. It is likely that these same processes cannot be observed in children and adults because of the networks of language-based associations that facilitate and speed retrieval.

Specificity of Retrieval Cues

Just as infants' memories 24 hours following training are highly specific to the training mobile, an effective reminder used in a prior cuing procedure is also highly specific to the original training context. A mobile containing more than a single novel object is not an effective retrieval cue 24 hours after training, and it also is not an effective reminder in a prior-cuing (direct-reactivation) procedure—in fact, it is no better than no reminder at all (Rovee-Collier, Patterson, & Hayne, 1985). Prefamiliarizing the infants with the to-be-substituted objects so that they were "different" (i.e., not represented in the memory of training) but not "novel" did not improve the efficacy of the altered reminder. Similarly, when infants were reminded with a mobile displaying a novel member of an alphanumeric form category that differed from the category members encountered during training (e.g., infants trained with different exemplars of an "A" category were reminded with an exemplar of the "2" category; see Fig. 8.7), the reactivation treatment was not effective; however, a reactivation treatment with a novel member of the training category was effective (Hayne, Rovee-Collier, & Perris, 1987). Even categorical reminders, therefore, are not generalized in the usual sense but are highly specific to the category boundaries established during original training.

Contextual Determinants of Retention

Infants' memories also include information about the physical environment in which an event occurs, and this information qualifies the efficacy of retrieval cues more closely associated with the contingency, both in simple forgetting and in reminder paradigms. Exposure of the original training mobile to infants as a reminder, for example, is highly effective in alleviating forgetting. In the presence of a distinctive crib bumper that differs from the one that was present during original training, however, the mobile reminder is not as effective for 3-month-olds as when the crib bumper during training and testing are identical (Butler, 1986); for 6-month-olds, the reminder is not effective at all if the bumper is different (Borovsky, 1987). When the mobile reminder was presented outside the crib in a familiar location where 3-month-olds usually ate (the kitchen or living room), or when it was presented in the bedroom but not in the crib, it was not an effective reminder: The memory remained inactive (Hayne & Rovee-Collier, 1985). In short, the infants *appeared not to recognize* the otherwise effective reminder out of context (see also Estes, 1973; Medin & Reynolds, 1985; Rovee-Collier, Griesler, & Earley, 1985). Similarly, Butler (1986) found that a change in the crib bumper during a retention test with the original mobile 3 days after training reduced test performance to operant level, while retention in the presence of the original bumper after the same delay was perfect. The fact that a change in the crib bumper after 24 hours—a delay after which the infants' memory for specific details of the training mobile is very precise—did not affect retention suggests that the context gates retrieval after the details of stimuli more closely associated with the focal task are forgotten.

The role of context in retention is currently a topic of great interest in animal research (for review, see Balsam, 1985) and has also been a focus of concern in the human adult verbal-learning and memory literature (e.g., Bower, 1981; Godden & Baddeley, 1975, 1980; Jenkins, 1974). The finding of robust context effects in infant retention, the demonstration that context can serve as a retrieval cue in its own right, the demonstration that contextual information facilitates discrimination, and the suggestion that contextual cues gate memory retrieval are unique in the literature on memory in early infancy. The ability to exploit contextual information has been described both as a hippocampal function (Nadel, Willner, & Kurz, 1984; Nadel & Zola-Morgan, 1984) and as a defining characteristic of episodic or declarative memory (Squire, 1986), both of which are presumed not to be implicated in the memory processing of infants as young as 3 months of age (see also Moscovitch, 1984). Because contextual information regarding the setting in which an event occurs clearly influences memory performance early in infancy, however, additional speculation regarding the neuroanatomical basis for the effects of situational cues on retention is obviously required.

The specificity of the reminder with respect both to its details and the context within which it is encountered suggests that infantile amnesia may also result, at least in part, from contextual changes, either real or perceived, that are increasingly likely to occur with time passage. We believe that the specificity of retrieval cues for memories acquired early in

infancy buffers against the possibility that those memories will be
retrieved in inappropriate situations where they might either "misguide"
behavior or become inappropriately modified (e.g., a predictive relation
could lose its predictive value). Moreover, for immature organisms with a
poorly developed inhibitory system, also a hippocampal function, the
requirement that retrieval cues be context-specific relieves the organism
of the need to withhold responding in an inappropriate context by
severely constraining the probability that retrieval will be instantiated in
the first place. In effect, the response constraints are contained in the
structure of the environment at a time when central inhibitory mechanisms are not fully functional. This same factor, however, reduces the
probability of retrieval after very long intervals.

Categorization and Memory Retrieval

Recently, we have found that retrieval specificity extends to categorical
responding, that is, the equivalent treatment of perceptually distinctive
events (Hayne et al., 1987; Greco, Hayne, & Rovee-Collier, 1986). After
training with a series of discriminably different mobiles in each of several
sessions, 3-month-olds generalized responding to novel mobiles that they
otherwise discriminate. Because novel stimuli cannot cue retrieval,
generalized responding to a novel test mobile must have been cued by the
features shared by the test and training stimuli. In fact, only a novel
member of the training category was an effective retrieval cue: During a
24-hour retention test, infants responded above operant level only to a
novel member of the original training category. Similarly, after forgetting
was complete, only a novel member of the original training category was
an effective reminder in a reactivation procedure.

It is generally thought that categorization is a higher level cognitive
process of which infants are incapable until the second half-year of life
(Olson & Strauss, 1984). This conclusion has been based on findings from
studies involving measures of visual attention. However, the ability of
infants so young to categorize suggests that this is a very basic skill (see
also Rosch, 1978). We propose that the relation between categorization
and memory is fundamental: Without the ability to remember, it would be
impossible to categorize successively encountered events; conversely,
without the ability to categorize novel events, retrieval by a similar but
discriminably different cue would not be possible. Furthermore, we think
it likely that categorization is a by-product of a selective retrieval process.

If this is the case, then the study of categorization may contribute to our
understanding of how memories are modified (e.g., chap. 3 in this volume;
Loftus & Loftus, 1980; Tulving, 1983). The problem centers on the
circumstances under which a subject will classify an unfamiliar event as a
constituent of a memory. If an event is classified as belonging to a
memory of an event, then it should be able to cue the retrieval of that

memory (Greco, Hayne, & Rovee-Collier, 1986; Hayne et al., 1987). There is considerable difference of opinion as to whether old memories are recoded by new information or whether new information and old information coexist in the same memory (for review, see Johnson & Hasher, 1987). If new information is classified as belonging to an old memory and can be shown to cue the retrieval of that memory, however, this could provide an opportunity for the new information to be incorporated into the memory of the original event, irrespective of whether it displaces the old information (Gordon, 1981).

Our studies of early categorization have confirmed findings with older infants that exposure to a series of perceptibly different events that share common properties is critical in order for a novel, discriminably different event with those same properties to be treated as a member of the original series (for review, see Olson & Sherman, 1983). Infants trained with only a single mobile over multiple sessions did not generalize to a discriminably different, novel mobile during a 24-hour test, nor was a novel mobile an effective reminder in a reactivation paradigm (Hayne et al., 1987; Rovee-Collier, Patterson, & Hayne, 1985). Infants trained with a different mobile per session, however, did generalize to another different, novel test mobile, and it also was an effective reminder after forgetting was complete (Greco, Hayne, & Rovee-Collier, 1986; Hayne et al., 1987). In all subsequent studies of classification, therefore, we have trained infants with a series of different block mobiles and have sought to define the particular conditions under which novel, physically different test stimuli might be classified as members of the series of training exemplars. We hypothesized that three factors might be important: (1) the contextual similarity between the training episode and the test with the novel stimulus event, (2) the time interval between successive events, and (3) the perceptible and functional similarity between successive events (see also Loftus, 1981).

1. *Contextual Similarity.* One of the functions of the context appears to be to identify the memory and distinguish it from conflicting memories of which the same cue is a part (Ackerman, 1987). A second function is to disambiguate an otherwise ambiguous test situation (Bouton & Bolles, 1985). We have found that a stimulus that is physically so dissimilar from the series of training exemplars that 3-month-olds unfailingly discriminate it for as long as 7 days following training will be responded to after this retention interval if presented in the original training context (Greco & Rovee-Collier, 1988; Greco, Hayne, & Rovee-Collier, 1986). When trained with a series of yellow-block mobiles bearing one of two types of alphanumeric characters (Fig. 8.7, top, center) in the presence of a red-and-blue crib bumper, infants generalized responding to a metal butterfly wind chimes (Fig. 8.7, bottom) to which they would otherwise not respond. However, this occurred *if and only if* generalization to the

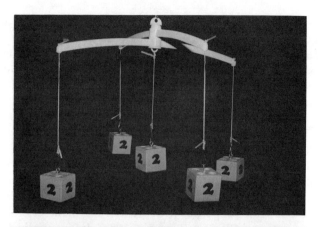

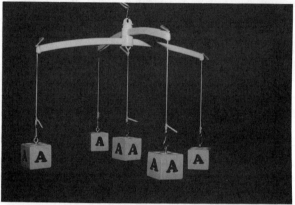

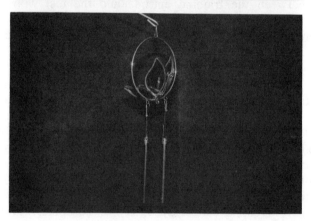

FIGURE 8.7. Stimuli used in studies of memory malleability. All characters on each yellow-block mobile were made of felt and were the same color, but the color differed from one session to the next during training. Three-month-olds, trained with different members of one of these alphanumeric categories for three sessions, typically do not generalize responding to the butterfly wind chimes, constructed of metal and colored glass, during a retention test 1 day after the end of training.

butterfly was tested in the presence of the red-and-blue bumper. The finding that physically different stimuli that 3-month-olds encounter in the same context are included as members of a common category is consistent with the report (Mandler, Fivush, & Reznick, 1987) that 14- and 20-month olds respond categorically to physically and functionally dissimilar objects (e.g., spoon and bowl) that were previously encountered at the same time or in the same place (e.g., in the kitchen). Categories formed in this manner are termed *contextual categories* (Mandler et al., 1987). This finding is also consistent with the fact that 3-month-olds do *not* respond to the same test object that had been present during training when the distinctive contexts of training and testing differ (Butler, 1986; Rovee-Collier, Griesler, & Earley, 1985).

2. *Temporal Contiguity.* In addition to common place information, it is likely that the temporal context within which events are encountered influences whether physically dissimilar events will be included as a part of the same memory. Presumably, the greater the time passage between two successive events, the greater the probability that the events will be perceived as separate and distinct occurrences, each with its own memory representation. The degree of temporal segregation between successive events plays a major role in a similar phenomenon described by Loftus (1981) as "mental bonding." We refer to the phenomenon in infancy as "postevent bonding" (Greco & Rovee-Collier, 1988).

In the absence of distinctive place information (i.e., the distinctive crib bumper) during training and testing, simple exposure to the nonmoving, physically dissimilar, metal butterfly wind chimes for 3 minutes immediately following training with the series of yellow-block mobiles was insufficient to produce generalized responding to the butterfly during the long-term retention test 24 hours later. When the functional similarity between the butterfly and the block mobiles was increased by demonstrating for the infants that the butterfly *moved,* however, infants did generalize responding to the butterfly 24 hours later (Greco, Hayne, & Rovee-Collier, 1986). To confirm whether the butterfly had been incorporated into the memory of the block mobiles, we asked whether it would cue retrieval of that memory in a reactivation paradigm 2 weeks later, when the memory of training is otherwise forgotten. We found that when the moving butterfly was exposed for only 3 minutes immediately following training, it subsequently was an effective reminder. Infants reminded with the butterfly exhibited complete retention when tested with a novel member of the training series of block mobiles 24 hours following the reactivation procedure. Conversely, a novel block mobile was an effective reminder for infants tested with the butterfly 24 hours later.

When the moving butterfly was first exposed for 3 minutes 6 days following the last training episode, however, infants did not generalize responding to the metal butterfly during a long-term retention test 24 hours later (a week after the end of training), in spite of the fact that the memory of the blocks was still strong at that time. Nor was it an effective reminder for the memory of the training series of block mobiles 2 weeks after training. Thus, when the interval between event 2 (exposure to the moving butterfly) and event 1 (exposure to the moving yellow-block mobile) was short to negligible, event 2 was integrated into the memory of event 1 and could serve as a retrieval cue for event 1 (and vice versa). This provides strong evidence of postevent bonding. When the temporal interval between successive events was substantial, however, the memory representations of these events were not integrated.

3. *Physical and Functional Similarity.* Events that are physically more similar (i.e., share more common elements) are usually treated more equivalently (stimulus generalization). However, form and function are highly correlated in the real world. In the preceding study, Greco, Hayne, and Rovee-Collier (1986) found that once physically dissimilar events were shown to be functionally similar, they were treated equivalently *if* the events were sufficiently temporally contiguous. In a subsequent manipulation involving the butterfly and block mobiles, Greco and colleagues exposed infants to additional functional information about the metal butterfly wind chimes. In addition to moving for 3 minutes immediately following the final training episode with the yellow-block mobiles, butterfly now rang (chimed). This additional manipulation, therefore, *decreased* the functional similarity between the two successively encountered events. Under these conditions, infants did not generalize to the butterfly 24 hours after training, nor was the ringing-and-moving butterfly an effective reminder in a reactivation paradigm for the memory of the training series after a 2-week delay. Therefore, when the functional dissimilarity between event 1 and event 2 was increased, the postevent bonding phenomenon was eliminated. The two events remained distinctive and separate memories.

Finally, Greco and co-workers introduced a third bit of functional information, this time designed to *increase* the net functional similarity between event 1 and event 2. Infants were allowed to move the ringable butterfly for themselves by kicking during the 3-minute exposure immediately following the end of operant training with the yellow-block mobiles. Under these exposure conditions, the infants did respond to the butterfly during the 24-hour long-term retention test, indicating that the memory of the ringing-and-moving-controllable butterfly had been included in the memory of the blocks. As convergent evidence for this conclusion, the ringing-and-moving butterfly also served as a reminder for the memory of the blocks in a reactivation paradigm 2 weeks later. However, under these conditions, *the blocks did not serve as a reminder* for infants tested with the butterfly, indicating that the category relation between the butterfly and the blocks was asymmetrical. Apparently the movement attribute of the moving-and-ringing butterfly could serve as a reminder for the movement attribute of the blocks; but the movement attribute of the blocks was insufficient to reactivate the memory attribute of ringing. Asymmetrical relations are commonly obtained in studies of adult categorization (Rosch, 1978). The reactivation procedure offers a potentially powerful means of probing not only the manner in which successive events are integrated but also the manner in which the integrated memories are organized.

As a result of her now-classic studies of eye-witness testimony, Loftus (1981) cited the interval between postevent information and the original event as well as the similarity of postevent information to the attributes in the original event as critical determinants of whether postevent information would be incorporated into the original memory or not. In addition, she viewed the amount of attention allocated to the postevent information as critical: If the second event were scrutinized, its perceived dissimilarity would be increased and the probability of postevent bonding would be reduced. At the other extreme, if the postevent information were not noticed at all, it also would not be included in the memory of event 1. This role of attention is virtually identical to the role accorded attention in Medin and Reynold's (1985) memory model of categorization. When this analysis is applied to the preceding findings, we see that the effect on postevent bonding of introducing the ringing to the moving butterfly could have been direct, increasing the functional differences between the butterfly and the mobile. Alternatively, the effect could have been indirect, increasing the infants' attention to the butterfly and thereby increasing its perceived distinctiveness along one of the previously exposed dimensions.

Studies with the butterfly and block mobiles have demonstrated that postevent bonding is one way in which memories of young infants, like memories of human adults, can be modified. At 3 months of age, the time window for postevent bonding of some types of postevent information extends for as long as 4 days after training (Greco & Rovee-Collier, 1988). We propose that postevent bonding may also occur immediately following retrieval of a memory representation in a reactivation paradigm. Depending upon the relative accessibility of the various memory attributes and the context at the time an original memory is actually accessed following a reactivation treatment, for example, a second event could interact with the active memory of the first event in different ways. These possibilities remain to be explored.

Conclusions and Implications for Interdisciplinary Research

Procedures that exploit the natural relation between learning and memory have necessitated a revision of the persisting notion that memories acquired in early infancy are highly transient. When motivated infants have a reason to remember, they do so by orders of magnitude longer than previously thought. Moreover, even when forgetting is complete and the memory appears to be no longer available (Tulving, 1983), it may still be accessed by an appropriate retrieval cue if the reminder is presented sufficiently in advance of the retention test. We concur with Campbell and Jaynes (1966) that memory reactivation is a strong candidate for the mechanism by which the effects of prior experience could influence behavior over extended developmental periods (see Hayne, 1988). Clearly, human infantile amnesia is not a result of the young infant's inability to encode, store, and retrieve information over the long term.

These findings challenge recent conclusions of memory authorities and child development specialists that long-term memory is a late-maturing capacity that does not emerge until the eighth or ninth month of life. In addition, the finding that early memories not only are highly organized but also are highly specific to the conditions under which they were originally acquired and *remain so* over the long term challenges the widely held belief that memories acquired prior to the eighth or ninth postnatal month are diffuse and undifferentiated. Finally, it is obvious that infants as young as 2 to 3 months of age must be endowed with neuroanatomical structures that can support the encoding, storage, and retrieval of memories over very long intervals. Because adult brain mechanisms for memory processing are presumably not functionally mature at this point in early development, future research is required to reveal how this behavior is mediated and what role the brain areas that process these early memories assume later in development (see Kucharski & Hall, 1987). Previous views regarding infant memory deficits will also have to be revised to account for the findings that (a) retrieval follows a different time course for different types of memory attributes, (b) retrieval is context dependent, (c) training with multiple, perceptibly different exemplars can result in memories that are categorically organized, and (d) the same principles that describe "mental bonding" in adult humans also apply to the modification of memories of human infants ("postevent bonding") as young as 2 to 3 months of age.

How the very young infant's recently discovered capacity for long-term memory contributes to cognitive development remains to be determined. It is likely that deficiencies in some component of memory processing very early in life will contribute to subsequent cognitive deficits. Conversely, it is possible that unusual facility in basic memory processing early in life may ultimately result in performance indicative of giftedness. These possibilities remain to be explored. As is evident in this volume, there has been little attempt to relate the theory and findings from studies of nonhuman species with those from studies of human adults. I believe that the study of early memory in nonverbal human infants provides an important bridge between the animal and adult-human memory traditions as well as a unique opportunity to provide an "infant model" of human memory.

Acknowledgments. The research described in this chapter was supported by Grant No. MH32307 from the National Institute of Mental Health and reflects the joint contribution of numerous students and colleagues, past and present. In particular, it is appropriate to recognize the substantive contributions, both theoretical and empirical, of Harlene Hayne, Carolyn Greco, Judy Butler, and Diane Borovsky. This chapter is dedicated to two former colleagues, John Santa and the late Marilyn Shaw, who valiantly struggled over a number of years to educate me about human memory and attentional allocation, respectively.

References

Ackerman, B.P. (1985). Children's retrieval deficit. In C. Brainerd & M. Pressley (Eds.), *Basic processes in memory development*. New York: Springer-Verlag.

Ackerman, B.P. (1987). Descriptions: A model of nonstrategic memory development. In H. W. Reese (Ed.), *Advances in child development and behavior* (Vol. 20). New York: Academic Press.

Balsam, P.D. (1985). The functions of context in learning and performance. In P. D. Balsam & A. Tomie (Eds.), *Context and learning*. Hillsdale, NJ: Lawrence Erlbaum Associates.

Bashinski, H., Werner, J., & Rudy, J. (1985). Determinants of infant visual fixation: Evidence for two-process theory. *Journal of Experimental Child Psychology, 39,* 580–598.

Bolles, R.C. (1976). Some relationships between learning and memory. In D. L. Medin, W. A. Roberts, & R. T. Davis (Eds.), *Processes of animal memory*. New York: John Wiley.

Borovsky, D. (1987). *Determinants of retention in 6-month-old infants*. Unpublished master's thesis, Rutgers University, New Brunswick, NJ.

Bouton, M.E., & Bolles, R.C. (1985). Contexts, event-memories, and extinction. In P. D. Balsam & A. Tomie (Eds.), *Context and learning*. Hillsdale, NJ: Lawrence Erlbaum Associates.

Bower, G.H. (1981). Mood and memory. *American Psychologist, 36,* 129–148.

Brody, L.R. (1981). Visual short-term cued recall memory in infancy. *Child Development, 52,* 242–250.

Bruner, J. (1964). The course of cognitive growth. *American Psychologist, 19,* 1–15.

Butler, J. (1986). *A contextual hierarchy in infant memory*. Unpublished master's thesis, Rutgers University, New Brunswick, NJ.

Campbell, B.A., & Coulter, X. (1976). Neural and psychological processes underlying the development of learning and memory. In T. J. Tighe & R. N. Leaton, (Eds.), *Habituation*. Hillsdale, NJ: Lawrence Erlbaum Associates.

Campbell, B.A., & Jaynes, J. (1966). Reinstatement. *Psychological Review, 73,* 478–480.

Campbell, B.A., & Spear, N.E. (1972). Ontogeny of memory. *Psychological Review, 79,* 215–236.

Caron, R.F. (1967). Visual reinforcement of head-turning in young infants. *Journal of Experimental Child Psychology, 5,* 489–511.

Cohen, L.B. (1973). A two-process model of infant visual attention. *Merrill-Palmer Quarterly, 19,* 157–180.

Cohen, L.B., & Gelber, E.R. (1975). Infant visual memory. In L. Cohen & P. Salapatek (Eds.), *Infant perception: From sensation to cognition* (Vol. 1). New York: Academic Press.

Cornell, E.H. (1974). Infants' discrimination of photographs of faces following redundant presentations. *Journal of Experimental Child Psychology, 18,* 98–106.

D'Amato, M.R., & Cox, J.K. (1976). Delay of consequences and short-term memory in monkeys. In D. L. Medin, W. A. Roberts, & R. T. Davis (Eds.), *Processes of animal memory.* Hillsdale, NJ: Lawrence Erlbaum Associates.

DeCasper, A.J., & Fifer, W.P. (1980). Of human bonding: Newborns prefer their mothers' voices. *Science, 208,* 1174–1176.

Enright, M.W. (1981). *A comparison of newly acquired and reactivated memories of three-month-old infants.* Unpublished doctoral dissertation, Rutgers University, New Brunswick, NJ.

Enright, M.K., Rovee-Collier, C.K., Fagen, J.W., & Caniglia, K. (1983). The effects of distributed training on retention of operant conditioning in human infants. *Journal of Experimental Child Psychology, 36,* 209–225.

Estes, W.K. (1973). Memory and conditioning. In F. J. McGuigan & D. R. Lumsden (Eds.), *Contemporary approaches to conditioning and learning.* New York: John Wiley.

Fagan, J.F. (1970). Memory in the infant. *Journal of Experimental Child Psychology, 9,* 217–226.

Fagan, J.F. (1984). Infant memory: History, current trends, relations to cognitive psychology. In M. Moscovitch (Ed.), *Advances in the study of communication and affect. Vol. 9: Infant memory.* New York: Plenum Press.

Fagen, J.W., Rovee, C.K., & Kaplan, M.G. (1976). Psychophysical scaling of stimulus similarity in 3-month-old infants and adults. *Journal of Experimental Child Psychology, 22,* 272–281.

Fagen, J.W., & Rovee-Collier, C. (1983). Memory retrieval: A time-locked process in infancy. *Science, 222,* 1349–1351.

Godden, D.R., & Baddeley, A.D. (1975). Context-dependent memory in two natural environments: On land and underwater. *British Journal of Psychology, 66,* 325–332.

Godden, D.R., & Baddeley, A.D. (1980). When does context affect recognition memory? *British Journal of Psychology, 71,* 99–104.

Gordon, W.C. (1979). Age: Is it a constraint on memory content? In N. E. Spear & B. A. Campbell (Eds.), *Ontogeny of learning and memory.* Hillsdale, NJ: Lawrence Erlbaum Associates.

Gordon, W.C. (1981). Mechanisms of cue-induced retention enhancement. In N. E. Spear & R. R. Miller (Eds.), *Information processing in animals: Memory mechanisms.* Hillsdale, NJ: Lawrence Erlbaum Associates.

Greco, C., Hayne, H., & Rovee-Collier, C. (1986, April). Category acquisition by 3-month-old infants. Paper presented at the meeting of the Eastern Psychological Association, New York.

Greco, C., & Rovee-Collier, C. (1988, April). Postevent bonding: The time window for the malleability of infant memory. Paper presented at the meeting of the International Conference on Infant Studies, Washington, DC.

Greco, C., Rovee-Collier, C., Hayne, H., Griesler, P., & Earley, L. (1986). Ontogeny of early event memory: I. Forgetting and retrieval by 2- and 3-month-olds. *Infant Behavior and Development, 9,* 441–460.

Groves, P.M., & Thompson, R.F. (1970). Habituation: A dual-process theory. *Psychological Review, 77,* 419–450.

Hasher, L., & Griffin, M. (1978). Reconstructive and reproductive processes in memory. *Journal of Experimental Psychology: Human Learning and Memory, 4,* 318–330.

Hayne, H. (1988). *The effect of multiple reminders on retention.* Unpublished doctoral dissertation, Rutgers University, New Brunswick, NJ.

Hayne, H., Greco, C., Earley, L., Griesler, P., & Rovee-Collier, C. (1986). Ontogeny of early event memory: II. Encoding and retrieval by 2- and 3-month-olds. *Infant Behavior and Development, 9,* 461–472.

Hayne, H., & Rovee-Collier, C. (April, 1985). Contextual determinants of reactivated memories in infants. Paper presented at the meeting of the Society for Research in Child Development, Toronto.

Hayne, H., Rovee-Collier, C., & Butler, J. (1986, November). Organization of reactivated memories. Paper presented at the meeting of the International Society for Developmental Psychobiology, Annapolis, MD.

Hayne, H., Rovee-Collier, C., & Perris, E.E. (1987). Categorization and memory retrieval by 3-month-olds. *Child Development, 58,* 750–767.

Hill, W.L., Borovsky, D., & Rovee-Collier, C. (1988). Continuities in infant memory development. *Developmental Psychobiology, 21,* 43–62.

Jeffrey, W.E. (1976). Habituation as a mechanism for perceptual development. In T. J. Tighe & R. N. Leaton (Eds.), *Habituation.* Hillsdale, NJ: Lawrence Erlbaum Associates.

Jenkins, J.J. (1974). Remember that old theory of memory? Well, forget it! *American Psychologist, 29,* 785–795.

Johnson, M.K., & Hasher, L. (1987). Human learning and memory. In M. R. Rosenzweig & L. W. Proter (Eds.), *Annual review of psychology* (Vol. 38). Palo Alto, CA: Annual Reviews.

Kagan, J. (1979). Growing by leaps: The form of early cognitive development. *The Sciences, 19,* 8–12, 39.

Kagan, J. (1984). *The nature of the child.* New York: Basic Books.

Kandel, E.R. (1979). Cellular insights into behavior and learning. *The Harvey Lectures, Series 73.* New York: Academic Press.

Kucharski, D., & Hall, W.G. (1987). New routes to early memories. *Science, 238,* 786–788.

Leaton, R.N. (1976). Long-term retention of the habituation of lick suppression and startle response produced by a single auditory stimulus. *Journal of Experimental Psychology: Animal Behavior Processes, 2,* 248–259.

Little, A.H., Lipsitt, L.P., & Rovee-Collier, C. (1984). Classical conditioning and retention of the infant's eyelid response: Effects of age and interstimulus interval. *Journal of Experimental Child Psychology, 37,* 512–524.

Loftus, E.F. (1981). Mentalmorphosis: Alterations in memory produced by the mental bonding of new information to old. In J. Long & A. Baddeley (Eds.), *Attention and performance IX.* Hillsdale, NJ: Lawrence Erlbaum Associates.

Loftus, E.F., & Loftus, G.R. (1980). On the permanence of stored information in the brain. *American Psychologist, 35,* 409–420.

Mactutus, C.F., Riccio, D.C., & Ferek, J.M. (1979). Retrograde amnesia for old (reactivated) memory: Some anomalous characteristics. *Science, 204,* 1319–1320.

Mandler, J.M. (1984). Representation and recall in infancy. In M. Moscovitch (Ed.), *Advances in the study of affect and communication. Vol. 9: Infant memory.* New York: Plenum Press.

Mandler, J.M., Fivush, R., & Reznick, J.S. (1987). The development of contextual categories. *Cognitive Development, 2,* 339–354.

McCall, R.B. (1971). Attention in the infant: Avenue to the study of cognitive development. In D. Walcher & D. Peters (Eds.), *Early childhood: The development of self-regulatory mechanisms.* New York: Academic Press.

Medin, D.L., & Reynolds, T.J. (1985). Cue-context interactions in discrimination, categorization, and memory. In P. D. Balsam & A. Tomie (Eds.), *Context and learning.* Hillsdale, NJ: Lawrence Erlbaum Associates.

Nadel, L., Willner, J., & Kurz, E.M. (1985). Cognitive maps and environmental context. In P. Balsam & A. Tomie (Eds.), *Context and learning.* Hillsdale, NJ: Lawrence Erlbaum Associates.

Nadel, L., & Zola-Morgan, S. (1984). Infantile amnesia: A neurobiological perspective. In M. Moscovitch (Ed.), *Advances in the study of communication and affect. Vol. 9: Infant memory.* New York: Plenum Press.

Olson, G.M., & Sherman, T. (1983). Attention, learning and memory in infants. In M. M. Haith & J. J. Campos (Vol. Eds.), *Handbook of child psychology. Vol. 2: Infancy and developmental psychobiology.* New York: John Wiley.

Olson, G.M., & Strauss, M.S. (1984). The development of infant memory. In M. Moscovitch (Ed.), *Advances in the study of communication and affect. Vol 9: Infant memory.* New York: Plenum Press.

Perlmutter, M. (1984). Continuities and discontinuities in early human memory: Paradigms, processes, and performance. In R. Kail & N. E. Spear (Eds.), *Comparative perspectives on the development of memory.* Hillsdale, NJ: Lawrence Erlbaum Associates.

Reeves, A., & Sperling, G. (1986). Attention gating in short-term visual memory. *Psychological Review, 93,* 180–206.

Revusky, S. (1971). The role of interference in association over a delay. In W. K. Honig & P. H. R. James (Eds.), *Animal memory.* New York: Academic Press.

Riccio, D.C., & Haroutunian, V. (1979). Some approaches to the alleviation of ontogenetic memory deficits. In B. A. Campbell & N. E. Spear (Eds.), *Ontogeny of learning and memory.* Hillsdale, NJ: Lawrence Erlbaum Associates.

Riccio, D.C., Richardson, R., & Ebner, D.L. (1984). Memory retrieval deficits based upon altered contextual cues: A paradox. *Psychological Bulletin, 96,* 152–165.

Roberts, W.A., & Grant, D.S. (1978). Interaction of sample and comparison stimuli in delayed matching to sample in the pigeon. *Journal of Experimental Psychology: Animal Behavior Processes, 4,* 468–482.

Rosch, E. (1978). Principles of categorization. In E. Rosch & B. B. Lloyd (Eds.), *Cognition and categorization.* Hillsdale, NJ: Lawrence Erlbaum Associates.

Rovee, C.K., & Fagen, J.W. (1976). Extended conditioning and 24-hr retention in infants. *Journal of Experimental Child Psychology, 21,* 1–11.

Rovee-Collier, C. (1987). Learning and memory in infancy. In J. D. Osofsky (Ed.), *Handbook of infancy* (2nd ed.). New York: John Wiley.

Rovee-Collier, C., Enright, M., Lucas, D., Fagen, J., & Gekoski, M.J. (1981). The forgetting of newly acquired and reactivated memories of 3-month-old infants. *Infant Behavior and Development, 4,* 317–331.

Rovee-Collier, C., Griesler, P.C., & Earley, L.A. (1985). Contextual determinants of retention in 3-month-old infants. *Learning and Motivation, 16,* 139–157.

Rovee-Collier, C., & Hayne, H. (1987). Reactivation of infant memory: Implications for cognitive development. In H. W. Reese (Ed.), *Advances in child development and behavior* (Vol. 20). New York: Academic Press.

Rovee-Collier, C., Patterson, J., & Hayne, H. (1985). Specificity in the reactivation of infant memory. *Developmental Psychobiology, 18,* 559–574.

Rovee-Collier, C.K., & Sullivan, M.W. (1980). Organization of infant memory. *Journal of Experimental Psychology: Human Learning and Memory, 6,* 798–807.

Rovee-Collier, C.K., Sullivan, M.W., Enright, M., Lucas, D., & Fagen, J.W. (1980). Reactivation of infant memory. *Science, 208,* 1159–1161.

Schacter, D.L., & Moscovitch, M. (1984). Infants, amnesics, and dissociable memory systems. In M. Moscovitch (Ed.), *Advances in the study of communication and affect. Vol. 9: Infant memory.* New York: Plenum Press.

Sokolov, E.N. (1963). *Perception and the conditioned reflex.* New York: Macmillan.

Spear, N.E. (1973). Retrieval of memory in animals. *Psychological Review, 80,* 163–194.

Spear, N.E. (1976). Retrieval of memories. In W. K. Estes (Ed.), *Handbook of learning and cognitive processes. Vol. 4: Memory processes.* Hillsdale, NJ: Lawrence Erlbaum Associates.

Spear, N.E. (1978). *The processing of memories: Forgetting and retention.* Hillsdale, NJ: Lawrence Erlbaum Associates.

Spear, N.E., & Parsons, P.J. (1976). Analysis of a reactivation treatment: Ontogenetic determinants of alleviated forgetting. In D. L. Medin, W. A. Roberts, & R. T. Davis (Eds.), *Processes of animal memory.* Hillsdale, NJ: Lawrence Erlbaum Associates.

Squire, L.R. (1986). Mechanisms of memory. *Science, 232,* 1612–1619.

Stinson, F.S. (1971). *Visual short-term memory in four-month infants.* Unpublished doctoral dissertation, Brown University, Providence, RI.

Strauss, M., & Carter, P. (1984). Infant memory: Limitations and future directions. In R. Kail & N. E. Spear (Eds.), *Comparative perspectives on the development of memory.* Hillsdale, NJ: Lawrence Erlbaum Associates.

Sullivan, M. (1982). Reactivation: Priming forgotten memories in human infants. *Child Development, 53,* 516–523.

Sullivan, M.W., Rovee-Collier, C.K., & Tynes, D.M. (1979). A conditioning analysis of infant long-term memory. *Child Development, 50,* 152–162.

Thompson, R.F., & Spencer, W.A. (1966). A model phenomenon for the study of neuronal substrates of behavior. *Psychological Review, 73,* 16–43.

Thompson, R., & Glanzman, D. (1976). Neural and behavioral mechanisms of habituation and sensitization. In T. J. Tighe & R. N. Leaton (Eds.), *Habituation.* Hillsdale, NJ: Lawrence Erlbaum Associates.

Timmons, C.R., Lapinski, K., & Worobey, J. (1986, April). Delayed matching-to-sample by young *Homo sapiens*. Paper presented at the meeting of the Eastern Psychological Association, New York.

Tulving, E. (1972). Episodic and semantic memory. In E. Tulving & W. Donaldson (Eds.), *Organization of memory*. New York: Academic Press.

Tulving, E. (1983). *Elements of episodic memory*. New York: Oxford University Press.

Tulving, E. (1985). How many memory systems are there? *American Psychologist, 40,* 385–398.

Tulving, E., & Thompson, D.M. (1973). Encoding specificity and retrieval processes in episodic memory. *Psychological Review, 80,* 352–373.

Vander Linde, E., Morrongiello, B.A., & Rovee-Collier, C. (1985). Determinants of retention in 8-week-old infants. *Developmental Psychology, 21,* 601–613.

Wagner, A.R. (1976). Priming in STM: An information-processing mechanism for self-generated or retrieval-generated depression in performance. In T. J. Tighe & R. N. Leaton (Eds.), *Habituation*. Hillsdale, NJ: Lawrence Erlbaum Associates.

Watson, J.S. (1984). Memory in learning: Analysis of three momentary reactions of infants. In R. Kail & N. E. Spear (Eds.), *Comparative perspectives on the development of memory*. Hillsdale, NJ: Lawrence Erlbaum Associates.

Werner, J.S., & Perlmutter, M. (1979). Development of visual memory in infants. In H. W. Reese & L. P. Lipsitt (Eds.), *Advances in child development and behavior* (Vol. 14). New York: Academic Press.

Wyers, E.J., Peeke, H.V.S., & Herz, M.J. (1973). Behavioral habituation in invertebrates. In H. V. S. Peeke & M. J. Herz (Eds.), *Habituation I*. New York: Academic Press.

CHAPTER 9

The Locus of Word-Finding Problems in Language-Impaired Children

Robert Kail

For the past decade and a half, it has taken much intestinal fortitude to conduct traditional memory research. Throughout that time, the Ebbinghaus tradition of memory experimentation has been criticized, even derided, by some of psychology's most respected scientists. Experimental psychologists have been admonished to leave the clear waters of verbal learning to probe the murky depths of ecological memory. Even the *Journal of Verbal Learning and Verbal Behavior* took a new name to reflect a changing focus.

Some of these changes can be traced to a well-known commentary by Tulving and Madigan that appeared in the *Annual Review of Psychology* in 1970. They wrote:

Many inventions and discoveries in other fields of human intellectual endeavour would bewilder and baffle Aristotle, but the most spectacular or counter-intuitive finding from psychological studies of memory would cause him to raise his eyebrows only for an instant. At the time when man has walked on the moon, is busily transplanting vital organs from one living body into another, and has acquired the power to blow himself off the face of the earth by the push of a button, he still thinks about his own memory processes in terms readily translatable into ancient Greek. (Tulving & Madigan, 1970, p. 437)

Near the end of the 1970s, Neisser (chap. 4 in this volume; 1978) expressed many of the same sentiments. He argued that

. . . the results of a hundred years of the psychological study of memory are somewhat discouraging. We have established firm empirical generalizations, but most of them are so obvious that every ten-year-old knows them anyway. We have made discoveries, but they are only marginally about memory; in many cases we don't know what to do with them, and wear them out with endless experimental variations. We have an intellectually impressive group of theories, but history offers little confidence that they will provide any meaningful insight into natural behavior.

My own interests have centered on the development of memory, and this work, too, has received some strong criticism. Ann Brown (1982), for example, argued that the prototype theory [of memory development] is open to the criticism that it is trivial. One reason it is open to this criticism is that the average child on the street would come up with a description very similar to the prototype.

Of course, the critics exaggerate; there are some success stories associated with the Ebbinghaus tradition of memory, successes in the sense that the research has allowed us to understand important memory phenomena that could not be explained by Aristotle or American 10-year-olds. Many of these successes were described in articles appearing in 1985 in the issue of the *Journal of Experimental Psychology: Learning, Memory, and Cognition* honoring the centennial of the publication of Ebbinghaus' *Memory: A contribution to experimental psychology.*

I want to describe another contribution of this tradition, one that may not be well recognized by experimental psychologists or social psychologists who study memory. Specifically, research in the Ebbinghaus tradition has been particularly useful in understanding how memory development goes awry. In capsule, my argument is simply that several fundamental distinctions associated with the Ebbinghaus tradition of memory research are useful in allowing us to determine the nature of memory deficit in various groups of handicapped individuals, and that, furthermore, they can be used to suggest possible ways to remediate memory.

Of course, in arguing for this contribution, I am not claiming that memory research should be exclusively the province of the Ebbinghaus tradition. The claim is simply that the Ebbinghaus tradition remains one of many legitimate ways to probe human memory and deficits therein.

Memory Deficits in Retarded Individuals

Probably the best known success story in which basic distinctions from modern memory theory have been used to isolate and remediate a memory deficit involves research on memory in retarded individuals. Memory deficits are commonly associated with mental retardation. Probably the first modern explanation for these deficits was Ellis' (1963) hypothesis that memory traces decay more rapidly in retarded than in nonretarded persons. If rate of decay is more rapid in retarded individuals, memory deficits should become more pronounced as the retention interval increases. Considerable effort was devoted to this hypothesis in the 1960s. In fact, the predicted pattern of results was not found often. Furthermore, when it was found, it seemed to be an artifact of group differences in acquisition. Retarded children seemed to be less able to learn materials to criterion, thereby leading to more rapid loss.

This phenomenon of differential acquisition actually contained the seed of the next theory of memory deficit in retarded persons. In the late 1960s, at about the time that the trace decay theory was falling on hard times,

Atkinson and Shiffrin (1968) proposed their influential theory of memory in which they distinguished control processes from structural features. In the late 1960s and early 1970s many developmental psychologists used this distinction to organize their efforts to understand the development of memory (Hagen, Jongeward & Kail, 1975). It became clear that developmental change was pronounced in Atkinson and Shiffrin's control processes, which constitute the strategic component of memory. In particular, it was proposed that preschool children and early elementary school children were unlikely to use strategies to improve their performance on memory tasks. On tasks in which the performance was less dependent upon such deliberate mnemonics, age differences were smaller and sometimes nonexistent.

This same distinction was also applied to research on memory in retarded children (Kail, 1984). It was claimed that the structural features of memory are unimpaired in individuals with cultural-familial forms of mental retardation. Their memory deficits were thought to reflect the strategic aspects of memory. This new hypothesis prompted a flurry of studies designed to show that retarded and nonretarded children differ in the likelihood and success with which they use mnemonic strategies. These investigations were fruitful, as it is now accepted that one basis for memory deficits in the educable mentally retarded is their failure to use memory strategies appropriately. That is, mentally retarded children do not seem to engage in the sort of planful, deliberate memory behavior that is typical of adults and older children.

The final part of this success story involves remediation. If memory strategies represent the source of memory deficits, those deficits should be eliminated if retarded individuals could be trained to use memory strategies. This turns out to be the case, although we are still trying to identify the precise conditions necessary to ensure that the newly acquired strategy is maintained following training and is transferred to approriate novel memory tasks.

Word-Finding Deficits Defined

In this chapter, I want to describe another instance in the literature that may represent a success of this sort. This is work that I have done in collaboration with a speech pathologist, Laurence Leonard, on language-impaired children. These children commonly have problems in "word finding." Such difficulties are often first suspected on the basis of particular behaviors exhibited during conversation: frequent and pronounced hestitations, circumlocution, the use of fillers such as *uh* and *let's see,* and the overuse of such indefinite terms as *stuff* and *thing.*

Word-finding difficulties are often measured with structured naming tasks, in which language-impaired children typically commit a greater number of errors and show longer naming latencies than their peers with normally developing language. For example, Wiig, Semel, and Nystrom (1982) found that language-impaired 8-year-olds made more errors on naming tasks involving pictured objects and colored shapes than did age-matched controls. The differences occurred even though all children, when given a name, could select the correct picture and could produce the correct name in delayed imitation of the investigator. Furthermore, even when impaired children name a picture correctly, they typically will take longer to do so than their peers. For example, Anderson (1965) found that language-impaired 8-year-olds named line drawings of common objects more slowly than did a group of age-matched normal children.

Using the term *word-finding deficit* to describe these problems implies that the child's difficulty rests specifically with accessing or retrieving a word that is present in memory. Indeed, the disorder has often been described as a "lexical look-up" problem (Menyuk, 1978) and as a problem involving "delayed speed of word retrieval" (Schwartz & Solot, 1980). Retrieval problems have been assumed because the words with which the child has difficulty are seemingly understood on comprehension measures and are often produced correctly, although not effortlessly, on naming tasks.

There are, however, other plausible explanations of word-finding problems. Consider, for example, the extent of language-impaired children's knowledge of words. In the modal theory of semantic memory, words vary in the elaborateness with which they are represented. Familiar words may be linked to many other nodes in memory by strong associations; less familiar words may have fewer and generally weaker links. The presence of many strong links is used to explain why retrieval is more rapid for better known words (Milianti & Cullinan, 1974). This in turn could explain why children's naming times decrease with increasing age (Denckla & Rudel, 1974): Compared with older children and adults, younger children may well have both fewer and generally weaker associations in semantic memory. In like manner, children with word-finding problems may name pictures more slowly because words are stored in a less elaborate manner. Word-finding problems would be by-products of the fact that impaired children's language develops more slowly and less elaborately than the norm. In other words, for language-impaired children, *all* retrieval is retrieval of relatively unfamiliar words.

Determination of whether word-finding problems represent a distinct disorder or are simply products of delayed language learning is important for applied as well as theoretical reasons. Word-finding problems related to inadequate or inappropriate retrieval strategies would presumably require instruction in the formulation and use of strategies for retrieving words that may be adequately represented in memory. In contrast, word-finding problems stemming from limited lexical knowledge would probably require instruction aimed at providing a richer base of information concerning a word's meaning, its semantic relations with other words, and its syntactic privileges of occurrence. Knowing the source of word-finding problems in language-impaired children would allow us to specify the more appropriate of two general approaches to remediation.

In the remainder of this chapter, I describe our efforts to discriminate these two explanations. We began by identifying several paradigms traditionally associated with the psychology of memory that could be used to discriminate specific retrieval deficits from less elaborated lexical knowledge. However, before proceeding to the tasks, let me describe the subjects of interest.

We tested 76 6- to 13-year-old language-impaired children who were enrolled in learning disability classrooms or in classrooms for communicatively disordered children. All had been diagnosed as language impaired by school personnel. All of the children had performance IQs of at least 85 on the WISC-R, but had composite language ages (reflecting comprehension and production abilities) at least 1 year below their chronological age.

There were also two control groups. Each of the children in these groups had a performance IQ of 85 or above on the WISC-R and had composite language ages that were at least equal to their chronological age. Half of the control children were matched to the language-impaired children by chronological age. The performance of children in this age-control group constituted the primary reference point for evaluating the performance of language-impaired children. We also tested children who were matched to language-impaired children by language age. Generally, comparisons involving these language controls were not particularly illuminating, and I will not discuss them further.

The first experiment I want to describe essentially represented an effort to determine if we could see, in the laboratory, the phenomenon itself. That is, could we see the delayed naming that clinicians observe in spontaneous conversation and on naming tasks? More important, could these word-finding deficits be seen on tasks that would allow us to begin to separate the retrieval component of performance from other components?

To answer these questions, we used a task introduced by Posner and Mitchell (1967) in which pairs of stimuli are presented. Some pairs consist of stimuli that are identical physically and in name. Others are physically dissimilar but have the same name. Still others differ physically and in name. With adults as subjects, judgments of physical similarity are approximately 75 ms more rapid than are judgments of name similarity. This difference is traditionally interpreted as representing the additional amount of time needed to retrieve letter names from memory, that is, beyond the time required to judge perceptual similarity.

The time to retrieve name information from memory, as measured in the Posner and Mitchell (1967) paradigm, declines systematically with age. For example, Bisanz, Danner, and Resnick (1979) presented pairs of familiar objects to 8-, 10-, 12-, and 19-year-olds. On some trials subjects judged if the objects were alike physically; on other trials they judged if the objects were alike in name. The difference in the time needed for these judgments was 122 ms for 8-year-olds, 191 ms for 10-year-olds, 98 ms for 12-year-olds, and 80 ms for 19-year-olds.

We (Kail & Leonard, 1986, exper. 3) tested 26 language-impaired children and their age controls on procedures similar to those used by Bisanz and colleagues. On 48 trials, subjects judged if pairs of common objects were identical physically; on 48 other trials, they judged if similar pairs were identical in name. As expected, the difference between name matching and perceptual matching was greater for language-impaired children than for children in the age-control group. In other words, apparently the language-impaired children were systematically slower in their retrieval of these object names.

Also informative are children's judgments of physical similarity. During matching on the basis of physical similarity, two types of stimuli lead to "no" responses. Some stimuli differ physically and in name. Others differ physically but have a common name. Both pairs differ according to the criterion of physical similarity, yet older children and adolescents often respond more slowly on the latter pairs. The common name in the latter pairs, though irrelevant to the matching criterion, slows the judgment that the stimuli differ physically. This interference was significant for children in our age-control group: Judgments of perceptual similarity were 70 ms slower for this group when the stimuli had a common name compared with pairs in which the names differed. For language-impaired children, the difference was not significantly different from zero and was backward from the expected direction. Irrelevant name information seems to interfere with age-control children's judgments of physical similarity but not with language-impaired children's judgments.

Thus, in terms of two measures, language-impaired children's performance was poorer than that of their age mates with normal language. This outcome is probably not particularly compelling to advocates of ecological approaches to memory. In using Posner's task, we had taken the word-finding problem out of its natural language context. Perhaps the results would differ if word-finding were studied in the course of such real-world language tasks as conversation or reading. In fact, it is well established that adults use relevant context in many cognitive tasks. More than 50 years ago, Carmichael, Hogan, and Walter (1932) showed that memory for a stimulus was distorted by the context in which the stimulus was presented. In the ensuing 50 years, and particularly in the last 10 to 15 years, the impact of context—both positive and negative—has been shown for lexical decision making, reading, recall, comprehension, and picture naming. For example, adults can read a word more rapidly if it follows a relevant context (such as a sentence) than if it follows a neutral context (e.g., Stanovich & West, 1981).

In the developmental literature, the typical and somewhat surprising result is that context effects are actually larger for younger individuals than for older ones. An outcome from an experiment by Schwantes (1985) is illustrative. In part of his experiment, Schwantes compared vocalization times for words presented in isolation to vocalization times for the same words when they completed a sentence. An example of the manipulation would be "Out in the rain he got cold and" as a context for the word "wet." As shown in Table 9.1, children and adults read words faster when the context was present. Furthermore, this effect was larger for children than for adults, whether the magnitude of the effect was measured in absolute time or in terms of percentage decrease in naming time relative to the no context condition.

One compelling explanation of contextual facilitation generally and its greater facilitation in younger individuals is the interactive-compensatory model of reading proposed by Stanovich and West (1981,1983). They argued that context effects of the sort discussed here stem from two sources: rapid, automatic spread of activation in semantic memory and slower activation that reflects the subject's conscious expectancies of what may follow. Any variable that slows word recognition allows more time for a subject's expectancies to influence performance. This line of reasoning is used to explain the fact that, for adults, context effects in word recognition are larger when words are degraded. Much the same argument applies to developmental work: Younger children are slower to recognize words, which allows more time for the (relatively slow) formation of expectancies.

Of course, the same logic could be applied to language-impaired children in a naming task: Retrieval of the name of a picture is slower for impaired children than for age controls, which allows more time for context effects to operate. Thus, the prediction is for a significant interaction, in which naming times are faster following an appropriate context, particularly for impaired children.

We (Kail & Leonard, 1986, exper. 6) evaluated this prediction by asking language-impaired children and their age controls to name pictures in each of three conditions that differed in the degree of contextual support they afforded. In one condition, presentation of a picture was

TABLE 9.1. Mean vocalization times (in ms) for words in isolation or in context.[a]

	No context	Context	Decrease in time MS	%
8-year-olds	825	650	175	21
19-year-olds	611	517	94	15

[1] From Schwantes, 1985.

preceded by a list of unrelated words. In another, the picture was an appropriate completion for a sentence. In the last, the picture again completed a sentence, but the sentence itself was embedded in a story context. Thus, in the first condition children had no basis for expecting a particular picture. In the sentence condition, children could benefit from syntactic privileges of occurrence and clues from the semantic features of the major constituents of the sentence. In the story condition, syntactic and semantic clues in the sentence were supplemented by additional story information that further constrained the range of appropriate pictures.

In each of the three conditions, 20 language-impaired children and 20 age controls named 20 pictures. As shown in Figure 9.1, both sentences and story contexts facilitated picture naming. The language-impaired children seemed to benefit more from the presence of context. Compared with the no context condition, language-impaired children named pictures 120 ms more rapidly following a sentence context and 150 ms more rapidly following the story context. Corresponding figures for age-control children were 50 and 80 ms. In fact, the interaction was not statistically reliable. What we can say, however, is that the deficits seen in the first study are not simply by-products of the fact that we forced children to perform language tasks in an environment that deprived them of their usual language aids.

Bases of Word-Finding Deficits

In the remaining experiments, our aim was to focus more directly on the contrast between the elaboration and retrieval explanations of word-finding deficits. That is, having determined that word-finding deficits could be seen in the laboratory, we wanted to examine whether the

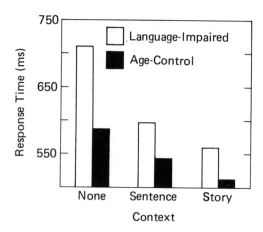

FIGURE 9.1. Mean response time as a function of context condition, separately for language-impaired and age-control children. From Kail & Leonard, 1986.

deficits were chiefly due to generally delayed language acquisition of the impaired children or involved specific retrieval deficits. We tested children on a number of tasks that allowed us to separate the retrieval components of performance from the elaborative or representational components. We also chose tasks according to two other criteria. First, we tried to select paradigms that had been used previously in developmental work, so that we had some expectations of the patterns of performance to be expected for unimpaired children. Second, we chose tasks so that, collectively, they would represent a reasonably wide range of retrieval demands.

Let me begin by describing an experiment in which we used Sternberg's (1966) well-known memory-scanning paradigm. Here subjects are asked to remember subspan sets of stimuli. Immediately thereafter, a probe stimulus is presented and subjects judge, as rapidly as possible, if the probe was a member of the memory set. Typically response time increases linearly as a function of the number of stimuli in the memory set, a result that has often been interpreted as meaning that the probe stimulus is compared serially with each member of the memory set. The slope of this function is used to estimate the time needed to retrieve each member of the memory set and compare it with the probe. The intercept provides an estimate of the time needed to encode the probe digit and respond.

We chose the Sternberg paradigm because it met the criteria described already and also because we thought it might be particularly sensitive to retrieval problems that might not be detected with measures of recognition or recall. That is, suppose that language-impaired children suffer retrieval problems much more frequently than even clinicians suspect. Retrieval by language-impaired children could be consistently slower than for their peers, but the deficits are detected only when the process is quite slow or breaks down completely. The Sternberg paradigm, in which memory scanning is typically on the order of 25 to 40 ms per digit, should be sufficiently sensitive to detect such small-scale but systematic deficits.

In the version of the Sternberg task that we (Kail & Leonard, 1986, exper. 2) used, the memory set consisted of two, four, and six pictures of familiar objects. Subjects were allowed to study the card for approximately 5 s. Twelve test trials followed in which individual pictures were shown and subjects judged if the picture had been a member of the immediately preceding memory set. Of the 12 test trials, 6 were of pictures from the memory set and 6 were of pictures not included in the memory set. Each child received 12 different memory sets, 4 at each of the three set sizes, yielding a total of 144 trials.

The reaction time data are shown in Table 9.2. As expected, reaction times increased systematically as a function of set size. Of particular interest is the fact that the slope of this function is virtually identical for language-impaired children and their age controls. That is, language-

TABLE 9.2. Mean response times in memory search experiment.

| | Mean response time (ms) according to set size[a] | | | | |
Group	2	4	6	Slope	Intercept
Language-impaired	1126	1207	1226	27	1080
Age-control	948	994	1052	26	894

[a] A "memory set" consisted of two, four, or six pictures.

impaired and age-control children apparently were comparable in their ability to retrieve members of the memory set and compare them with the probe. In contrast, there were group differences in the intercept of the memory set function; overall, response times for language-impaired children were nearly 200 ms slower. This difference could reflect slower encoding of the probe, slower motor times, or both. The important result, however, is that in a task in which speed of retrieval is the key element, language-impaired children performed at exactly the same rate as their peers. Impaired children in fact do not suffer from a systematic but subtle retrieval deficit that is detectable with the Sternberg task.

In another experiment the retrieval demands were of a different sort. We used a free recall paradigm, one in which the focus is on accuracy rather than speed of retrieval. The specific variant of free recall that we used, a repeated free recall task developed by Wilkinson, DeMarinis, and Riley (1983), was chosen because storage and retrieval components of performance can be separated. A list of words is presented to children. Following presentation of the last word in the list, the child is asked to recall the words. When the child is unable to recall additional words, the child performs a distracting task briefly. Then the child is asked to recall, once again, all of the words in the list—those that had been recalled previously and any additional words. After the child completes recall, the procedure is repeated one more time, yielding one presentation of the list but three recall attempts.

The rationale behind this task is as follows. Suppose one child recalls only half of the words in the list on the first attempt, and retrieves exactly those same words on the second and third attempts. Suppose another child recalls all of the words on the first attempt, half of the list on the second, and a third of the list on the last attempt. The first child apparently stored fewer words initially, but was quite consistent in retrieving items thereafter. The second child apparently stored more items initially but was less able to retrieve them consistently on subsequent occasions.

To be more specific, in this task a word can be either recalled or forgotten on each of three recall attempts, resulting in eight possible recall patterns. Typically, most words are consistently recalled or consistently forgotten. Other words, however, are recalled on some attempts but not others. To account for these various patterns of recall, Wilkinson and colleagues (1983) proposed a strengthen-and-discard model of repeated free recall that involves three processes: (a) *Naming-storage* refers to the processes whereby a presented item is identifed and tagged in memory as a member of the list to be recalled. (b) *Retrieval* of a word on one trial strengthens the association between that word and the list, thereby increasing the likelihood that the word will be recalled on a subsequent trial. (c) In complementary fashion, *forgetting* of a word on one trial decreases the strength of the association between the word and the list, thereby decreasing the probability of its recall on subsequent trials.

According to the strengthen-and-discard model, presentation of a given word will result in successful storage with probability s. The probability of successful retrieval on the first attempt is given as r_0, where the subscript indicates the number of previous retrievals. Such an item will be recalled on the first attempt with probability sr_0. Let us further define r_1 and r_2 as the probabilities of successful retrieval on the second and third attempts, respectively, given successful retrieval on the first and second attempts, respectively. Hence, the likelihood that an item will be recalled on all three attempts is simply $sr_0r_1r_2$.

Probabilities for the remaining seven recall patterns are shown in Table 9.3. Consider, for example, the probability that a word is never recalled, that is, pattern FFF. This can occur in two ways. First, the item may not be stored successfully, with probability $1 - s$. Alternatively, the word may be stored, but the initial attempt at retrieval is unsuccessful. Because the word was forgotten on the first attempt, the associative link is weakened, such that the word will be forgotten with probability f_1 on the second recall attempt and f_2 on the third attempt. That is, f_1 denotes the probability of forgetting given that an item was not retrieved on the immediately preceding trial; f_2 denotes the probability of forgetting given nonretrieval on the two immediately preceding trials.

TABLE 9.3. Probabilities of recall patterns for the strengthen-and-discard model. From Kail et al., 1984.

Pattern[a]	Probability
RRR	$s\,r_0\,r_1\,r_2$
RRF	$s\,r_0\,r_1\,(1 - r_2)$
RFR	$s\,r_0\,(1 - r_1)\,(1 - f_1)$
RFF	$s\,r_0\,(1 - r_1)\,f_1$
FRR	$s\,(1 - r_0)\,(1 - f_1)\,r_1$
FRF	$s\,(1 - r_0)\,(1 - f_1)\,(1 - r_1)$
FFR	$s\,(1 - r_0)\,f_1\,(1 - f_2)$
FFF	$s\,(1 - r_0)\,f_1 f_2 + (1 - s)$

[a] R and F indicate recall or forgetting, respectively, of a word during repeated free recall. Parameters are defined in the test.

Wilkinson and colleagues (1983) tested 10-, 12-, and 14-year-olds on the repeated free recall task. The key result was that age differences in performance were localized in the storage parameter, s. That is, adolescents were more likely than children to store a word initially. However, given that a word was stored successfully, subjects at all ages were equally likely to retrieve the word, and, furthermore, the impact of forgetting on subsequent recall was age invariant.

We (Kail, Hale, Leonard, & Nippold, 1984) tested 20 language-impaired children and their age controls on the repeated free recall procedure. A list of 16 words was presented, followed by three recall attempts separated by 20 s of counting backward. Frequencies of different recall patterns are shown in Table 9.4. Patterns RRR and FFF are far and away the most common. Language-impaired children were much less likely than age controls to recall a word on all three attempts, and much more likely to forget a word on all three attempts. To account for these patterns, we first fitted the recall data to a version of the model in which we assumed that values for all six model parameters differed for language-impaired children and their peers. This model was consistent with the data. The problem here is that the model includes 12 free parameters and is not a parsimonious description of data that contain only 14 degrees of freedom.

To generate a more parsimonious account of the data, we created versions of the strengthen-and-discard model in which some parameters were assumed to be the same for the two groups, but others differed. For example, in a model corresponding to the assumption that differences in performance were localized in retrieval, the r parameters were free to vary across groups but s and f were not. Another model embodied the complementary assumption that performance differences were localized in storage; here only s was allowed to vary across groups. Neither of these models was consistent with the data. That is, estimated values of

TABLE 9.4. Frequency of different patterns of repeated free recall. From Kail et al., 1984.

| Pattern[a] | Frequency of recall | |
	Language-impaired	Age controls
RRR	79	135
RRF	8	4
RFR	7	7
RFF	23	12
FRR	3	11
FRF	3	0
FFR	4	5
FFF	193	146

[a] R and F indicate recall or forgetting, respectively, of a word during repeated free recall. Thus, RRR indicates a word recalled on each of three attempts.

TABLE 9.5. Estimated values of parameters.
From Kail et al., 1984.

Parameter[a]	Language-impaired children	Age controls
s	0.43	0.59
r_0	0.85	0.84
r_1	0.73	0.89
r_2	0.91	0.97
f_1	0.71	0.71
f_2	0.80	0.80

[a] Parameters are defined in the text.

the frequencies of the different patterns of recall generated from the parameter estimates differed consistently from those in Table 9.4.

A third model that we considered was one in which the s parameter was free to vary across groups, as were the r parameters. Only the f's were fixed. This model was consistent with the data. Furthermore, this model fit the data as well as the original "full" version of the model. As can be seen in Table 9.5, age-control children were more likely to store words than were language-impaired children. In addition, given that a word was stored successfully, language-impaired children were less likely than normal children to retrieve it successfully.

Group differences in the storage parameter are readily interpretable in terms of differences in the elaborateness of lexical representations in memory. For language-impaired children, lexical representations are less elaborate, which can be used to explain why words are less likely to be tagged as list members. Group differences in the retrieval parameter are not as straightforward. One possibility is that language-impaired children use less efficient retrieval algorithms, the natures of which are left unspecified by these procedures. Another possibility is that their retrieval algorithms may be the same qualitatively as that of the age controls, but these algorithms yield less when operating on relatively unelaborated lexical representations. I prefer this latter interpretation simply because it allows us to wrap up all of the parameter differences with a single explanation.

A final experiment complemented the others. In the previous experiments, the target of retrieval was an explicit item or set of items. Such explicit targets probably characterize much extralaboratory retrieval. Reading comprehension, for example, depends in part on retrieval of meanings for specific words. At the same time, the target of children's recall is defined less precisely in many extralaboratory experiences. Consider, for example, deciding who to invite to a birthday party or what to do after school. In both cases the retrieval target is a class of items rather than specifically designated exemplars. Furthermore, the number of potentially appropriate exemplars may be quite large.

Evidence regarding retrieval of this sort of information comes principally from the free emission paradigm devised by Bousfield and Sedgewick (1944), in which an individual simply names, over several minutes, as many members of a large category, such as animals, as he or she can. In this procedure, individuals typically retrieve several items, pause, then retrieve more items. The general interpretation of this phenomenon is that information in semantic memory is organized as clusters of related items. Pauses in the retrieval protocol reflect search for such clusters; when a cluster is found, the items are emitted in close succession.

In our work (Kail & Leonard, 1986, exper. 4), we tested samples of language-impaired and age-control children in the free emission paradigm, asking them to recall as many animals, pieces of furniture, or occupations as possible in a 5-minute interval. The mean number of words retrieved is shown in Table 9.6. In three of the four categories, age-control children retrieved 5 to 10% more words than did the language-impaired children, but these differences are not reliable. Of course, in a task like this, the mean number of words retrieved over several minutes is a gross and potentially misleading measure. More informative are two supplementary analyses. First, we grouped the words in the retrieval protocol into clusters. The procedures used were too lengthy to be described here, but they were based on two assumptions: first, that the distribution of pause times—times between successive retrievals—includes pauses associated with retrieval of new clusters and pauses associated with the rapid emission of words from the same cluster, and second, that the mean pause time for retrieval of a new cluster is greater than the mean time associated with emission of successive items from the same cluster.

These procedures were applied with equal success to the retrieval protocols of language-impaired and age-control children. For both groups, pauses of less than 5 or 6 s signified retrieval of items within

TABLE 9.6. Characteristics of unconstrained free recall.

	Number of words	Number of clusters	Cluster size
Sample 1			
Animals			
Language-impaired	30.93	13.38	2.37
Age controls	32.73	13.62	2.65
Furniture			
Language-impaired	20.09	13.74	1.67
Age-controls	22.18	12.94	1.80
Sample 2			
Animals			
Language-impaired	33.46	19.4	2.11
Age controls	31.91	17.4	2.04
Occupations			
Language-impaired	23.80	17.6	1.58
Age controls	26.40	16.5	1.82

clusters; longer pauses, retrieval of new clusters. Segregating words with this criterion, we determined that impaired and unimpaired children recalled the same number of clusters. Language-impaired children's clusters were slightly smaller, but the difference was not reliable.

A potential shortcoming in these analyses is that they ignore qualitative differences in the items retrieved. In fact, most children would begin retrieval with prototypic category members like dog or cat, then mention familiar but not prototypic instances such as sheep or rat and, as time progressed, retrieve more obscure members, such as chameleon. To analyze this characteristic of retrieval formerly, we had adults rate all of the retrieved words on a 4-point scale in which 4 corresponded to a prototypic category member and 1 was a nonmember. For both impaired and unimpaired children, typicality declined over successive minutes of retrieval, most rapidly for furniture and least rapidly for animals. However, only for occupations did the groups differ: The mean rated typicality was approximately 3 for children in the age-control group, meaning that these items were definitely category members, but not prototypic ones. Mean rated typicality was 2.5 for language-impaired children, which meant that the words were halfway between the nonprototypic category members and border line members.

What is striking about these results is the absence of group differences in performance. Language-impaired children retrieve many of the same category members as their peers and do so in much the same manner as their peers. In short, in this experiment, like the others that I have described in this chapter, we find no consistent evidence of pervasive deficits in performance that can be linked explicitly to retrieval processes. To the contrary, in these experiments as well as in others that Leonard and I have done (e.g., Leonard, Nippold, Kail, & Hale, 1983), language-impaired children's retrieval is usually similar to that of age-control children. Thus, we see little evidence to suggest language-impaired children's word-finding problems must be attributable to some specific retrieval deficit. Instead, our results seem to demonstrate that these problems are simply one more manifestation of the fact that language-impaired children learn words more slowly than their peers with normal language, which makes many words less accessible to retrieval algorithms that function normally. More specifically, we assume that semantic memory is qualitatively similar for language-impaired children and age-control children, consisting of many of the same entries organized in fundamentally the same way. However, we suggest that this knowledge is, quite simply, less elaborate in language-impaired children, consisting of fewer and weaker leaks between entries in semantic memory.

This explanation, however straightforward it may seem after the fact, was not obvious at the outset. Recall that the prevailing view among professionals dealing with these children is that word-finding problems represents a disorder distinct from delayed language acquisition, that they reflect inefficient or inappropriate retrieval processes, and that the best hope for remediation lies in training retrieval skill. To evaluate this view, we began with the basic distinction between storage and retrieval of information, a distinction that has a long history in the verbal learning tradition. We instantiated this distinction in a number of different experimental paradigms, with the results converging on the same conclusion. The conclusion is nontrivial in the sense that it is exactly opposite the explanation offered by the speech pathologists. It is relevant in the that we can help to specify appropriate contents of therapeutic programs for these children.

Acknowledgment. The research described in this chapter was supported by NINCDS grant 17663. I wish to acknowledge the important contributions to this work of my collaborator, Laurence B. Leonard.

References

Anderson, J.D. (1965). Initiatory delay in congenital aphasoid conditions. *Cerebral Palsy Journal, 26,* 9–12.

Atkinson, R.C., & Shiffrin, R.M. (1968). Human memory: A proposed system and its control processes. In K.W. Spence & J.T. Spence (Eds.), *The psychology of learning and motivation* (Vol. 2). New York: Academic Press.

Bisanz, J., Danner, F.W., & Resnick, L.B. (1979). Changes with age in measures of processing efficiency. *Child Development, 50,* 132–141.

Bousfield, W.A., & Sedgewick, H.W. (1944). An analysis of sequences of restricted associative responses. *Journal of General Psychology, 30,* 149–165.

Brown, A.L. (1982). Learning and development: The problem of compatibility, access, and induction. *Human Development, 25,* 89–115.

Carmichael, L., Hogan, H.P., & Walter, A. (1932). An experimental study of the effect of language on the reproduction of visually perceived form. *Journal of Experimental Psychology, 15,* 73–86.

Denckla, M. & Rudel, R. (1974). Rapid "automatized" naming of pictured objects, colors, letters, and numbers of normal children. *Cortex, 10,* 186–202.

Ellis, N.R. (1963). The stimulus trace and behavioral inadequacy. in N.R. Ellis (Ed.), *Handbook of mental deficiency.* New York: McGraw-Hill.

Hagen, J.W., Jongeward, R.H., & Kail, R.V. (1975). Cognitive perspectives on the development of memory. In H.W. Reese (Ed.), *Advances in child development and behavior* (Vol. 10). New York: Academic Press.

Kail, R. (1984). *The development of memory in children.* (2nd. ed.). New York: W.H. Freeman.

Kail, R., Hale, C.A., Leonard, L.B., & Nippold, M.A. (1984). Lexical storage and retrieval in language-impaired children. *Applied Psycholinguistics, 5,* 37–49.

Kail, R., & Leonard, L.B. (1986). Word-finding abilities in language-impaired children. *ASHA Monographs,* No. 25.

Leonard, L.B., Nippold, M.A., Kail, R., & Hale, C.A. (1983). Picture naming in language-impaired children. *Journal of Speech and Hearing Research, 26,* 609–615.

Menyuk, P. (1978). Linguistic problems in children with developmental dysphasia. In M. Wyke (Ed.), *Developmental dysphasia*. London: Academic Press.

Milanti, F., & Cullinan, W. (1974). Effects of age and word frequency in object recognition and naming in children. *Journal of Speech and Hearing Research, 17*, 373–385.

Neisser, U. (1978). Memory: What are the important questions? In M.M. Gruneberg, P.E. Morris, & R.N. Sykes (Eds.), *Practical aspects of memory*. London: Academic Press.

Posner, M.I., & Mitchell, R.F. (1967). Chronometric analysis of classification. *Psychological Review, 74*, 392–409.

Schwantes, F.M. (1985). Expectancy, integration, and interactional processes: Age differences in the nature of words affected by sentence context. *Journal of Experimental Child Psychology, 39*, 212–229.

Schwartz, E., & Solot, C. (1980). Response patterns characteristic of verbal expressive disorders. *Language, Speech, and Hearing Services in the Schools, 11*, 139–144.

Stanovich, K.E., & West, R.F. (1981). The effect of sentence context on ongoing word recognition: Tests of a two-process theory. *Journal of Experimental Psychology: Human Perception and Performance, 7*, 658–672.

Stanovich, K.E., & West, R.F. (1983). On priming by a sentence context. *Journal of Experimental Psychology: General, 112*, 1–36.

Sternberg, S. (1966). High-speed scanning in human memory. *Science, 153*, 652–654.

Tulving, E., & Madigan, S.A. (1970). Memory and verbal learning. *Annual Review of Psychology, 21*, 437–484.

Wigg, E., Semel, E., & Nystrom, L. (1982). Comparison of rapid naming abilities in language-learning-disabled and academically achieving eight-year-olds. *Language, Speech, and Hearing Services in the Schools, 13*, 11–23.

Wilkinson, A.C., DeMarinis, M., & Riley, S.J. (1983). Developmental and individual differences in rapid remembering. *Child Development, 54*, 898–911.

Part IV   Perspectives from Social Psychology

CHAPTER 10

Three Catechisms for Social Memory

Thomas M. Ostrom

All human existence is social. Life for the individual starts off dyadically, regardless of whether the beginning is marked at the moment of conception or at the time of birth, and increases in social complexity over the entire life course. Since earliest times, physical and emotional needs have been met through social exchanges. It is reasonable to assume, then, that the human cognitive system has evolved to accommodate this social reality. Memory structures and mechanisms, along with their neurological substrata, must be capable of dealing with (as well as drawing upon) the social agents in their environment.

This point has been made by a number of authors, including two of the contributors to this volume (Nelson, 1981; Ostrom, 1984). But it has not been taken very seriously by most cognitive psychologists who study memory. For most of them, the basic theoretical issues remain the same for a person stimulus (e.g., one's mother) as for a nonperson stimulus (e.g., a teacup). Or in the more complicated case of text comprehension, no important differences are seen between understanding a story about a boulder rolling down a hill and a story about a man committing murder. From this perspective, there is little reason to regard the study of social memory as anything special. This chapter disputes that conclusion. It shows that many new fundamental questions arise when the social context of memory is examined closely.

Most of the existing work on social memory has been conducted by developmental and social psychologists. Unfortunately, not a great deal of research has yet accumulated on this problem; the chapters in this book that were prepared by developmental and social psychologists cover a substantial portion of the advances to date.

The field of social memory is still trying to identify its major questions. Most current researchers have adopted the strategy of selecting a narrowly defined problem they find interesting and tractable, and devoting their energies to advancing our understanding of that set of issues. Their work provides exemplars, but doesn't yet adequately represent the entire domain of issues relevant to social memory. It is difficult, therefore, for researchers working on different problems to identify how their work fits into the mosaic of social memory or what makes their work uniquely informative. The present set of catechisms should enable social memory researchers to better understand their place in the sun.

In addition to cognitive psychologists and social memory researchers, there is a third readership to whom this chapter is addressed. There are persons just becoming interested in the study of memory, whether they be students formally enrolled in a course or researchers in allied fields (such as the other cognitive sciences), who seek an overview of the role of memory in human behavior. Most treatments of memory focus on how cognitive systems deal with narrow laboratory tasks. Reading such reports provides only a few hints about the role of memory in complicated social contexts. This chapter offers the nontechnical reader a more comprehensive perspective regarding the rich and diverse character of memory.

A trinity of catechisms is presented. The catechisms are intended not as statements of religious orthodoxy, but rather as glimpses at what lies before us. We are like explorers of a new planet who in their first weeks have spent one part of their time testing some explicit ideas (e.g., about rock formations and biological life forms) and another part of their time musing about the unknowns yet to be studied. Both activities raise new questions and offer some guidance for future exploration. Yet we know that in the future those questions inevitably will change as new facts are accumulated and current horizons are passed. The present catechisms must be regarded in the same way. They are the questions that seem most pressing at this early stage in the exploration of social memory.

The First Catechism: Social Stimuli

The first catechism deals with questions about the nature of the stimuli in our social world, and how those stimuli are represented cognitively. The concept of the stimulus has made great strides since the early research in psychophysics and learning theory. In most psychophysical research, for example, the stimulus was an undifferentiated event that was varied experimentally on one dimension alone. The weight of an object or intensity of a light was the theoretical focus, and the cognitive representations of these stimuli were usually in the form of a point on a subjective continuum. Thurstone made this assumption explicit and referred to mental representations as "discriminal processes" when outlining his law of comparative judgment (Thurstone, 1927).

Both cognitive and social psychologists have come to realize that people go far beyond such primitive representations. Social psychologists, especially those in the field of social cognition, have widely adopted the term *schema* as a generic label for the complex cognitive representation evoked by social stimuli. For example, Fiske and Taylor (1984) identified four kinds of schema (person, self, role, and event), emphasizing that the key difference among them is one of content. The labels of the four designate the domain of content to which each applies. However, the four were not viewed as differing in terms of their influence on such cognitive activities as the perception of incoming information, retrieval of stored information, and generation of inferences.

In contrast to this undifferentiated view of schemas, there is considerable work in cognitive psychology on identifying different forms of cognitive representation that are used for different classes of stimuli (e.g., Anderson, 1985; Wyer & Gordon, 1984). A variety of structures have been identified, such as images (e.g., geometric forms), linear orderings (e.g., a sequence of consonants from the alphabet), hierarchies of propositions (e.g., *Airedale is a dog* and *dog is an animal*), scripts (e.g., restaurant dining consists of the scenes: entering, ordering, eating, and exiting), and if–then production units (e.g., if the traffic light is green, then proceed through the intersection). It is clear, then, that the more primitive, undifferentiated view of schema will not capture the diversity of structures potentially available to the perceiver in social settings. The first catechism for social memory concerns the forms of representation that exist for different social spheres.

Question I. *Are traits and behaviors represented differently?* .
Nearly all existing research in person memory has employed either traits or behaviors as stimulus items. It could be argued that presenting a trait (e.g., cruel) spontaneously evokes one or more behavioral exemplars (e.g., kicked the old lady). Similarly, presenting a behavior may activate its corresponding trait category. If this were true, then presenting either would activate comparable trait-exemplar structures in memory.

Alternatively, the two types of stimulus items may lead to very different representations. Traits will usually be processed in the context of semantic memory, and consequently should activate semantically similar traits (e.g., *cruel* may activate *vicious* and *sadistic*). No behavioral exemplars would necessarily become part of this structure. Early research on implicit personality theory (e.g., Rosenberg & Sedlak, 1972) was based on this assumption. No doubt exemplars of a trait can be generated upon request, but this does not mean they are always activated spontaneously at encoding.

There is some reason to believe that a behavior may spontaneously evoke a trait. Several investigators (Smith & Miller, 1983; Winter & Uleman, 1984) offered data in support of the prediction that merely reading a behavior makes its coordinate trait category more accessible. Srull, Lichtenstein, and Rothbart (1985) have shown that in the absence of any advance expectancy, presenting a series of behaviors will activate a trait category that is congruent with a majority of the behaviors. The trait category, once activated, then serves as an expectancy for the later

behaviors, and leads to superior recall for the later behaviors that are
incongruent with that expectancy.

Behaviors encountered in a coherent social context (e.g., going to the
movies) may activate nontrait structures. The very concept of a script
(Schank & Abelson, 1977) derives from the premise that in many contexts
behaviors are represented in a temporal sequence. Behaviors serve to
identify the current scene being enacted and trigger expectancies for the
subsequent behaviors of self and others. As another example, sets of
behaviors, such as ones encountered in courtroom testimony, can evoke
story structures (Pennington & Hastie, 1986).

Question II. *Are static displays represented differently from dynamic displays?*

Social interaction is dynamic. It rides the rails of time, never coming to a
halt or reversing itself. It doesn't provide the participant the luxury of
stop-action snapshots, with which the perceiver can leisurely compare
one person's facial expression with that of another person to see how they
differ in response to a suggestion just made. And with few exceptions,
such as televised sports events, instant replays are rarely available to
reevaluate tacit inferences made in the course of ongoing interaction.

Most research on cognition has employed fairly static stimulus displays. Three types of stimulus presentation are in common usage:

1. The subject may be given a page with a list of traits on it to memorize
or from which to form an impression. This allows the subject to go back
and reread each information item as often as necessary within the time
limits provided. This hardly reflects the moment-to-moment shifts that
occur in the stimulus field in natural social interaction.

2. A second category of research presents memory items sequentially,
with each item displayed for less than 10 s. Chapter 12 in this volume
shows that the form of representation changes when its presentation is of
sufficient duration to allow a thorough search for linkages to previous
items. Although time is allowed to move in sequential presentations, the
perceiver is still deprived of the kinds of control normally available in
interpersonal interaction. The perceiver is forced to spend an equal
amount of time attending to each stimulus item and is deprived of any
ability to request clarification or elaboration of the information items.

3. A third type of research employs repeated presentation of the
stimulus items (as when learning the list to a criterion of accuracy). This
literally puts the person in a nonvolitional videotape replay mode, where
the inexorable quality of time is negated.

To understand social memory, then, it is necessary to discover how
time constrains the structures formed in dynamic interaction settings.

Question III. *Do different representations result from active versus passive unitization of stimuli?*

Propositions such as *the man kicked the dog* represent one of the smallest
and most fundamental cognitive units. They connect elements like *man,*

kicked, and *dog* into a single chunk, one that can act cognitively as a single unit.

A basic problem in understanding social interaction resides in knowing how people form these units. Observing a scene in which a man kicks a dog need not be automatically encoded as the proposition *the man kicked the dog.* Numerous alternative possibilities exist, even for this simple example: the man is angry, the man is cruel, the man is frustrated, the man kicks things, the man is punishing the dog, the man is defending himself, the man hates dogs, everyone kicks the dog, the dog is attacking the man, the man will kick you, and so on.

Most current research on cognitive processes employs units that are predetermined by the experimenter and passively accepted by the subject. The reasoning behind this practice is twofold. First, it is necessary for the experimenter to know what the units are in advance when using methodologies such as recall and response time. Otherwise, it is impossible to score recall protocols or to assess response times in tasks such as those involving lexical decision making.

Second, many have implicitly assumed that the unitization process is independent of the processes involved in cognitively operating on those units (e.g., the activities of storage and retrieval). This assumption should be questioned. In the midst of an interaction episode, persons seem to simultaneously arrive at propositional units and a way of structuring those units. A structure that does not satisfy current goals may lead to a revision in the qualitative character of the subsequent propositional units, which in turn would yield a more suitable structure. Such phenomena cannot be uncovered by adopting passive unitization methodologies.

One approach to the unitization problem was initiated by Newtson (e.g., Newtson, Rinder, Miller, & LaCross, 1978). He used the methodology of asking subjects to observe a sequence of behaviors presented on a videotape. Subjects were asked to press a button at the completion of each meaningful unit. He was primarily interested in the duration of the segments. His approach focused primarily on unit size. Consequently, it has not informed us about the propositional content of the units or the manner in which they are cognitively structured.

Question IV. *Does the number of coparticipants affect the cognitive representation of each participant?*

Social interactions always involve one or more coparticipants. Most past research in social memory has focused only on the dyadic context, a setting that involves just the perceiver and one partner. This point is well illustrated by the research reported in Chapters 11 and 12 in this volume. In a dyadic context, the perceiver is able to focus attention exclusively on the other person. This permits the perceiver to develop a well-differentiated cognitive representation of the interaction partner and to more easily interpret the partner's current behavioral reactions.

Many social interactions, such as family gatherings, luncheons, parties, and business meetings, involve more than one coparticipant. In these contexts it is often necessary for the perceiver to develop separate representations of each of the other group members. A series of studies by Pryor and Ostrom (e.g., Ostrom, Pryor, & Simpson, 1981) has established that perceivers can develop separate categories for representing information about the different interaction participants. However, their research has also shown that social factors such as communication structure, processing goals, social roles, and unfamiliarity can lead to avoidance of person categories when cognitively representing multiperson social encounters.

One important concern raised by this question has to do with the separate cognitive representations formed of each individual in the group. First, it would seem that from attentional concerns alone, the perceiver would not be able to develop as differentiated a structure for one person when many others are present as when interacting with that person alone. This question has yet to be studied.

Second, there is the need to develop new structures beyond those required to separately represent each participant. In group settings it becomes important to represent the set of relationships that bind the group members to one another. For example, we need to know about the sociometric structure of likes and dislikes, the role interrelations, and the dominance hierarchy that governs interpersonal influence. Work has been done showing that some sociometric structures are cognitively balanced (e.g., Heider, 1958; Picek, Sherman, & Shiffrin, 1975) and that some dominance structures are linearly ordered (e.g., Tsujimoto, Wilde, & Robertson, 1978). But in this research, persons are designated simply by names, with no possibility of concurrently forming individuated person categories representing ongoing behavior. We still do not know what kinds of changes take place in the representation of each person when these interpersonal structures are being formed on-line.

Question V. *Does the self as participant-versus-observer affect the representation of the other?*

One principal difference between being a participant versus being an observer is that a participant must respond to the other. That is, conversations consist of people taking turns talking to one another. A second principal difference is that as a participant, one's responses become a stimulus to the other. Agreement versus disagreement with a partner's religious preferences will yield very different consequences. Third, people adopt self-presentational strategies when in a face-to-face context (e.g., Baumeister & Hutton, 1987). Individual differences in self-presentation should influence representations more when acting as a participant than when acting as an observer.

A primitive stimulus-response analysis of participant interaction implies that you listen to your partner (the stimulus information), then formulate and communicate your reply (the response). That is, the representation of your partner's actions is completed prior to the production of a response. The need to formulate a reply and the concern over how the companion will react is addressed only subsequent to the representation of the other's actions. This suggests that concerns about responding have no effect on how people represent the other's behaviors. From this viewpoint, it makes little difference whether the subject is a participant or an observer when the research focus is on studying mental representations. All the important differences produced by these two roles are confined to postrepresentation mental activities.

This simplistic model appears to characterize contemporary approaches to understanding the cognitive representation of stimulus information. Nearly all research puts the subjects in the role of observers. Subjects passively receive the stimulus information, which is most often presented in a predictably structured fashion (e.g., sentences given one at a time for 8 s each). The decision of when to respond is determined by the experimenter, and the response options are also experimenter designated. Further, rarely does the response affect the nature of the subsequent information about the stimulus object. Most often, subjects know that no further information will be provided. In those cases where more information will appear, the subjects know that their responses will have no effect on the character of that information.

This simplistic model does not hold up to the reality of being a participant in social interaction. If the representation must be completed prior to formulating a response, the person would have to engage in an enormous amount of cognitive activity during the brief turn-taking interval (rarely longer than 5 or 6 s) between the end of the partner's utterance and the start of the person's reply. Among the demands on the participants are the need to (a) be sure they accurately understood the partner's prior utterance, (b) relate that utterance to their own (and to the partner's) previous utterances, (c) relate that utterance to other background information that they know the partner has about them (and they have about the partner), (d) relate the utterance to their own goals, (e) deduce intentions and goals held by the partner that are implied by the utterance, (f) identify and evaluate their response alternatives, (g) project the partner's reaction to each of the alternatives, and (h) deal with any personal affect that may have been aroused by the partner's utterance (see also Ostrom, 1984).

It is absurd to assume that all these cognitive events occur subsequent to forming the representation of the partner's utterance. There simply would not be time, given the normal duration of the turn-taking interval. And in fact, on many occasions conversational transitions occur with either no gap or with a brief period during which both parties speak simultaneously (Clark, 1985). This means that these other cognitive events must occur concurrently with the construction of a representation of the partner's actions and utterances. Nothing is currently available in the social memory literature about the interdependence of such concurrent activities, even though this problem is central to the understanding of social discourse.

Question VI. *Do self actions become part
of the stimulus representation?*

As an interaction participant, one may be called upon to respond to the partner at any moment. The partner may stop in midsentence and ask "What do you think?" A third person may interrupt the discussion and ask an entirely irrelevant question. Even when taken aback, we usually manage to provide a timely response. We are an action-oriented species, and so it seems reasonable to assume that our cognitive system is constructed to facilitate action in social contexts.

One type of cognitive unit that has proven conceptually useful, especially in the context of understanding problem-solving behavior, is the production rule (Anderson, 1983; Newell & Simon, 1972). This refers to if–then contingency units such as *if I turn the ignition key, the car will start* or *if I smile at the student, she will smile back.* Such units are clearly properties of the stimulus object (i.e., the car and the student), and so are eligible for inclusion in the representation formed of the interaction partner. The activation of such productions may well be the immediate cognitive precursor of overt behavior.

The production rules we employ in interaction contexts are special in that they link an action of the self to an action of the partner in a contingent, cause-effect manner. Specific production rules will evolve for each interaction partner (e.g., when I smile at Tammy-the-sourpuss, she stares blankly at me). Interestingly, some research has shown that people do not spontaneously identify such production rule knowledge as important to their impressions of others. Ostrom (1975) asked people to indicate the kinds of information they would want to form an impression of another person. No subjects sought if–then contingency information. Instead, they asked for information about demographic features, physical appearance, traits, attitudes, and group memberships.

The inclusion of such production rules into the representation of the partner automatically incorporates the actions of the self into that cognitive structure. This calls into question the traditional practice of separating stimulus from response. The cognitive representation of stimulus information very likely includes response information. Accessing representations of this type during interaction would allow individuals to enact reasonably appropriate responses in a timely manner, even under the most unexpected of circumstances.

The Second Catechism: Social Behavior

People do more than think, they behave. Indeed, from the early part of this century, psychology has been defined as the study of human behavior. Many in the field still do not hold the cognitive revolution in high regard. One of their primary reservations is that, to them, the study of cognition appears not to inform us about the determinants of overt behavior. They view the theoretical focus as being exclusively within the head, with little or no attention being devoted to understanding such complex overt behavior as that displayed in social interactions.

The kind of theorizing adopted by most social psychologists before the advent of information-processing constructs adopted a fairly simplistic view of the relation between cognition and behavior. As has been argued elsewhere (e.g., Devine & Ostrom, 1988; Ostrom, 1987), almost all of the earlier theories were dimensional in nature. Theorists would select a problem such as attitude, aggression, or morale and begin their theoretical attack by positing a continuum. People were known to vary in terms of how pro or anti their attitude was, how much or little aggression they would display, or how supportive or antagonistic their morale was.

A threefold set of theoretical tasks emerged from this conceptual framing of the problem domain. One was to establish the *antecedents* of a person's location on the continuum. What made the person change an attitude in the pro or anti direction? The second theoretical task was to establish the *consequences* of the person's location on the theoretical dimension. For example, how do political attitudes affect voting behavior? The third task was to measure *individual differences* on the dimension, and to see how they related to other characteristics of the person. For example, are prejudiced people more likely to be dogmatic than nonprejudiced people?

Of these three theoretical tasks, it is the second that dealt with getting out of the head and predicting social behavior. The conceptual approach adopted by most theorists (often implicitly) was very straightforward. The behavioral alternatives would be located on the same theoretical continuum as was the person. For example, attitudinal behaviors themselves will range from favorable to unfavorable toward the attitude object, and each can be located as a unique point on that continuum. Overt behavior, then, involved the person adopting the action closest to the person's own location on the dimension. This solution was inexact and did not have much theoretical depth, but it did allow theorists to get on with the business of empirically and theoretically probing a problem domain.

This dimensional approach led theorists to ignore large sectors of important phenomena within the chosen problem domain. In the case of attitudes, for example, this approach could not predict which behavioral alternatives were most salient, what activated the attitude in the first place, when and why attitudinally discrepant behaviors would be enacted, or which of two attitudinally equivalent behaviors would be selected. These inadequacies of the dimensional approach coincide with potential strengths of the information-processing approach. The symbolic character of cognitive structures enables that conceptual orientation to deal with the qualitative features of overt behavior. Instead of actions being represented as points on a continuum, they are embedded (possibly in the form of production rules) in structures representing the current interaction context and the individuals populating it.

Question I. *How does the cognitive system enable decision making?*
The traditional decision-making literature provides an excellent illustration of the dimensional approach to the understanding of overt responses. The prime exemplars of these traditional theories are the bayesian approach (Peterson & Beach, 1967), expectancy-value models (Feather, 1982), and information integration theory (Anderson, 1981). In all cases, the key theoretical constructs (i.e., subjective probability, expectancy, value, weight, and scale value) are represented as points on a continuum.

Researchers in the field of social memory are just beginning to turn to the question of how judgments, choices, inferences, and decisions are derived from cognitive representations. They reject the dimensional approach, preferring to construe these phenomena within the set of constructs provided by the information-processing approach. Wyer (Chapter 12 in this volume) argues that this shift is at the heart of the social memory approach. And further, that this focus on inferences and decisions serves to distinguish the field of social memory from cognitive psychology in general.

One illustration of this new approach is provided by Ostrom (1987). He outlined one way people could make bipolar judgments (e.g., liberal-conservative, friendly-unfriendly) without assuming they access a point on a subjective bipolar continuum. His approach assumes that two kinds of representations are activated when a person is requested to make a bipolar rating of a stimulus.

As an illustration, assume that a man is asked to rate his wife on a 9-point scale of introversion (1) to extroversion (9). One representation that is activated by the rating task involves his wife's characteristics. The representation will contain some elements that are introverted, some that are extroverted, and many that are neither.

The second representation corresponds to the set of response alternatives that are actively considered. In this example they would be the nine categories in the rating scale. Most people will not have separate representations for each of the nine categories. Probably they will only have three, a category for introvert, a category for extrovert, and a category for undecided. Each of these response categories has its own defining features.

The actual selection of one rating category presumably involves a matching process. The man compares his representation of his wife to the features of each of the three categories. This matching process may follow principles comparable to those outlined by Tversky (1977; Tversky & Gati, 1982) in his contrast model for similarity judgments. A perfect match with one of the three would lead to a rating of 1 (for introvert), 5 (for undecided), or 9 (for extrovert). Intermediate ratings may be chosen on the basis of relative quality of match. For example, a rating of 3 would be given when the fit to the introvert category equaled the fit to the uncertain category.

Ostrom provided only the outlines of such a model. The specific details of the model and its empirical exploration have yet to be undertaken. But it does serve to illustrate how the information-processing approach differs from the dimensional approach in explaining judgments and decisions. A similar approach has been taken by Pennington and Hastie (1986) in their story model approach to understanding the processes of juror decision making.

Question II. *How does the cognitive system enable conversations?*
A great deal of our waking hours are spent in conversations with other people. It is through language that we convey our likes and dislikes, acquire and dispense information, and develop and solidify intimate relationships. Most of the basic phenomenon in social psychology (see the chapter titles in an introductory textbook) occur through the medium of language in social interactions. Attributional explanations, persuasive communications, aggressive verbal exchanges, and altruistic offers of assistance are all linguistic acts.

Despite the prominent role of language in social interaction, social psychologists have stubbornly resisted the study of language. Chapters on language were included in the last two editions of the *Handbook of Social Psychology* (Clark, 1985; Miller & McNeill, 1969), but almost none of the citations in either chapter were from the core journals in social psychology. The same lack of attention to language is found in the field's introductory textbooks. One gets the impression from reading these texts that life is like a television show with the sound turned off, where the actors communicate through making check marks on rating scales.

Most work on language has been done by cognitive psychologists, developmental psychologists, linguists, philosophers, and computer scientists. Three stages of language generation can be identified. *Construction* refers to determining what needs to be communicated. *Transformation* refers to converting the intended meaning into subjective linguistic units. And *execution* refers to the overt expression of the linguistic units in spoken or written form.

A number of discussions of this extensive literature exist (e.g., Anderson, 1985; Clark & Clark, 1977; Foss & Hakes, 1978). Of special concern here is how the language generation process operates in social interaction contexts. This focus is necessary if we are to understand the role of language in social phenomena such as interpersonal persuasion (e.g., salesmanship and jury decision making) or aggression (e.g., employee hostility and domestic violence). Modeling interactive exchanges is very difficult, but one area in which advances have been made is that of question answering (e.g., Graesser & Clark, 1985; Lehnert, 1978).

Question III. *How does the cognitive system enable social actions?*
Social interaction consists of more than just deciding and talking—it also
involves doing. Voters don't just say they like President Reagan, they
send him campaign contributions. Drivers don't simply decide to be altruistic to a hitchhiker, they stop and give him a ride. Parents don't merely
say to their child they are angry, they spank the brat. The information-
processing approach is obligated to provide an answer to how people
produce these molar, socially meaningful actions.

There is a second set of social actions that also requires explanation,
actions of a much less molar character. These are the nonverbal and
paralinguistic displays that occur in the course of social interaction. We
may smile or frown, maintain a relaxed or alert posture, and make eye
contact or avert our gaze. All these are significant forms of social
behavior that affect those with whom we interact. Under some circumstances these actions may be even more influential than information
conveyed directly through the spoken word.

Little, if any, work has been done by social psychologists on how the
cognitive system relates to these social actions. However, research
relevant to these concerns is being undertaken by workers in the fields of
motor control and robotics (e.g., Prinz & Sanders, 1984). The relevant
work starts from the premise that motor behavior (which is fundamental
to enacting both molar and paralinguistic responses) is centrally represented in the cognitive system.

The tasks that face the theorists in this area include understanding the
cognitive representation of motor behavior (e.g., is it in the form of
production rules?), understanding the control structures that select and
sequence muscle movements, and understanding the mechanics of the
different muscle systems. To be of use in understanding complex social
actions, this work will have to go beyond explaining simple actions such
as a smile. We will need to know how the control system constructs the
complex and time-extended sequence of motor movements involved in
such molar actions as donating money to a candidate. Here the intention
(or goal) to donate may have been formed during a conversation with
someone at work. But the behavioral enactment may involve driving
home, finding the checkbook and pen, writing the check, finding an
envelope and stamp, addressing the envelope, driving to the post office,
and depositing the envelope in the mail box.

The Third Catechism: Collective Memory

This catechism takes its focus from a book by one of the world's first
social memory advocates, a man whose formal education was as a
philosopher and mathematician. Maurice Halbwachs wrote *La Mémoire
Collective* before his death in Buchenwald, a World War II concentration
camp. The volume was published posthumorously in 1950, with the

English edition appearing in 1980. In this and several earlier books, Halbwachs distinguished between individual memory and collective memory.

Halbwachs made the strong argument that there is no such thing as individual memory; all memory is collective. At the heart of this argument is the thesis that memory cannot be understood without simultaneously understanding the social milieu in which the person resides. There is no such thing as an individual memory that exists in social isolation. The operation of our cognitive system always involves other people. When we are with other people, we use them "to corroborate or invalidate as well as supplement what we somehow know already about an event that in many other details remains obscure" (p. 22). And even when we are physically alone other people are integral to memory:

> Our memories remain collective, however, and are recalled to us through others even though only we were participants in the events or saw the things concerned. In reality, we are never alone. Other men need not be physically present, since we carry with us and in us a number of distinct persons. (p. 23)

Concern over these issues has recently surfaced in social psychology. Wegner (1987) published a mostly speculative chapter titled "Transactive Memory." Although he was apparently unfamiliar with Halbwachs' works, he raised many of the concerns addressed in this third catechism. However, he offered very few new data on these issues. Nor did he tie these ideas to issues in information processing.

Halbwachs' views have not yet gained ascendancy among contemporary researchers in memory. One reason is that he did not document his ideas with empirical evidence, leading those familiar with his arguments to dismiss them as irrelevant. Another reason was that Bartlett (1932), who was a contemporary of Halbwachs, explicitly rejected Halbwachs' views (see Bartlett, 1932, chap. 18). However, as Douglas (1980) showed, this rejection was based on a misreading of Halbwachs.

This third catechism will document that, in contrast to Bartlett's criticisms, Halbwachs' ideas about memory are fully congruent with contemporary information-processing conceptions. His ideas make us aware of the fact that memory is socially distributed; namely, that other people serve as satellite memory stores that the individual can access upon need. Halbwachs' ideas add an entirely new dimension to the research agenda challenging the field of social memory.

Question I. *How do others influence encoding and retrieval?*
Several avenues need to be explored. There is abundant research to show that people preferentially encode and access information relevant to their current goals (e.g., Ostrom, Lingle, Pryor, & Geva, 1980). In an interaction context, personal goals are formed and altered as a function of the goals of the other participants. The nature of this goal interdependence is not yet well understood.

Perhaps of greater interest, people use others as an extension of their own memories. People who know one another well also come to know the kinds of things the other tends to remember and forget (i.e., the other person's selective foci of encoding and retrieval). It is common for a traveling couple to divide up the memory load while on vacation. For example, one will keep track of the travel itinerary (e.g., when does the flight leave tomorrow?) and the other will keep track of financial resources (e.g., how many Deutschmarks do they have left?). Sometimes these memory roles are negotiated and other times they emerge spontaneously. Both partners seem effortlessly to selectively encode and quickly retrieve the information from their assigned domains. Wegner (1987) reported data from dating couples that clearly demonstrate this phenomena.

One of the more fascinating consequences of this arrangement is the knowledge structure retrieved by one partner regarding the other partner's domain. For example, both partners may have been present the day before when the desk clerk told them the airport bus leaves at 3:45 p.m. Upon awakening, the nonresponsible partner may wonder when the bus is to leave. He does not recall the time was 3:45 p.m. Instead, as the nonresponsible partner, he recalls a far more complicated structure: (a) that he and his partner obtained the information the day before, (b) that it was obtained from the room clerk in the hotel lobby at a particular time of day, (c) that he does not remember the information, (d) and that his companion should remember it. Often this tacit memory-sharing agreement is so strong that the man will become angry if his companion is unable to recall the information, or does so inaccurately. Such memory differences must derive in part from differences in processing goals, which in turn are doubtlessly affected by each person's interests, occupation, hobbies, past responsibilities in the relationship, and cultural experiences.

One approach researchers might take to this problem area builds on past research on stereotypes. Work on gender stereotypes, for example, might suggest that after a couple looks at a shirt in a shopping center, the woman may more accurately recall the design and material whereas the man may more accurately recall the price. Furthermore, members of each group may hold comparable assumptions about the selective memory biases of the two groups. A synthesis of the stereotyping approach with work on metamemory (e.g., Flavell & Wellman, 1977; Wellman, 1983) is needed. This work has typically concentrated on persons' beliefs about the operation of their own memory. It needs to be extended to the study of assumptions made about other people's memories if we are to understand the operation of collective memory.

Question II. *How do others influence the longevity of memories?*
How do we account for the perseverance of detailed memories over long time intervals? At a class reunion, you might meet an old friend who

relates an amusing escapade from your school days that you hadn't thought about in years. The narrative is filled with small details, like facial expression and quips made during the event, all of which ring true, but none of which you could have recalled on your own. Is it simply that your friend has a better memory than you? As another example, how is it that some members of primitive tribes can talk for days about events and tribal geneology from hundreds of years ago, and do so in great detail? These examples seem inconsistent with the idea that as memory fades over time, the details are lost.

The strength of an association is determined by the recency and frequency of activation. The more often we rehearse an idea, the easier it is to retrieve it later. Interpersonal encounters may provide the primary basis for rehearsing social memories. Your classmate may have told this amusing story over and over again in the intervening years (ask the spouse!), fully rehearsing the details on each occasion. The tribal historian is called upon continually to retrieve this historical knowledge to provide precedents in tribal decision making and for entertainment purposes. Again we have repeated rehearsal evolving out of our social milieu.

A key issue in this area is whether the nature of the rehearsal process is different for passive rehearsal than for rehearsal that takes place in the context of linguistic exchanges. Does speaking an idea strengthen it more than just thinking it? That is, is a cognitive bond that is accessed in the act of communication strengthened differently than one silently accessed? It is possible that the communicative act involves repeated accessing activity, whereas passive rehearsal does not.

Research in impression formation has shown that impressions are more crystalized when in a transmission set than when in a reception set (Zajonc, 1960). The information items about the stimulus person become more coherently interlinked when subjects anticipate communicating the information (the transmission set) than when they anticipate the receipt of new information (the reception set) about the person. This suggests that there would also be better recall under transmission- than under reception-processing goals.

Another property of overt communication is that people will often engage in precommunication rumination. For example, we often try to put our thoughts in order before speaking (Bond, 1985). There is also postcommunication rumination. People do not like to be misleading or inarticulate, and so will review their earlier statements for accuracy or appropriateness. This allows them to repair misimpressions or to reorganize the way they structure a presentation for future use. This often occurs after telling a joke or giving a lecture for the first time. Such forms of rumination emerge primarily from social interactions, and so raise a set of issues unique to the field of social memory.

Since social rehearsal can have such an impact on the longevity of memories, it becomes important to learn the social conditions under which active versus passive rehearsals occur. Both recall and recognition demands exist in social settings. Recall is required in cases where one is explicitly asked questions about past experiences. But it also occurs when people are asked to defend their decisions, opinions, past actions, and attributions. Recognition processes occur when people listen to a partner relate a shared experience or a communicator make claims about historical facts with which the perceiver is familiar. Other issues include whether rehearsal is affected by the person's role in the group or by current social goals.

Question III. *How do others modify our memories?*

Despite what we may tell others about the accuracy of our memory, most of us are aware that our memory is fallible. Most retrieved information is tinged with a bit of uncertainty. People will even show uncertainty when retrieving well-learned facts like their age, birthplace, and own name, at least under some hypnotic conditions (Rokeach, 1972).

This uncertainty doubtless leads people to query the memories of others for purposes of corroboration, refutation, and elaboration. People use others to evaluate the quality of their own recall—to validate the accuracy of their memory, to detect any errors that have distorted their memory, and to fill in details they have lost.

This raises the question of how people buttress and repair their memory representations. In the case of buttressing shaky beliefs through obtaining consensual support, we must ask how the original structure is modified by this new information. Does the person have a "truth" node to which the fact is attached, and the pathway to that node becomes strengthened through social verification? Or does the person link the confirming episode (along with source, place, and time information) to the fact? Similar issues must be raised in the case of repairs to the structure that are made as a result of encountering refutation and/or elaboration of prior beliefs during conversations with others.

Social psychologists have long been interested in social comparison processes (Goethals & Darley, 1987; Festinger, 1954). The theory of social comparison is based on the assumption that people prefer accuracy over inaccuracy. It was developed to account for how people evaluate the correctness of their attitudes and the competence of their abilities. It is a small step to extend the principles of this theory to the social processes underlying the validation and modification of memory structures in general.

Discussion

No argument has been made above that the basic information-processing stages, structures, or mechanisms are different for social memory than for traditional memory research. Indeed, at least one search for empirical documentation of such differences proved futile (Ostrom, 1984). The kinds of social memory research proposed here fully adopt the theoretical and methodological advances that characterize the modern cognitive revolution.

What separates social memory from traditional memory is the commitment to understand social behavior. The questions raised in these three catechisms result from taking the constructs of cognitive psychology seriously and using them in this quest for understanding. The chapter has shown how face-to-face interaction places extraordinary demands on the information-processing system, and the chapter raises questions about the adequacy of currently proposed mechanisms to handle these demands. The chapter also identified a number of ignored and poorly understood phenomena that become visible in the light of the social memory beacon.

The chapter expressly focused on social behavior and the information-processing mechanisms that are linked to it. In the process, a set of topics was ignored. These are the subjective states that people experience when with others. Prominent among these are mood and affect. But beyond experiencing such positive and negative feelings, people also manifest subjective states such as hope, pride, embarrassment, doubt, anger, anxiety, dismay, jealousy, and longing. Such qualitative states are squarely in the domain of social memory. This is because they can only be understood by understanding the interplay between the cognitive system and social experience. Subjective experiences like these emerge naturally as a byproduct of the processes discussed in all three of the catechisms described in this chapter.

As argued by Wyer (Chapter 12 in this volume), it is usually wasteful, and ultimately futile, to try to define the boundaries of a discipline like social memory. A functional definition is probably the best. Social memory is defined by the research and theory developed by workers currently identified with the field. Chapters 11 and 12 in this volume offer excellent exemplars of work in social memory. The present chapter forecasts the types of empirical and theoretical issues that will absorb the interest of social memory researchers in the near future. But as the field matures, this research agenda will surely change in its composition. Even the three catechisms identified in this chapter are not immutable. They, too, will be transformed by the wisdom of time.

Acknowledgment. This chapter benefited from excellent comments on an earlier draft from Robert Fuhrman, Al Goethals, Reid Hastie, Maria Nowakowska, Alan Ogburn, Constantine Sedikides, John Skowronski, and Thomas Srull.

References

Anderson, J.R. (1983). *The architecture of cognition.* Cambridge, MA: Harvard University Press.

Anderson, J.R. (1985). *Cognitive psychology and its implications* (2nd ed.). New York: W. H. Freeman.

Anderson, N.H. (1981). *Foundations of information integration theory*. New York: Academic Press.

Bartlett, F.C. (1932). *Remembering: A study in experimental and social psychology*. New York: Cambridge University Press.

Baumeister, R.F., & Hutton, D.G. (1987). Self-presentation theory: Self-construction and audience pleasing. In B. Mullen & G.R. Goethals (Eds.), *Theories of group behavior* (pp. 71–87). New York: Springer-Verlag.

Bond, C.F. (1985). The next-in-line effect: Encoding or retrieval deficit? *Journal of Personality and Social Psychology, 48,* 853–862.

Clark, H.H. (1985). Language use and language users. In G. Lindzey & E. Aronson (Eds.), *Handbook of social psychology* (Vol. 2, pp. 179–232). (3rd ed.). Reading, MA: Addison-Wesley.

Clark, H.H., & Clark, E.V. (1977). *Psychology and language*. New York: Harcourt Brace Jovanovich.

Devine, P.G., & Ostrom, T.M. (1988). Dimensional vs. information processing approaches to social knowledge: The case of inconsistency management. In D. Bar-Tal & A. Kruglanski (Eds.), *The social psychology of knowledge*. Cambridge: Cambridge University Press.

Douglas, M. (1980). Introduction: Maurice Halbwachs (1877–1945). In M. Halbwachs, *The collective memory* (pp. 1–19). New York: Harper & Row.

Flavell, J.H., & Wellman, H.M. (1977). Metamemory. In R.V. Kail, Jr., & J.W. Hagen (Eds.), *Perspectives on the development of memory and cognition* (pp. 3–33). Hillsdale, NJ; Lawrence Erlbaum Associates.

Feather, N.T. (1982). *Expectations and actions: Expectancy-value models in psychology*. Hillsdale, NJ: Lawrence Erlbaum Associates.

Festinger, L. (1954). A theory of social comparison processes. *Human Relations, 7,* 117–140.

Fiske, S.T., & Taylor, S.E. (1984). *Social cognition*. Reading, MA: Addison-Wesley.

Foss, D. J., & Hakes, D.T. (1978). *Psycholinguistics*. Englewood Cliffs, NJ: Prentice Hall.

Goethals, G.R., & Darley, J.M. (1987). Social comparison theory: Self-evaluation and group life. In B. Mullen & G.R. Goethals (Eds.), *Theories of group behavior* (pp. 21–48). New York: Springer-Verlag.

Graesser, A.C., & Clark, L.F. (1985). *Structure and procedures of implicit knowledge*. Norwood, NJ: Ablex.

Halbwachs, M. (1980). *The collective memory*. New York: Harper & Row.

Heider, F. (1958). *The psychology of interpersonal relations*. New York: John Wiley.

Lehnert, W.G. (1978). *The process of question answering: A computer simulation of cognition*. Hillsdale, NJ: Lawrence Erlbaum Associates.

Miller, G.A., & McNeill, D. (1969). Psycholinguistics. In G. Lindzey & E. Aronson (Eds.), *The handbook of social psychology* (Vol. 3, pp. 666–794). (2nd ed.). Reading, MA: Addison-Wesley.

Nelson, K. (1981). Social cognition in a script framework. In J. Flavell & L. Ross (Eds.), *Social cognitive development: Frontiers and possible futures*. Cambridge, MA: Cambridge University Press.

Newell, A., & Simon, H.A. *Human problem solving*. Englewood Cliffs, NJ: Prentice-Hall.

Newtson, D., Rinder, R., Miller, R., & LaCross, K. (1978). Effects of availability of feature changes on behavior segmentation. *Journal of Experimental Social Psychology, 14,* 379–388.

Ostrom, T.M. (1975, September). Cognitive representation of impressions. Paper presented at the meeting of the American Psychological Association, Chicago.

Ostrom, T.M. (1984). The sovereignty of social cognition. In R. Wyer & T. Srull (Eds.), *Handbook of social cognition* (Vol. 1, pp. 1–38). Hillsdale, NJ: Lawrence Erlbaum Associates.

Ostrom, T.M. (1987). Bipolar survey items: An information processing perspective. In H. Hippler, N. Schwarz, & S. Sudman (Eds.), *Social information processing and survey methodology* (pp. 71–85). New York: Springer-Verlag.

Ostrom, T.M., Lingle, J.H., Pryor, J.B., & Geva, N. (1980). Cognitive organization of person impressions. In R. Hastie, T. Ostrom, D. Hamilton, E. Ebbesen, R. Wyer, & D. Carlston (Eds.), *Person memory: The cognitive basis of social perception* (pp. 55–88). Hillsdale, NJ: Lawrence Erlbaum Associates.

Ostrom, T.M., Pryor, J.B., & Simpson, D.D. (1981). The organization of social information. In E. Higgins, C. Herman, & M. Zanna (Eds.), *Social cognition: The Ontario symposium* (Vol. 1, pp. 3–38). Hillsdale, NJ: Lawrence Erlbaum Associates.

Pennington, N., & Hastie, R. (1986). Evidence evaluation in complex decision making. *Journal of Personality and Social Psychology, 51,* 242–258.

Peterson, C.R., & Beach, L.R. (1967). Man as an intuitive statistician. *Psychological Bulletin, 68,* 29–46.

Picek, J.S., Sherman, S.J., & Shiffrin, R.M. (1975). Cognitive organization and coding of social structure. *Journal of Personality and Social Psychology, 31,* 758–768.

Prinz, W., & Sanders, A.F. (Eds.) (1984). *Cognition and motor processes*. Berlin: Springer-Verlag.

Rokeach, M. (1972). *Beliefs, attitudes, and values: A theory of organization and change*. San Francisco, CA: Jossey-Bass.

Rosenberg, S., & Sedlak, A. (1972). Structural representations of implicit personality theory. In L. Berkowitz (Ed.), *Advances in experimental social psychology* (Vol. 6). New York: Academic Press.

Schank, R.C., & Abelson, R.P. (1977). *Scripts, plans, goals, and understanding: An inquiry into human knowledge structures*. Hillsdale, NJ: Lawrence Erlbaum Associates.

Smith, E.R., & Miller, F.O. (1983). Mediation among attributional inferences and comprehension processes: Initial findings and a general method. *Journal of Personality and Social Psychology, 44,* 492–505.

Srull, T.K., Lichtenstein, M., & Rothbart, M. (1985). Associative storage and retrieval processes in person memory. *Journal of Experimental Psychology: Learning, Memory, and Cognition, 11,* 316–345.

Thurstone, L.L. (1927). A law of comparative judgment. *Psychological Review, 34,* 273–286.

Tsujimoto, R.N., Wilde, J., & Robertson, D.R. (1978). Distorted memory for exemplars of a social structure: Evidence for schematic memory processes. *Journal of Personality and Social Psychology, 36,* 1402–1414.

Tversky, A. (1977). Features of similarity. *Psychological Review, 84,* 327–352.

Tversky, A., & Gati, I. (1982). Similarity, separability, and the triangle inequality. *Psychological Review, 89,* 123–154.

Wegner, D.M. (1987). Transactive memory: A contemporary analysis of the group mind. In B. Mullen & G.R. Goethals (Eds.), *Theories of group behavior* (pp. 185–208). New York: Springer-Verlag.

Wellman, H.M. (1983). Metamemory revisited. In M.T. Chi (Ed.), *Trends in memory development research.* New York: Karger.

Winter, L., & Uleman, J.S. (1984). When are social judgments made? Evidence for the spontaneousness of trait inferences. *Journal of Personality and Social Psychology, 47,* 237–252.

Wyer, R.S., & Gordon, S.E. (1984). The cognitive representation of social information. In R.S. Wyer & T.K. Srull (Eds.), *Handbook of social cognition* (Vol. 2, pp. 73–150). Hillsdale, NJ: Lawrence Erlbaum Associates.

Zajonc, R. (1960). The process of cognitive tuning in communication. *Journal of Abnormal and Social Psychology, 61,* 159–167.

CHAPTER 11

Understanding Impression Formation: What Has Memory Research Contributed?

David L. Hamilton

At some point in the future, those who comment on the shifting tides in the history of social psychology will view the current era as quite remarkable. As we are all well aware, social cognition has been the major conceptual force impacting upon social psychological thought and empirical work for the last decade (Fiske & Taylor, 1984; Lachman & Manis, 1983). This orientation is characterized by an emphasis on understanding how the individual, as a participant in a complex social world, processes information available about the self, others, and the social environment; how that information becomes represented in memory; and how that memory representation is used later in the course of making judgments, interacting with others, and the like. And as social psychology has adopted this approach to understanding its subject matter, it has borrowed heavily from the repository of theoretical concepts and experimental techniques that have been of use in cognitive psychology. As a consequence, it is now commonplace in the social psychological literature to find, for example, discussions of how information is stored in associative networks, and reports of experiments that have used free recall, recognition, or response latency as the primary dependent measure (see, for example, Fiske & Taylor, 1984; Hamilton, 1981a; Hastie et al., 1980; Higgins, Herman, & Zanna, 1981; Sorrentino & Higgins, 1986; Wyer & Srull, 1984). None of this was true as few as 10 years ago. And this change is not restricted to a selected subset of topics in social psychology, but rather is quite pervasive throughout the subject matter of the field. As Markus and Zajonc (1985, p. 137) recently commented:

This adoption of the cognitive view among social psychologists has been so complete that it is extremely difficult for most of the workers in the field to conceive of a viable alternative. Given a problem, the tendency to frame it in cognitive terms . . . is nearly automatic. The result is that one can no longer view today's social psychology as the study of social behavior. It is more accurate to define it as the study of the social mind.

Whether this aspect of social psychology's evolution is a good or bad thing is a matter of some debate. I recently heard one well-known social psychologist, in a talk on the rise and fall of various movements in the history of social psychology, predict that we are almost to the end of what he referred to as "the social cognition episode." Still, it is difficult to find clear evidence of a waning of interest in the approach, and as the Markus and Zajonc comment suggests, in many respects it has become second nature as a way of thinking about problems and issues. If anything, I see this orientation expanding rather than receding as it is applied in new domains (cf. Ostrom, 1984). Such extension may reveal some of the limits of the approach, but identifying its boundary conditions does not mean that it has outlived its usefulness.

Social Psychology's Interest in the Study of Memory

At the core of social psychology's interest in cognitive processing has been the study of memory. Why would social psychologists be interested in memory? The answer, I think, lies in the fact that many of the phenomena that are central to social psychology's concerns involve mental representations that are influential in guiding social behavior. Attitudes and belief systems, stereotypes of social groups, first impressions of others—all of these concepts can be thought of as cognitive structures that represent the individual's knowledge, beliefs, and inferences pertinent to some domain. They are cognitive representations that are stored in memory. The recent surge of interest in social cognition reflects in part a recognition that our understanding of both the nature and the functioning of these concepts can be enhanced by investigating directly the role of these structures in information processing. Given this perspective, it is a natural consequence that memory research has become a central part of this effort.

One implication of what I have said is that, compared with cognitive psychologists who study memory, social psychologists who use memory measures in their research are not primarily interested in understanding the memory system per se. Rather, they study memory because it is a useful means of learning more about some social psychological topic of interest, such as the role of attitudes in persuasive communication or the nature of first impressions of strangers. Recognition of this point has a number of implications. First, it suggests that there may be topics and issues that are of considerable importance for understanding the memory system and its functioning, but which will be of little interest to the social cognition researcher. That is, for any given social psychological phenomenon that is the primary focus of inquiry, not all aspects of the memory system will be relevant or important for understanding that topic. In this respect, the study of memory is a useful tool that provides diagnostic information about the nature and functions of some substantive topic of social psychological importance.

Second, it follows that in social psychology a focus on memory, either conceptually or for research purposes, will encounter limits as a means for understanding the subject matter of interest. That is, a cognitive analysis based on investigation of relevant memory structures and processes, however informative, is likely to provide only a partial account of what social psychologists want and need to know about complex topics like the nature of attitudes, stereotyping, and impression formation. The questions and issues of concern to social psychology cannot be understood fully in cognitive terms alone.

In view of these points, it follows that social psychologists who investigate memory for socially relevant information are making use of the conceptual and empirical tools of cognitive psychology in order to enlighten themselves about the *cognitive components* of phenomena that are inherently complex and multifaceted. Any singular focus on these cognitive components alone will therefore be incomplete. The last 10 years of social cognition research have been characterized by such a singular focus, and it is this feature of the current literature that causes distress for some members of the discipline. It is important, I think, that social cognition research be viewed in its appropriate context, that is, a systematic exploration of one, but only one, component of the subject matter under investigation. It is also important to recognize that, in this respect, social cognition researchers differ from some other memory researchers for whom an understanding of memory systems per se is, quite legitimately, an end in itself.

Despite the limitations implied in these remarks, it is now clearly evident that the recent emphasis on information processing, including the study of memory for socially relevant information, has been an extremely useful development for the understanding of topics of social psychological interest (cf. Hastie, Park, & Weber, 1984; Wyer & Gordon, 1984). In the remainder of this chapter I will discuss one of these topics and illustrate how the study of memory has increased our understanding of one particular topic, namely, the nature of impression formation.

Early Conceptions of Impression Formation

Contemporary research on first impression formation had its origins in the now classic paper by Solomon Asch (1946), published some 40 years ago. According to Asch, the process of impression formation begins immediately when we first encounter information about another person. As we learn more and more about the person, this new information becomes incorporated into the evolving impression. The new information is not simply tacked onto the impression, but is incorporated and integrated into it. In this process, each new piece of information is interpreted in the context of what is already known about the person, as represented in the emerging impression. Asch talked about a "dynamic interaction" between the existing impression and incoming items of information as an important part of the process. Underlying and directing these processes is the perceiver's tendency to develop a unified, coherent impression of the target person's personality. According to Asch, the perceiver implicitly assumes that personalities are organized, and therefore one's impression of another person should reflect the coherence and systematic nature of the target person's character. Thus the dynamic interaction that Asch described as occurring among informational elements is aimed at uncovering and understanding the organized and thematic aspects of the person's personality.

In his article, Asch (1946) reported a series of relatively simple experiments, the results of which, he argued, supported his conceptualization of the impression formation process. Over the years, the main empirical findings Asch presented have proven to be remarkably stable. The warm-cold effect, primacy effects, context effects on evaluations of individual attributes—these and other findings first reported by Asch have been replicated numerous times (see Schneider, Hastorf, & Ellsworth, 1979, for a discussion of this literature). The proper interpretation of these effects, however, has been another matter. Some aspects of Asch's findings were challenged immediately (Luchins, 1948), and two decades later, Anderson's information integration model provided a serious alternative framework for understanding many of these now established effects (Anderson, 1981). Despite these challenges, Asch's (1946) views on the impression formation process have persisted and still, I suspect, constitute the prevailing theoretical account of how impressions are formed.

Asch's thinking, and hence his theoretical discussions and terminology, was guided largely by the tenets of Gestalt psychology. Nevertheless, several of the key elements of his theoretical argument can easily be translated into more contemporary, information-processing terms. For example, it is clear from his discussions of the dynamic interaction among informational elements that occurs as information is received that, in some sense, items of information become associated with each other as they are encoded. Thus the developing impression, as a cognitive representation in memory of the information processed about the target person, can be thought of as consisting of a network of associations among representations of various informational items previously acquired. It is also clear in Asch's writing that this cognitive representation is organized as a result of the perceiver's attempt to identify the coherent elements of the target's personality, to understand the major themes that characterize this person as an individual. As a consequence, the network of associations among items of information would be neither random nor complete, but rather should reflect the perceiver's efforts to impose some structure on the assortment of descriptive facts he or she has received.

One likely prospect is that an impression would be organized around the various prominent themes of personality content reflected in the information available about the person, although other organizational schemes might also be viable.

As these examples illustrate, many of the classic ideas about the nature of impressions can be reconstrued in terms of their implications for what a memory representation ought to look like. During the last 10 years, social cognition researchers have pursued these implications empirically with, I think, impressive success. In the remainder of this chapter I will indicate how, both in my own research program and in the work of others, social psychologists have used memory-based analyses to increase our understanding of how information about persons becomes represented in memory as a part of what we mean by a personality impression.

Organization of Information in Impression Formation

One of the hallmarks of person impressions, as posited by Asch and others, is that that they are organized, coherent conceptions of what other persons' personalities are like. Information acquired about another person is not simply deposited in memory but is the basis for considerable cognitive activity in which the perceiver develops and elaborates on that information. This involves a number of processes, including trait inferences that go beyond the information available and evaluative judgments that flavor our reactions to the individual. Here I will limit concern to another aspect of this process, namely, how the items of information themselves become represented in memory.

Several years ago we set out to study whether and how subjects organize behavior-descriptive information they learn about another person (Hamilton, 1981b; Hamilton, Katz, & Leirer, 1980a,b). Our general hypothesis was that, given the task of forming an impression of an individual, perceivers would attempt to organize the available information in terms of whatever personality-relevant themes are conveyed in that information, and that the behavior descriptions would be stored in memory in categories corresponding to those themes.

The paradigm we used to investigate this question in a number of studies was straightforward. Subjects were presented a series of sentence predicates, typically 16 or so, each of which described a single behavioral act. Within the set of behavior descriptions, each of several categories of personality content was represented by several items. For example, some of the items might describe social behaviors, such as "went to the movies with some friends" and "had a party at his apartment last weekend." Another category might pertain to intellectual or academic activities (e.g., "got the highest grade on a chemistry test"; "is working on a research project with a professor"), and another might reflect an interest in sports ("jogs 5 miles every morning"; "plays in a city softball league"). In a typical study, the stimulus set would consist of 16 sentence predicates, with four items representing each of four categories. The 16 items were always presented to subjects in a random order, with the constraint that items from the same category not occur in adjacent positions in the stimulus list.

All subjects received the identical set of behavior descriptions. Before this information was presented, two groups of subjects were established through instructions defining the purpose of the experiment and what the subject's task was. Half of the subjects were told that the study concerned the impression formation process and that they were to form an impression of the person described by the sentence predicates. To create a comparison group, the other half of the subjects were told that the study concerned memory for descriptions of actions and that they were to try to remember as many of the behavior descriptions as they could. Following a brief filler task, all subjects were given a free recall task in which they were to write down as many of the behavior descriptions as they could remember. Our predictions were that subjects who were forming an impression of a target person would organize the information in memory according to the four personality content categories represented in the behavior descriptions, and that this organization would facilitate later recall of the behavior descriptions.

In a series of experiments we analyzed both the amount and the organization of subjects' recall, and the results supported our hypotheses. First, with regard to the amount of recall, our results consistently showed that subjects given impression formation instructions recalled significantly more behavior descriptions than did subjects given the memory instructions (Hamilton et al., 1980a,b). Figure 11.1 shows the mean recall performance for subjects in these two conditions for seven different experiments (Hamilton, 1981b, p. 142). In each case the impression group significantly outperformed the memory group. This finding has now been replicated in numerous experiments by other investigators (Srull, 1981,1983; Srull, Lichtenstein, & Rothbart, 1985; Wyer, Bodenhausen, & Srull, 1984; Wyer & Gordon, 1982).

Second, in our analyses of the organization of subjects' free recall protocols, we found that subjects who formed an impression based on the behavior descriptions had organized this information in terms of the four categories of personality content to a greater extent than had subjects in the memory condition. This conclusion was based on analyses of categorical clustering in the subjects' recall protocols, that is, the extent to which items reflecting the same content category, which were dispersed in the stimulus sequence, were grouped together when they were recalled. Figure 11.2 shows these results for one experiment in which the stimulus items were presented either once or twice before the recall task was administered (Hamilton, 1981b, p. 144). The right-hand panel shows this

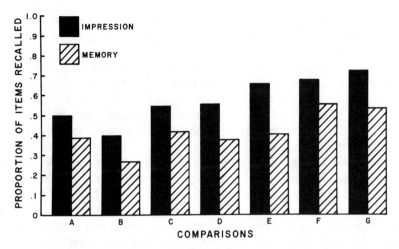

FIGURE 11.1. Proportion of items recalled by impression and memory groups in seven different comparisons. From Hamilton, 1981b, p. 142.

difference between the impression and memory conditions in amount of clustering, for both the one- and two-presentation cases.

As an aside, I might mention that measures of clustering tend to be related to the number of items recalled, and that this can sometimes pose interpretation problems. The left panel of this figure shows that, when the stimulus items were presented twice before recall was assessed, the difference between impression and memory conditions in amount of recall almost disappeared. Yet the right panel indicates that the difference in clustering, if anything, increased as a result of having two exposures to

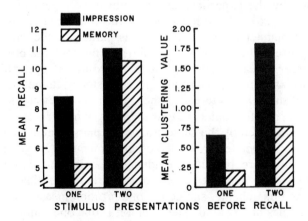

FIGURE 11.2. Mean recall and clustering values for impression and memory groups following one or two stimulus presentations. From Hamilton, 1981b, p. 144.

the stimulus information. Thus the two dependent measures are not inextricably related to each other and do not necessarily produce identical patterns of results.

This point was also made in another experiment in which we used a multitrial presentation and recall procedure (Hamilton et al., 1980b). In this case the same set of items was presented in a different order on each trial, and subjects' recall was assessed following each presentation. Again, the list of stimulus items included behaviors corresponding to four categories of personality content. Consistent with the previous results, the impression group recalled significantly more items than the memory group on the first trial, and this difference persisted for several additional trials. With repeated exposures to the same list of behaviors, this initial superiority in recall performance of the impression group gradually faded, and eventually the memory group achieved comparable levels of recall. Similarly, analyses of clustering in recall showed that, from the first trial, impression formation subjects organized the descriptive behaviors in terms of the categories of personality content to a significantly greater extent than did subjects in the memory condition, again replicating the earlier findings. However, in contrast to the results for recall performance, this difference between impression and memory conditions in categorical clustering did not decrease across trials. The impression group organized the descriptive information in terms of the prominent personality themes represented in the behavior sentences, and their recall consistently reflected this categorization.

The design of this experiment also permitted an analysis of Sternberg and Tulving's (1977) subjective organization measure. Whereas the clustering measures determine the extent to which subjects organize the information according to certain a priori categories built into the stimulus presentation by the experimenter, the subjective organization measure determines the extent to which subjects' recall is consistently organized in the same manner across trials. In this paradigm, the same stimulus items are presented on each of several trials, but they are presented in a different order on each trial. Therefore, if two items appear together on the recall lists for successive trials, this consistency cannot be due to the proximity of those items to each other in stimulus presentation. Rather, consistency in recall of pairs of items together, across trials, would reflect organization imposed by the subject in which pairs of items have become systematically associated with each other in memory. Subjective organization measures are based on evidence of this kind of consistency. Whereas clustering measures assess organization according to a particular categorization scheme, subjective organization measures reflect consistent groupings of any kind. The trade-off is that one cannot know what was the basis of the subject's organization that produced these consistencies. Analyses of this measure of organization in recall showed that the impression and memory groups were generally comparable. Although the impression group showed a slight advantage in the early trials, probably because of the relevance of the four personality categories to their task, the two groups were for the most part quite similar in degree of subjective organization across the set of trials (see Hamilton et al., 1980b).

Taken together, these results lead us to several conclusions.

1. We know from the subjective organization findings that both impression and memory groups achieve some form of organization in processing and storing these behavior descriptions.
2. We know from the clustering results that the impression and memory groups differ substantially in *how* they organize that information. Specifically, we know that the impression subjects, but not the memory subjects, organize the information in memory in terms of certain broad personality themes.
3. We know that these categories are immediately available to subjects whose task is to form an impression, as evidenced in their clustering values following one exposure to the information.
4. Although the subjective organization results suggest a comparable degree of organization in the two groups, the impression group's use of the personality categories appears to be a more effective means of organizing the information, at least for purposes of retention. This conclusion is based on the fact that impression subjects were able to recall more of the behavior descriptions than the memory subjects—a difference that persisted until subjects had had several presentations of the stimulus items.

In the studies I have reported thus far, all of the stimulus items described socially desirable behaviors and, in developing these stimulus sets, we avoided instances of inconsistency between behaviors describing the same person. Yet in forming an impression of another person we often encounter information that is inconsistent with other information we have already learned about the person. We are then faced with the task of either incorporating that information into the evolving impression or discounting it as somehow unimportant or irrelevant. In either case the perceiver must deal with this inconsistency, and how this is done has been the focus of a considerable amount of research in the recent social cognition literature. I want to turn now to a consideration of how inconsistent information is included in a cognitive representation of another person that develops during impression formation.

Memory Representation of Information Consistent and Inconsistent with an Impression

One of the most stable findings to emerge from research on person memory is that an item of information that is *inconsistent* with an initial impression is more likely to be recalled than an item that is *consistent* with that impression. This finding, first reported by Hastie and Kumar

230   David L. Hamilton

(1979), has been replicated in numerous subsequent experiments (Bargh & Thien, 1985; Crocker, Hannah, & Weber, 1983; Hamilton et al., 1980a; Hastie, 1980,1984; Hemsley & Marmurek, 1982; Srull, 1981; Srull et al., 1985; Stern, Marrs, Millar, & Cole, 1984; Wyer et al., 1984; Wyer & Gordon, 1982).

Much of the recent work on this topic has been conducted within the framework of a simple network model designed to account for this result. The model, first proposed by Hastie (1980; Hastie & Kumar, 1979) and later extended by Srull (1981), is shown in Figure 11.3. According to the model, the stimulus person is represented in memory by a "subject node," and information acquired about that person becomes attached to the node for storage in memory (indicated in Figure 10.3 by the vertical connecting lines). An expectancy or initial impression that the person possesses some dispositional characteristic—for example, that he is friendly—may be established either by presenting at the outset a set of homogeneous trait terms (Hastie & Kumar, 1979) or through the subject's accumulation of several behavior descriptions that convey that quality (Srull et al., 1985). The behavioral information describing the person includes some items that are consistent with that impression, some that are inconsistent with it, and some that are irrelevant to the trait dimension represented in the impression. The model proposes, and evidence supports, that information inconsistent with an impression spends more time in working memory as it is processed (Bargh & Thein, 1985; Hemsley & Marmurek, 1982; Stern et al., 1984), at which point it forms associations with other items of information already known about the person

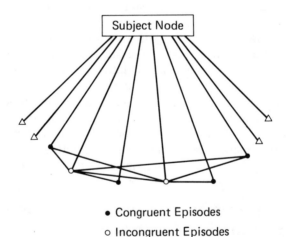

● Congruent Episodes
○ Incongruent Episodes
△ Irrelevant Episodes

FIGURE 11.3. An associative network representation of various tyeps of behavioral information describing the same person. From Srull et al., 1985, p. 319.

(indicated in Figure 11.3 by the horizontal connecting lines). This increased associative activity for inconsistent items probably involves attributional analysis directed at a causal understanding of the unexpected behaviors (Clary & Tesser, 1983; Hamilton, 1988; Hastie, 1984). In contrast, expectancy-congruent information is easily processed, spends less time in working memory, and does not form associative links with other items. Thus the horizontal connections shown in the model arise during the encoding of inconsistent items; they do not form as consistent items are processed.

An impressive amount of support for the implications of this model has accumulated in recent years (see Hamilton, 1988; Hastie, Park, & Weber, 1984; Wyer & Gordon, 1984, for reviews). I want to mention two findings in particular as a basis for discussion of some recent research of my own. First, Srull (1981) calculated the conditional probabilities associated with various kinds of item sequences in subjects' recall protocols. He found, for example, that recall of a *consistent* item was more likely to be followed by recall of an inconsistent item than by that of another consistent item, supporting the model's contention that consistent items do not become associated with each other during encoding. In contrast, recall of an *inconsistent* item was about equally likely to be followed by either type of item, supporting the notion that inconsistent behaviors form associations with both consistent and other inconsistent items. These conditional probabilities, then, parallel the pattern of inter-item connections represented in the model.

A second set of noteworthy findings comes from an experiment reported by Srull et al. (1985). The unique feature of this study was that subjects spoke their recall of the behavior sentences into a tape recorder, rather than writing down those they could remember. The experimenters then measured the time intervals between recall of successive items—that is, the amount of time that lapsed between speaking the last word of one recalled item and speaking the first word of the next recalled item. The idea being tested was that two items that are directly connected to each other in memory can be recalled quickly in succession, whereas if getting from one item to the next requires going back up to the subject node, the interrecall intervals should be longer. That is, transitions along horizontal pathways in the model should be quicker than vertical transitions. The model specifies that these horizontal connections will always include an inconsistent item as one of its end points. It therefore follows that interrecall intervals should be shorter when either the preceding or the following item is an inconsistent behavior. Srull and colleagues' (1985) results are shown in Table 11.1 They are consistent with the model's predictions. Successive recalls involving an inconsistent item occurred more quickly than did transitions where neither item was incongruent, presumably because these latter transitions required going through the subject node.

TABLE 11.1. Mean interresponse time(s) between
successively recalled items.[a]

Type of item subsequently recalled	Type of item previously recalled		
	Congruent	Incongruent	Irrelevant
Congruent	7.9	5.6	9.1
Incongruent	5.4	6.1	8.7
Irrelevant	9.4	8.8	9.3

[a] Data from Srull, Lichtenstein, and Rothbart, 1985.

Most of this research, however, has used a paradigm in which all information describing the target person, aside from a few irrelevant items, pertains to a single trait concept. There has been much less work investigating the effects of consistent and inconsistent information when subjects acquire information about *multiple* categories of personality content (for exceptions, see Wyer et al., 1984; Wyer & Gordon, 1982; Wyer & Martin, 1986).

In the research described earlier in this chapter we found that, in the process of forming an impression, subjects organized the behavior descriptions into meaningful personality categories, as reflected in their clustering of items in free recall. In those experiments there were no expectancy-inconsistent items in the stimulus list, so all of the behaviors presumably were consistent with the impression that evolved as the information was processed. One way (though not the only way) of thinking about these results is that such clustering reflects inter-item associations that formed among behavior descriptions within the same category as the information was organized and represented in memory. If this interpretation is viable, it conflicts with the assumption of the Hastie–Srull model that inter-item associations are *not* formed between pairs of items that are consistent with impression-based expectancies. There are, however, a number of differences between the paradigms used in our work and in the research on the Hastie model, as well as other findings in the literature, so that a definitive interpretation of this issue cannot be drawn at this point.

To investigate these issues more directly, Leila Worth and I conducted an experiment that combined features of the two paradigms. The basic features of the experiment are shown in Table 11.2. All subjects received 24 statements describing a person's behaviors. Three different trait concepts were represented in these behaviors, in ways shown in the table. There were always six items that were positive instantiations of the trait, which I have referred to as consistent items. In the first experimental condition these were the only behaviors representing these categories, and there were six irrelevant behaviors as well. In the next condition, the stimulus set also included two inconsistent behaviors pertinent to one of

TABLE 11.2. Distribution of stimulus items in various experimental conditions.

Experimental condition	Type of stimulus behavior						
	Friendly		Intelligent		Adventurous		Irrelevant
	−	+	−	+	−	+	
Consistent items only in all categories	6	0	6	0	6	0	6
Inconsistent items in one category	6	2	6	0	6	0	4
Inconsistent items in two categories	6	2	6	2	6	0	2

the personality categories. To keep the total number of items constant, only four irrelevant items were included. (Although the table shows inconsistent items occurring in the "friendly" category, there were actually three replications of this condition such that the inconsistencies occurred in each of the three categories.) The third condition extended this to the case where two categories included inconsistent items.

After subjects had completed a filler task, they were asked to recall as many of the behaviors as they could by speaking them into a tape recorder. These recall data were analyzed in several ways to explore the organization of the information in memory.

As in previous research, our results indicated that the proportion of inconsistent items recalled was significantly greater than the proportion of consistent items recalled. Our primary interest, however, was in how these consistent and inconsistent behaviors are organized in memory in relation to the three categories of personality content represented in this information. To investigate this question, it is necessary to go beyond analyses of the numbers of items of various types that subjects recalled and to examine other kinds of evidence that are potentially more diagnostic of how information is represented in memory.

In one analysis we calculated conditional probabilities to determine the following: Given that a consistent or an inconsistent item was just recalled, what was the probability that a consistent or an inconsistent item would be recalled next? These conditional probabilities were calculated separately for recall sequences in which both of the items in question came from the same personality category and in which they came from different categories. These values are shown in Table 11.3. Several aspects of these data are noteworthy. Consider first the top row, for the condition in which no inconsistent items were presented. This corresponds directly to the clustering studies I described earlier. It is clear that subjects' recall was organized by trait categories—that is, when an item from one category was recalled, the next item recalled was more likely to be from the same category than from one of the other categories. This finding essentially replicates our earlier results based on analyses of clustering in free recall.

TABLE 11.3. Conditional probabilities of recall

Condition	Item sequence[a]	Probability	
		Within category	Between category
Consistent items only			
in all categories	C–C	.47	.19
Inconsistent items in one			
category	C–C	.46	.17
	C–I	.18	.07
	I–C	.28	.19
	I–I	.22	—
Inconsistent items in two			
categories	C–C	.43	.19
	C–I	.13	.07
	I–C	.31	.20
	I–I	.15	.12

What happens when inconsistent behaviors are also presented in the stimulus descriptions? It is clear in these data that inconsistent items were organized within these trait categories as well. That is, regardless of the type of item sequence, the within-category conditional probabilities were uniformly higher than the between-category probabilities.[1] Thus, inconsistent items were more likely to become associated in memory with consistent items reflecting the same personality dimension than with consistent items representing other trait categories. Although this finding may not seem surprising, it does contradict some viewpoints represented in the literature. For example, Wyer and Gordon (1982,1984) have argued that inter-item associations are based on evaluative properties of the behaviors, and not on their descriptive content (see also Wyer & Martin, 1986). Our data did not support this interpretation.

Moreover, our results showed that, even when inconsistent items were present in the descriptive material, consistent items reflecting the same trait category were associated with each other. That is, given that a consistent item had just been recalled, it was quite likely that the next item recalled was a consistent item from the same category. This finding implies that consistent items within a category were more closely associated with each other than the Hastie–Srull model would suggest (Hastie, 1980; Srull, 1981).

The interpretive question then arises, why do we find this evidence of inter-item association between pairs of consistent items when other

---

[1] Given the distribution of consistent and inconsistent items in the stimulus sets (cf. Table 11.2), the various types of transitions indicated in Table 11.3 were not equally probable. We therefore compared the obtained conditional probabilities with values that would be expected on the basis of chance. In all cases the obtained within-category conditional probabilities were substantially higher than chance expectation, and the obtained between-category conditional probabilities were lower than the corresponding expected values.

researchers (e.g., Srull, 1981) have not? At this point we can only speculate, but we believe an important element may be that our experiment included behavioral information pertinent to multiple personality concepts, whereas in most previous studies all stimulus sentences have been consistent or inconsistent with a single trait concept. Intuitively, it seems that this difference would have an important influence on the subject's processing task. When all information is relevant to one personality dimension, processing an expectancy-consistent behavior simply requires matching it to the trait concept. Its "fit" with other consistent items need not be determined. In contrast, when the behavioral information includes descriptions reflecting several different concepts, the subject may not only match a consistent item to its appropriate trait, but also think about this behavioral fact in relation to other previously acquired items that were interpreted as manifesting that trait, as if to verify that the behavior has been construed in the most appropriate manner. Because any given behavior can be interpreted in alternative ways, it may be important to determine that it "fits" with other information already stored in that category. This latter step would result in the formation of inter-item associations between the consistent items. In other words, there may be processing differences for consistent items in the one-category and multiple-category cases.

Another analysis we conducted on these data was based on the interresponse times between successively recalled items. Following Srull et al. (1985), a shorter response interval between two items as they are recalled is assumed to reflect closer association between these items as they are organized and stored in memory. In particular, short intervals are interpreted as reflecting direct links between items, whereas longer intervals presumably reflect a retrieval process that included going back to the subject node between two successively recalled items. Table 11.4

TABLE 11.4. Mean interresponse times for different types of recall sequences

Condition	Item sequence	Mean response time(s)	
		Within category	Between category
Consistent items only in all categories	C–C	5.29	13.05
Inconsistent items in one category	C–C	4.94	8.41
	C–I	5.04	7.14
	I–C	10.11	7.60
	I–I	2.34	—
Inconsistent items in two categories	C–C	3.77	8.69
	C–I	6.91	9.30
	I–C	4.22	11.36
	I–I	4.10	5.79

[a] C, consistent item; I, inconsistent item.

shows the average interresponse times for the various conditions of our experiment.[2] The pattern of these results is quite similar to what we just saw for the conditional probabilities. Again, several aspects of the data are theoretically meaningful.

First, within-category response intervals were clearly shorter than those for between-category transitions. Despite one odd reversal of this pattern, both the consistency and the magnitude of this difference clearly indicate that behavior descriptions pertaining to the same personality category were organized and stored together in memory. Between-category transitions generally took much longer, indicating that distinct clusters of items were differentiated in memory.

Second, within-category transitions between two *consistent* items took about the same amount of time as other kinds of within-category transitions. In contrast to the predictions of some models (Hastie, 1980; Srull, 1981; Wyer & Gordon, 1984), this finding indicates that consistent items within a category may be linked directly with each other in memory. Of particular importance is the fact that, within the same descriptive category, these intervals between two consistent items were not meaningfully longer than transitions involving inconsistent items.

Third, the associations that inconsistent items formed with consistent items were limited to those consistent items in the same trait category. There has been some suggestion in the literature that an evaluatively inconsistent item may develop linkages with consistent items in both its

---

[2] Many subjects did not have complete interresponse time data because their recall protocols did not include all possible types of inter-item transition. For example, given the infrequency of both inconsistent items and between-category recall sequences, not all subjects would have a between-category C–I transition in their recall protocol. For purposes of data analysis, then, it was necessary to combine data from several individuals to form what Srull et al. (1985) called "pseudosubjects"—subgroups of subjects whose data are merged to form a complete set with values in all cells of the design. To do this, we first identified the type of transition that occurred with the least frequency (between-category I–I transitions). There were 11 subjects who had interresponse times for this transition. This value determined the maximum number of pseudosubjects we could have in the condition in which two categories had inconsistent items. We then created 11 pseudosubjects in each condition in the following manner. First, for each of the three stimulus conditions, 11 subjects were randomly selected from those who had interresponse time values for the least frequently occurring transition type in that condition. These subjects' data were combined with the data from 11 randomly selected subjects who possessed interresponse times for the next most infrequent transition type. This process continued until all 11 pseudosubjects in each condition included data for all possible types of transition. At that point all remaining subjects were randomly assigned to the 11 subgroups. For each of these 11 pseudosubjects (in each condition) the average interresponse time was determined for each transition type. The resulting data for these 33 pseudosubjects were then used in the analyses of interresponse times.

own and other trait categories (e.g., Wyer & Gordon, 1984). These data suggest that this is not the case.

Finally, there is some tentative evidence that *inconsistent* items from different categories may form direct associations with each other. This possibility is suggested by the bottom-right entry in Table 11.4—the mean interresponse interval for transitions between two inconsistent items from *different* personality categories. The average interresponse interval in this case was noticeably shorter than any other between-category transition, and it approached the values typical of within-category transitions. Because there were only two inconsistent items in each category and instances of their successive recall were infrequent, this mean is based on a relatively small number of data points. Hence this result must be viewed with caution. If reliable, however, this finding would suggest that, at least under some conditions, between-category inter-item associations are formed.

Person Memory and Impression Formation: A Recapitulation

At the beginning of this chapter I said that social psychologists study memory in order to understand more complex phenomena. In the case of the research I have discussed, memory data have been used to help us understand at least some aspects of the impression formation process. Let me try to put some closure on the various experiments I've presented by asking the following question: What have we learned about the nature of first impressions from studying memory for a target person's behaviors?

Taken together, the findings I have summarized indicate several features that must be included in any model of how information about another person becomes represented in memory. First, given that the perceiver's goal is to form an impression of the person, the information will be interpreted and organized in memory in terms of the meaningful personality categories conveyed by that information. Thus, items of information are grouped on the basis of trait concepts. I am *not* saying that this is the *only* way this information can be organized in memory (Hoffman, Mischel, & Mazze, 1981; Ostrom, Pryor, & Simpson, 1981; Pryor & Ostrom, 1981; Smith, Branscombe, & Zarate, 1986; Srull & Wyer, 1986; Trzebinski, McGlynn, Gray, & Tubbs, 1985). I *am* saying that the impression formation task often, and perhaps typically, inclines the perceiver to organize it in this way. This conclusion seems well justified by both the clustering results from the early studies and the conditional probability and interresponse interval findings shown in Tables 11.3 and 11.4.

Second, items in the same trait category become directly associated with each other as they are represented in memory. Several previous models have proposed that an *inconsistent* item will be linked with both consistent and inconsistent items, but these models have generally assumed that pairs of consistent items are not directly associated with each other. Our data indicate that this is not the case. Interresponse intervals for pairs of consistent items in the same category were as short as intervals between pairs that included an inconsistent item. Thus, *any* items *within* a category may be associated with any other item.

Third, these within-category associations are stronger and/or more extensive for inconsistent than for consistent items. This assumption is necessary to account for the higher probability of recall of inconsistent items than consistent items.

Fourth, there is little evidence that items reflecting one trait concept become directly associated with items representing another trait concept. Between-category transitions in recall probably require a retrieval route that goes from one category up to the subject node, and from there to another category. The one possible exception to this statement is that two items that are inconsistent with different trait concepts may themselves become directly linked to each other.

And finally, all of the properties I have just described about the representation of behavior-descriptive information in memory pertain to the case where the subject's task is to form an impression of the target person. The same information may be organized and stored in different ways when some other task or processing goal is engaged, as shown in the memory conditions of some of our experiments as well as in other task conditions used in other research (Cohen, 1981; Hoffman et al., 1981; Pryor & Ostrom, 1981; Srull & Wyer, 1986).

These findings illustrate effectively that the study of memory can help us understand certain aspects of how first impressions are formed. However, at the beginning of this chapter I also stated that a focus on memory alone will not be sufficient to provide a full accounting of complex social psychological phenomena, such as impression formation. This point is illustrated simply by thinking about the distinction between what we empirically investigate and the conceptual phenomenon we seek to understand. In person memory research we study subjects' memory for factual information they have acquired about another person's behaviors. Conceptually, we want to understand the nature of impressions. But impressions of others include more than the retention of facts that one has learned about them. An impression includes inferences about a person's dispositions, attitudes, interests, limitations, quirks and idiosyncracies, and so forth. An impression includes intuitive explanatory ideas about why the person is the way he is. An impression includes an evaluative sense of whether we like this person or not. None of these aspects of impressions is a part of what we typically study in person memory research.

From an information-processing perspective, an impression is a cognitive representation of what one knows and believes about another person—the perceivers's conception of what that person is like. Thus it includes both the factual information that has been acquired and the perceiver's inferential and evaluative elaborations on that information. In the history of social psychological research on impression formation, each of these components of impressions has been the focus of inquiry at one time or another. Asch's (1946) early work emphasized the importance of trait inferences that are made as first impressions develop, and impression formation research during the 1960s and 1970s focused specifically on the evaluative aspects of impressions (Anderson, 1981). As we have seen, the more recent period of person memory research has investigated memory for the actual information on which an impression is based. The complexity of the impression formation process will not be understood by limiting our attention to one or another of these components. Memory research therefore plays an important role in the study of impression formation, but the continuing challenge is to include all aspects of impressions in the models of these cognitive representations we develop.

Acknowledgment. Preparation of this chapter was supported in part by National Institute of Mental Health Grant MH 40058. I wish to thank Leila T. Worth for her contributions to the research reported in this chapter and for her comments on a preliminary version of the manuscript. I am also grateful to George R. Goethals, Diane M. Mackie, James M. Olson, Thomas M. Ostrom, Robert S. Wyer, Jr., and the participants at the 1986 Nags Head Conference on Social Cognition for their useful feedback in discussions of the issues addressed in this chapter.

References

Anderson, N.H. (1981). *Foundations of information integration theory.* New York: Academic Press.

Asch, S.E. (1946). Forming impressions of personality. *Journal of Abnormal and Social Psychology, 41,* 258–290.

Bargh, J.A., & Thein, R.D. (1985). Individual construct accessibility, person memory, and the recall-judgment link: The case of information overload. *Journal of Personality and Social Psychology, 49,* 1129–1146.

Clary, E.G., & Tesser, A. (1983). Reactions to unexpected events: The naive scientist and interpretive activity. *Personality and Social Psychology Bulletin, 9,* 609–620.

Cohen, C.E. (1981). Goals and schemas in person perception: Making sense out of the stream of behavior. In N. Cantor & J. Kihlstrom (Eds.), *Personality, cognition, and social behavior.* Hillsdale, NJ: Lawrence Erlbaum Associates.

Crocker, J., Hannah, D.B., & Weber, R. (1983). Person memory and causal attributions. *Journal of Personality and Social Psychology, 44,* 55–66.

Fiske, S.T., & Taylor, S.E. (1984). *Social cognition*. New York: Random House.

Hamilton, D.L. (Ed.) (1981a). *Cognitive processes in stereotyping and intergroup behavior*. Hillsdale, NJ: Lawrence Erlbaum Associates.

Hamilton, D.L. (1981b). Organizational processes in impression formation. In E.T. Higgins, C.P. Herman, & M.P. Zanna (Eds.), *Social cognition: The Ontario Symposium* (Vol. 1, pp. 135–159). Hillsdale, NJ: Lawrence Erlbaum Associates.

Hamilton, D.L. (1988). Causal attribution viewed from an information processing perspective. In D. Bar-Tal & A.W. Kruglanski (Eds.), *The social psychology of knowledge* (pp. 359–385). Cambridge, England: Cambridge University Press.

Hamilton, D.L., Katz, L.B., & Leirer, V.O. (1980a). Cognitive representation of personality impressions: Organizational processes in first impression formation. *Journal of Personality and Social Psychology, 39,* 1050–1063.

Hamilton, D.L., Katz, L.B., & Leirer, V.O. (1980b). Organizational processes in impression formation. In R. Hastie, T.M. Ostrom, E.B. Ebbesen, R.S. Wyer, Jr., D.L. Hamilton, & D.E. Carlston (Eds.), *Person memory: The cognitive basis of social perception* (pp. 121–153). Hillsdale, NJ: Lawrence Erlbaum Associates.

Hastie, R. (1980). Memory for behavioral information that confirms or contradicts a personality impression. In R. Hastie, T.M. Ostrom, E.B. Ebbesen, R.S. Wyer, Jr., D.L. Hamilton, & D.E. Carlston (Eds.), *Person memory: The cognitive basis of social perception* (pp. 155–177). Hillsdale, NJ: Lawrence Erlbaum Associates.

Hastie, R. (1984). Causes and effects of causal attribution. *Journal of Personality and Social Psychology, 46,* 44–56.

Hastie, R., & Kumar, P.A. (1979). Person memory: Personality traits as organizing principles in memory for behavior. *Journal of Personality and Social Psychology, 37,* 25–38.

Hastie, R., Ostrom, T.M., Ebbesen, E.B., Wyer, R.S., Jr., Hamilton, D.L., & Carlston, D.E. (Eds.) (1980). *Person memory: The cognitive basis of social perception*. Hillsdale, NJ: Lawrence Erlbaum Associates.

Hastie, R., Park, B., & Weber, R. (1984). Social memory. In R.S. Wyer, Jr., & T.K. Srull (Eds.), *Handbook of social cognition* (Vol. 2, pp. 151–212). Hillsdale, NJ: Lawrence Erlbaum Associates.

Hemsley, G.D., & Marmurek, H.H.C. (1982). Person memory: The processing of consistent and inconsistent person information. *Personality and Social Psychology Bulletin, 8,* 433–438.

Higgins, E.T., Herman, C.P., & Zanna, M.P. (Eds.) (1981). *Social cognition: The Ontario Symposium* (Vol. 1). Hillsdale, NJ: Lawrence Erlbaum Associates.

Hoffman, C., Mischel, W., & Mazze, K. (1981). The role of purpose in the organization of information about behavior: Trait-based versus goal-based categories in person cognition. *Journal of Personality and Social Psychology, 40,* 211–225.

Lachman, J., & Manis, M. (1983). Social cognition: Some historical and theoretical perspectives. In L. Berkowitz (Ed.), *Advances in experimental social psychology* (Vol. 16, pp. 49–123). New York: Academic Press.

Luchins, A.S. (1948). Forming impressions of personality: A critique. *Journal of Abnormal and Social Psychology, 43,* 318–325.

Markus, H., & Zajonc, R.B. (1985). The cognitive perspective in social psychology. In G. Lindzey & E. Aronson (Eds.), *Handbook of social psychology,* 3rd Edition (Vol. 1, pp. 137–230). New York: Random House.

Ostrom, T.M. (1984). The sovereignty of social cognition. In R.S. Wyer, Jr., & T.K. Srull (Eds.), *Handbook of social cognition* (Vol. 1, pp. 1–38). Hillsdale, NJ: Lawrence Erlbaum Associates.

Ostrom, T.M., Pryor, J.B., & Simpson, D.D. (1981). The organization of social information. In E.T. Higgins, C.P. Herman, & M.P. Zanna (Eds.), *Social cognition: The Ontario Symposium* (Vol. 1, pp. 3–39). Hillsdale, NJ: Lawrence Erlbaum Associates.

Pryor, J.B., & Ostrom, T.M. (1981). The cognitive organization of social information: A converging-operations approach. *Journal of Personality and Social Psychology, 41,* 628–641.

Schneider, D.J., Hastorf, A.H., & Ellsworth, P.C. (1979). *Person perception.* Reading, MA: Addison-Wesley.

Smith, E.R., Branscombe, N.R., & Zarate, M.A. (1986). Traits, roles, and goals as organizing principles in person memory. Unpublished manuscript, Purdue University.

Sorrentino, R.M., & Higgins, E.T. (Eds.) (1986). *Motivation and cognition: Foundations of social behavior.* New York: Guilford Press.

Srull, T.K. (1981). Person memory: Some tests of associative storage and retrieval models. *Journal of Experimental Psychology: Human Learning and Memory, 7,* 440–463.

Srull, T.K. (1983). Organizational and retrieval processes in person memory: An examination of processing objectives, presentation format, and the possible role of self-generated retrieval cues. *Journal of Personality and Social Psychology, 44,* 1157–1170.

Srull, T.K., Lichtenstein, M., & Rothbart, M. (1985). Associative storage and retrieval processes in person memory. *Journal of Experimental Psychology: Learning, Memory, and Cognition, 11,* 316–345.

Srull, T.K., & Wyer, R.S., Jr., (1986). The role of chronic and temporary goals in social information processing. In R.M. Sorrentino & E.T. Higgins (Eds.), *Handbook of motivation and cognition* (pp. 503–549). New York: Guilford Press.

Stern, L.D., Marrs, S., Millar, M.G., & Cole, E. (1984). Processing time and the recall of inconsistent and consistent behaviors of individuals and groups. *Journal of Personality and Social Psychology, 47,* 253–262.

Sternberg, R.J., & Tulving, E. (1977). The measurement of subjective organization in free recall. *Psychological Bulletin, 84,* 539–556.

Trzebinski, J., McGlynn, R.P., Gray, G., & Tubbs, D. (1985). The role of categories of an actor's goals in organizing inferences about a person. *Journal of Personality and Social Psychology, 48,* 1387–1397.

Wyer, R.S., Jr., Bodenhausen, G.V., & Srull, T.K. (1984). The cognitive representation of persons and groups and its effect on recall and recognition memory. *Journal of Experimental Social Psychology, 20,* 445–469.

Wyer, R.S., Jr., & Gordon, S.E. (1982). The recall of information about persons and groups. *Journal of Experimental Social Psychology, 18,* 128–164.

Wyer, R.S., Jr., & Gordon, S.E. (1984). The cognitive representation of social information. In R.S. Wyer, Jr., & T.K. Srull (Eds.), *Handbook of social cognition* (Vol. 2, pp. 73–150). Hillsdale, NJ: Lawrence Erlbaum Associates.

Wyer, R.S., Jr., & Martin, L.L. (1986). Person memory: The role of traits, group stereotypes, and specific behaviors in the cognitive representation of persons. *Journal of Personality and Social Psychology, 50,* 661–675.

Wyer, R.S., Jr., & Srull, T.K., (Eds.) (1984). *Handbook of social cognition.* Hillsdale, NJ: Lawrence Erlbaum Associates.

CHAPTER 12

Social Memory and Social Judgment

Robert S. Wyer, Jr.

One of the most frequent questions that social cognition researchers are asked by their colleagues (and to me one of the most irritating) is what distinguishes social cognition from cognitive psychology in general. My own reaction to this question is typically, "What difference does it make?" The categorization and subcategorization of disciplines is an exercise for the philosopher or linguist. It is of little concern to investigators themselves, whose work is guided by the specific phenomenon they consider important regardless of the label that someone else wishes to assign to it. Perhaps another source of my irritation at being asked the question is that I have never heard a very good answer to it, and have been frustrated in trying to come up with an answer myself.

However, there may indeed be an answer that has some more general implications, at least insofar as it pertains to research and theory in the area of memory. Memory research in cognitive psychology has typically evolved from a desire to understand learning and comprehension. If a lay person were to ask most memory researchers why their work is important, the researchers would probably point out its possible implications for understanding how people learn and retain what they read, and for knowing how to present material in a way that facilitates the acquisition of knowledge.

In contrast, social cognition psychologists come from a tradition that has been concerned primarily with how people make judgments and behavioral decisions. Thus, the researchers' ultimate objective is not learning per se, but rather how information acquired is actually used. Memory measures were initially introduced into social psychological research in the somewhat naive hope that the amount and type of information that people recall might provide insight into the cognitive bases of their judgments and behavior.

This distinction between the goals of memory research in cognitive psychology and the goals of memory research in social cognition may seem obvious. However, it is useful in understanding the sort of experiments that are conducted in the two areas and the scope of their theoretical and empirical implications. Investigators whose objective is to understand the determinants of learning are likely to study memory under conditions in which subjects are told explicitly to learn and remember the material they are presented. Theoretical formulations of memory that emerge from this work are therefore applicable primarily under conditions in which information is received and processed with this particular objective in mind.

In contrast, a social cognition researcher is likely to present information to subjects with instructions that they should use it to make some judgment or decision (to form an impression of the person it describes, to determine the person's suitability for a particular occupation, etc.). Thus, learning the material is not the subjects' primary objective, if it is an objective at all. The memory task that is later presented usually comes as a surprise.

If there is one thing we have learned from social cognition research over the past decade, it is that the goals people have at the time they receive information have enormous impact on their processing of this information, the cognitive representations that they form from it, and consequently, the aspects of the information that they retain (for a review of the role of goals in all phases of social information processing, see Srull & Wyer, 1986b). Thus, the conclusions based on this research, and the theoretical formulations of social memory that evolve from it, are likely to differ considerably from those that emerge from the memory research performed in many areas of cognitive psychology.

There is another implication of this discussion. That is, to the cognitive psychologist who is interested in learning and retention, an understanding of memory is often an end in itself. That is, recall and recognition indices provide the *criteria* for learning. When judgment tasks are used (as in the study of semantic memory, for example; see Collins & Loftus, 1975; Smith, Shoben, & Rips, 1974), this is done as a means of understanding the content and structure of memory.[1] To the social cognition psychologist, on the other hand, an understanding of memory is the means and not the end. Specifically, memory indices are tools in understanding one step of the judgment process, namely, the type of cognitive representations that are formed from information that people receive with a particular

---

[1] This discussion is not intended to imply that *no* research in cognitive psychology is concerned with judgment and with the relation between memory and judgments or behavior. A substantial body of research on inference and decision processes clearly exists (cf. Einhorn & Hogarth, 1981; Kahneman, Slovic, & Tversky, 1982). Moreover, research on problem solving is explicitly concerned with the factors that determine when different subsets of prior knowledge are retrieved and brought to bear on problem solutions (cf. Gick & Holyoak, 1980; Ross, 1984). In most of this research, however, the focus has been on retrieval processes and not with the structure and organization of memory.

goal in mind. An equally important question, but one that can be investigated only after the first question is answered, is how these cognitive representations, once they are constructed, are actually used.

The general framework within which social cognition psychologists operate is conveyed somewhat simplistically in Figure 12.1, which describes different components of the judgment process and how they are related. (For a more formal theoretical statement of these relations within the framework of a specific formulation of social information processing, see Wyer & Srull, 1986.) For clarity, independent and dependent variables are enclosed in solid lines, and the hypothetical constructs that mediate the relations among these variables are enclosed by dashes. Each pathway connecting two variables reflects a relation that msut be theoretically specified by a formulation of either memory or judgment.

The diagram is incomplete in many respects. For one thing, it does not recognize the important role that general world knowledge plays in all aspects of processing. Some observations based on this diagram are nevertheless worth making.

1. The sort of information processing that occurs, and the structure and content of the cognitive representations that are formed, are a function of *both* the type of stimulus information presented and the goals or objectives of the information processor at the time the information is

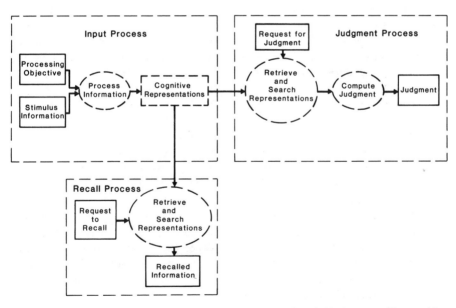

FIGURE 12.1. Relations among various components of social judgment. Observable (independent and dependent) variables are enclosed by solid lines and mediating variables by slashed lines. Rectangles denote "states" and ovals denote "processes."

received. The processes that occur may often be idiosyncratic to a particular combination of these variables. For example, subjects clearly process a set of trait adjectives and behavior descriptions differently if they are asked to form an impression of the person to whom they refer than if they are asked to learn and remember the information (Hamilton, Katz, & Leirer, 1980; Srull, 1981; Wyer, Bodenhausen, & Srull, 1984; Wyer & Gordon, 1982). By the same token, subjects with an impression formation objective may process this sort of information differently than they would process an episodic sequence of observed behaviors a person manifests in a particular situation (Allen & Ebbesen, 1981; Cohen & Ebbesen, 1979; Newtson, 1976; Wyer & Bodenhausen, 1985).

2. The mediator denoted "cognitive representation" is free floating. That is, it is bounded on all sides by other mediating variables. In one sense, then, it is simply a convenient metaphor for describing the results of information processing in a way that facilitates theoretical statements concerning the consequences of this processing for memory and judgment. There may, in fact, be several functionally equivalent metaphors for conceptualizing the cognitive representation of information. Nevertheless, whatever metaphor is chosen must be tied explicitly to the other mediating variables to which it is theoretically linked.

3. There is a clear parallel between the generation of "memory" responses and the generation of "judgment" responses. In both cases, subjects presumably retrieve and use some aspects of the cognitive representations they have formed of the information they received in order to generate an output. However, the particular aspects of the representation that are retrieved, and how they are used, depend on which type of output is requested. There is no a priori reason to believe that the cognitive material retrieved when subjects are asked to make a judgment, and the way it is operated on to arrive at this judgment, are in any way similar to the material retrieved and the operations performed when the same subjects are asked to recall as much information as possible. Therefore, there is no necessary relation between the implications of recalled information and judgments. In fact, the existence of such a relation appears to be more the exception than the rule (cf. Anderson & Hubert, 1963; Dreben, Fiske, & Hastie, 1979; Loken, 1984; Riskey, 1979; Wyer, Srull, & Gordon, 1984; for recent theoretical analyses of the conditions in which such a relation should and should not exist, see Hastie & Park, 1986; Lichtenstein & Srull, 1986; Wyer & Srull, 1986).

More generally, Figure 12.1 makes salient the fact that a comparable theoretical formulation of social information processing requires three models:

1. An input model, which specifies the way in which information is encoded and organized under different processing objective conditions.
2. A recall model, which specifies the manner in which these representations are retrieved and used in the course of recalling the information.
3. A judgment model, which specifies how the representations are used to make different types of judgments.

The second, recall, model may depend on the type of metaphor selected to describe the cognitive representations that are formed (e.g., an associative network metaphor, a push-down stack metaphor, etc.). However, it may be applicable under all conditions in which subjects are asked to recall information. Therefore, models of information retrieval developed in cognitive psychology may potentially be adapted for use in the present context. The input and judgment models, however, are likely to be specific to the type of input information presented and the goals of the receiver both at the time of information acquisition and the time of judgment. The formulations typically developed by cognitive psychologists interested in information acquisition per se are *not* likely to be applicable in the development of these latter models.

The goal of the social cognition psychologist is therfore to specify the nature of the relations between the various components of Figure 12.1. To attain this goal, memory data are typically used to infer the cognitive representations that are formed from information and the processes that underlie their construction. Once the nature of these representations is established, the ways in which the representations are used to make judgments can be conceptualized and empirically investigated.

The remainder of this chapter provides some specific examples of theoretical and empirical work in social cognition that fit into the general framework outlined above. These examples are drawn primarily from work done in our own laboratory. This is primarily for convenience, and not because equally good examples do not exist elsewhere. I will provide examples from two domains, one in the area of person impression formation and one in the area of event memory and judgment. The general issues of concern are the same in both domains. The specific conclusions to be drawn nevertheless depend very substantially on the processing objectives investigated, the type of information presented, and the type of judgments made.

Person Memory and Judgment

In the first area of research and theory to be described, the information that subjects are given typically describes a set of behaviors of a person in various situations. Sometimes, this information is preceded by a set of trait adjective descriptions of the person, and sometimes it is not.

Subjects receive this information for the purpose of forming a general impression of what the person described is like. As a result of numerous studies performed over the past several years, we have gained a reasonably clear picture of the sorts of cognitive activities that are likely to be involved in the formation of a person impression on the basis of this type of information and the cognitive representations that are formed as a result of these activities. We are now in the process of specifying how these representations are used to make different types of judgments of the persons to which these representations refer.

A complete description of the formulation we have developed and the research bearing on its validity is available elsewhere (Srull & Wyer, in press). Here I will try to provide a more informal description of the cognitive processes we believe underlie the formation of a person impression. Then I will give some examples of recent research that bears on these processes and when they occur. Finally I will discuss some of the research we are doing on judgment processes.

To convey what we think is going on when subjects form an impression of someone on the basis of trait adjective descriptions and individual behaviors, a concrete example will be helpful. Suppose subjects receive information about a person consisting of trait adjectives describing the person as kind and honest, followed by a series of behaviors of the person. Some of these behaviors are kind, others are unkind, some are honest, still others are dishonest. The representations we postulate as being formed from this information are conceptualized in terms of an associative network metaphor in which person, trait, and behavior concepts are represented by nodes and associations between them are represented by pathways. However, these pathways are presumably the result of specific cognitive processes that lead the concepts to be thought about in relation to one another.

The following processes are postulated to occur:

1. *Descriptive encoding.* First, subjects attempt to interpret each of the behaviors presented in terms of a trait that it exemplifies. In our example, if the target person is described as carrying groceries for an elderly woman, reading bedtime stories to his neighbor's children, and cheating on an exam, subjects would presumably interpret the first two behaviors as kind and the last one as dishonest. This cognitive activity presumably establishes an association between each behavior and the trait concept used to interpret it, or, to use our associative network metaphor, establishes a pathway connecting the trait and the behavior. If several behaviors are encoded in terms of the same trait, this results in a cluster of behaviors, all associated with the same trait concept. These trait-behavior clusters are independent, as the encoding process outlined above does not require thinking about the traits in relation to one another. Thus, the trait-behavior clusters formed from reading

three "kind" behaviors and three "dishonest" behaviors are shown in Figure 12.2 (top right). (Trait-behavior clusters pertaining to other attributes would of course be formed as well.)

2. *Concept formation.* Second, subjects extract a more general concept of the person as likeable or dislikeable. This concept is typically based on the first information presented. In our example, this information consists of trait-adjective descriptions of the person as kind and honest. Therefore, a concept of the person as likeable is formed. However, although this concept is primarily evaluative, it retains certain descriptive features of the traits on which it is based. Thus, the concepts of a likeable, kind person and a likeable, honest person may be evaluatively similar, but some descriptive features of these concepts may differ.

3. *Evaluative encoding.* Once the evaluative person concept is formed, the person's behaviors are interpreted in terms of their consistency with this concept. This interpretation is based primarily on evaluative

**Steps of Person
Impression Formation**

**Resulting
Representations**

1. Descriptive Encoding

a. Trait-behavior clusters

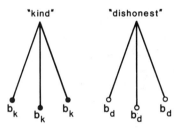

2. Concept Formation

b. Evaluative person representation

3. Evaluative Encoding

4. Inconsistency Resolution

5. Bolstering

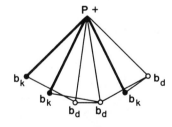

FIGURE 12.2. Cognitive representations formed on the basis of trait adjectives describing a person as kind and honest, followed by three kind behaviors (b_k) and three dishonest behaviors (b_d). P+ denotes a favorable evaluative person concept formed on the basis of the initial trait adjective descriptions. Wider pathways denote strong associations between the concepts they connect.

considerations (e.g., whether the behaviors are similar or dissimilar in favorableness to the general concept of the person who performed them). As a result of this cognitive activity, an association is established between each behavior and the person concept. The strength of this association is likely to depend on the features they have in common. Thus, behaviors that are evaluatively consistent with the central concept become more strongly associated with the concept than behaviors that are inconsistent with it. The result of this processing is an evaluative person representation that is independent of the trait-behavior clusters that were formed as a result of the encoding behaviors in terms of traits. Consequently, each behavior is typically contained in two representations: one trait-behavior cluster and the evaluative person representation.

4. *Inconsistency resolution.* As noted above, behaviors that are evaluatively inconsistent with the evaluative person concept do not form as strong associations with this concept as do evaluatively consistent ones. However, when an inconsistent behavior is encountered, subjects attempt to reconcile its occurrence (e.g., to understand why a bad person might do a good thing, or why a nice person might do something despicable). In doing so, they think about the behavior in relation to other behaviors the person has manifested, and this leads associations between these behaviors to be established. (For a similar assumption in other models of person memory, see Hastie, 1980.)

The implications of steps 3 and 4 in combination can be seen with reference to our example. As noted above, the evaluative person concept is based on the initial trait adjective description, and therefore should be favorable (P+). If these adjectives are followed by three kind (b_k) and three dishonest (b_d) behaviors in the order $b_k b_k b_d b_d b_k b_d$, the subject should form the two trait-behavior clusters noted earlier but also an evaluative person representation of the sort shown at the bottom right of Figure 12.2. Note that the kind behaviors, which are consistent with the evaluative concept, are more strongly associated with it than the dishonest behaviors, as indicated by the wider associative pathways. However, the dishonest behaviors, which are inconsistent with the evaluative person concept, stimulate thought that leads associations to be formed between these behaviors and others. For simplicity, the diagram assumes that each dishonest behavior becomes linked to the two behaviors that immediately precede it. However, assuming that the presented behaviors are often still in working memory when subsequent ones are presented, forward associations may occur as well.

5. *Bolstering.* Finally, subjects review the behaviors they have read about in an attempt to confirm the validity of the central person concept they have formed on the basis of the initial information presented. In doing so, they pay primary attention to confirming behaviors, thus further

strengthening the association of these behaviors with the central concept.

These, then, are the processes that we postulate to be involved in impression formation, and the cognitive representations that are formed as a result of them. Note that the *structure* of these representations is intimately tied to the *processes* that theoretically lead to them. Specifically, each pathway contained in these representations represents the consequence of thinking about the behaviors or concepts involved in relation to one another in order to attain some impression-related processing objective. The representations themselves, which are not thought about in relation to one another, are consequently stored independently at a memory location (e.g., "bin"; see Wyer & Srull, 1986) pertaining to the person to whom they are relevant.

Free recall data have typically been used to validate our assumptions about the nature of these representations and the processes that underlie their construction. (For support of the model using reaction time data, see Srull, Lichtenstein, & Rothbart, 1985.) Because these efforts have been successful, we have also begun to look at the way these representations are used to make judgments. Examples of each type of resarch are provided below (for a more complete summary, see Srull & Wyer, in press).

Recall

Suppose subjects are asked to recall the information they have read. To do so, they presumably retrieve one or more of the representations they have formed of the person from the memory location pertaining to this person, and search its contents for the information to be recalled. If the representation they happen to retrieve is a trait-behavior cluster, they should report the behaviors contained in it before retrieving and reporting the contents of a second representation. One implication of this is that recalled behaviors may often be clustered in terms of the trait concepts they exemplify, as found empirically to be the case by Hamilton et al. (1980; see also chapter 10 in this volume). A second implication is that if subjects are asked to recall both behaviors and trait adjective descriptions, their recall of the name of a trait concept should cue the recall of those behaviors that have become associated with this concept. That is, the likelihood of recalling a given behavior should be greater if an adjective describing the trait concept it exemplifies is also recalled than if this adjective is not recalled. Wyer and Gordon (1982) found this to be true as well.

Suppose, however, that subjects retrieve the evaluative person representation and use this as a basis for recall. Then things become more complicated, but also more interesting. The retrieval of behaviors in this representation is assumed to be the result of a sequential search process. Specifically, subjects presumably start at the central concept node and progress down a pathway to a behavior node, report this behavior, continue along a pathway to a second behavior, and so on, returning to the central node and repeating the process whenever they reach a dead end (i.e., a behavior that is not connected to any behaviors other than the one from which it is accessed). Some subtle implications of this sequential search process have in fact been supported in resarch by Srull (1981), and Srull, Lichtenstein, and Rothbart (1985). For example, note that as a result of the process we postulate as underlying the formation of interbehavior associations, inconsistent behaviors become associated with both consistent behaviors and other inconsistent ones. In contrast, consistent behaviors become associated with only inconsistent behaviors. This means that the likelihood of recalling a consistent behavior should be much greater immediately following an inconsistent behavior than immediately following a consistent behavior. This is in fact the case.

More generally, the conceptualization assumes that the recall of a given behavior is a function of two factors: (a) the strength of its association to the central person concept and (b) the number of ways of accessing it (i.e., the number of pathways leading into it). Considered in isolation, the first factor should give consistent behaviors a recall advantage. However, the second factor by itself should give inconsistent behaviors a recall advantage, as more pathways are typically connected to inconsistent behaviors than to consistent ones. The net recall advantage of consistent and inconsistent behaviors depends on which of these factors predominates.

Note that the factors that influence the recall of consistent and inconsistent behaviors are localized in different components of the overall process we are postulating. Specifically, the ease of recalling consistent behaviors is primarily the result of evaluative encoding and bolstering, whereas the recall of inconsistent behaviors is primarily a result of inconsistency resolution. Thus, the relative recall advantage of consistent and inconsistent behaviors should be influenced by variables that affect the likelihood of engaging in one or another of these processes.

Results support this line of reasoning. Many studies performed in this research paradigm have found a recall advantage of inconsistent behaviors. In a study by Srull (1981), however, subjects were presented behaviors serially, and were required to repeat each behavior aloud several times during the time interval between presentation of this behavior and presentation of the next one. Although this rehearsal might seem to facilitate learning, it also prevents subjects from thinking about the behaviors presented in relation to one another. Therefore, it should interfere with inconsistency resolution. As expected, the recall of inconsistent behaviors was greatly reduced in this condition relative to normal presentation conditions. In fact, it was nonsignificantly less than the recall of consistent behaviors.

In a more recent study (Wyer & Martin, 1986), some subjects were given a 5-minute distractor task after the behaviors were presented (a standard procedure that is used in most studies to eliminate short-term memory effects). Other subjects, however, were told to think more carefully about the information they had received and the person they were to judge. This latter condition was expected to increase bolstering. This appeared to be the case. Whereas inconsistent behaviors enjoyed their usual recall advantage over consistent behaviors in the first (distraction) condition, consistent behaviors gained a recall advantage over the inconsistent ones in the second condition.

One indirect implication of this analysis is that a priority system underlies the processes involved in impression formation. That is, it seems unlikely in many instances that people will have the time or inclination to engage in all of the various types of processing we have postulated. Therefore, when processing demands are high, certain activities may take priority over others. In fact, we postulate that the priorities given to these activities are reflected in the sequence of processing steps we outlined earlier, with one refinement. That is, descriptive encoding and concept formation take highest priority, followed by evaluative encoding, inconsistency resolution, and finally bolstering. However, in the case of inconsistency resolution and bolstering, subjects give priority to behaviors that are descriptively related to the central person concept over behaviors that are only evaluatively related to this concept. (Thus, if a person's likeableness is based on the fact that the person is kind, reconciling the occurrence of an unkind behavior takes priority over reconciling the occurrence of a dishonest one, and bolstering the concept of the person with a kind behavior takes priority over bolstering it with an honest one.)

The priorities given to the various processes involved in impression formation can be inferred from the rate at which the recall of each type of behavior increases with the amount of time that subjects are given to consider it. Specifically, if the recall of one type of behavior increases to asymptote more rapidly than the recall of another type, it means that the process that theoretically underlies the recall of the first type of behavior has relatively greater priority than the process that underlies the recall of the second. This logic was applied in a study by myself, Lee Budesheim, and Leonard Martin (1986). Subjects were given expectancies that a person had a particular trait (e.g., kind), followed by 36 behaviors that were either kind (i.e., both evaluatively and descriptively consistent with the trait), unkind (both evaluatively and descriptively inconsistent with the trait), honest (only evaluatively consistent with the trait), or dishonest (only evaluatively inconsistent with the trait). Each of these behaviors was presented for either a short (4 s), moderate (8 s) or long (12 s) time. In addition, we gave subjects the expectation they would receive either a small number of behaviors (20) or a large number (90). This was done because we thought that the processing strategies subjects might adopt would depend on how much information they thought they would have to consider. This turned out to be the case.

Figure 12.3 shows the effect of study time on the recall of each type of behavior. The top two panels present the results obtained when subjects anticipated receiving only a small amount of information. In this case, the recall of descriptively inconsistent behaviors increased to asymptote much more quickly with an increase in study time than did the recall of any other type of behavior. This suggests that descriptive inconsistency resolution took priority over both evaluative inconsistency resolution and bolstering, as we expected.

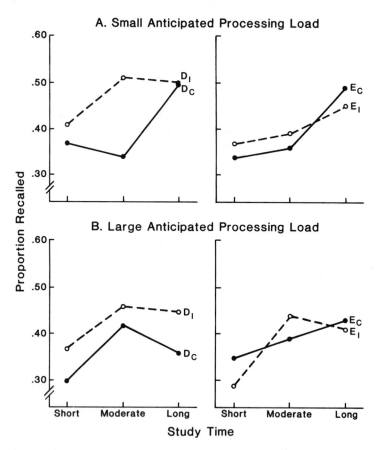

FIGURE 12.3. Proportion of behaviors recalled as a function of study time under conditions in which (A) subjects anticipated receiving a small number of behaviors and (B) subjects anticipated receiving a large number of behaviors. D_C and D_I denote behaviors that are descriptively consistent and the descriptively inconsistent with the central person concept, respectively, and E_C and E_I denote behaviors that are only evaluatively consistent and evaluatively inconsistent with this concept, respectively.

Note that the results confirm our interpretation of earlier research. That is, the recall advantage of inconsistent over consistent behaviors is appreciable only when behaviors are presented for a moderate length of time, and so subjects engage in inconsistency resolution but not bolstering. When study time is very short, subjects do not engage in either bolstering or inconsistency resolution, and so their recall of both consistent and inconsistent behaviors is low. When the behaviors are presented for a long time, subjects engage in bolstering as well as inconsistency resolution, and so their recall of both consistent and inconsistent behaviors is high.

The question arises as to whether these results reflect differences in subjects' ability to perform all of the cognitive activities we postulate within the time period available, or whether they reflect a processing strategy that subjects apply intentionally at the time they receive the information. Subjects who anticipate receiving only a small amount of information may believe that their task is a simple one, and that it is unnecessary to engage in extensive on-line processing of the behaviors as they are presented. Consequently, they may typically defer low priority activities until all of the information is in, engaging in these activities only if they have a lot of time available and nothing else to do. If this is so, the likelihood of engaging in these activities on-line may increase when subjects anticipate receiving more information than they can keep in mind. The data obtained under large anticipated load conditions, shown in the bottom of Figure 12.3, suggest that this is the case. That is, descriptively consistent and evaluatively inconsistent behaviors both increase much more quickly with a moderate increase in presentation time than they did under small anticipated load conditions. In other words, evaluative inconsistency resolution and descriptive bolstering appear to be given increased priority under these conditions. In contrast, evaluative bolstering, which presumably has the lowest priority of those activities we have identified, does not seem to be performed extensively at all.

These results tell us several things. First, they confirm the fact that person impression formation is not a unitary process. Rather, it involves several different component processes, each of which may have a different effect on the cognitive representations formed of a person. Second, the number and type of impression-directed cognitive activities that subjects perform not only may depend on the time and effort that they are able to devote to these activities, but also may be the result of intentional information-processing strategies that subjects believe will best attain their objectives under the conditions in which they find themselves.

An analysis of impression formation into different component processes permit a variety of questions to be raised that are of both theoretical and empirical interest. Many individual and situational differences in people's memory for information may reflect differences in the strategies they used to process this information at the time it was first presented. As but one example, suppose people recall different amounts and types of information about members of social or ethnic groups to which they belong than about outgroup members. This could be due in part to differences in the expectancies held for ingroup and outgroup members, which lead different behaviors to be regarded as inconsistent or consistent. However, it could also result from differences in the priorities given to inconsistency resolution or bolstering, independently of expectations. Procedures similar to those employed in the study described above could potentially be used to investigate this question.

Judgment Processes

The above results exemplify our use of recall data to understand the processes that underlie impression formation and the cognitive representations that result from them. Given that the nature of these representations is reasonably well established, it is now possible to ask the next question, namely, how these representations are used as a basis for judgments. Our judgment model is fairly simple, and consists mainly of three postulates:

Postulate 1. When subjects are asked to judge a person, they first attempt to identify a representation of the person whose central concept has direct implications for this judgment.

Postulate 2. If subjects find a representation whose central (defining) concept has direct implications for the judgment they wish to make, they use this concept as a basis for their judgment without reviewing the individual behaviors that are associated with it.

Postulate 3. If subjects do not find such a representation, they default to the general evaluation-based person representation and base their judgment on both (a) the evaluative implications of the central concept defining this representation and (b) the descriptive implications, if any, of a subset of the associated behaviors, identified as the result of a partial review of these behaviors.

On the basis of these postulates, one can see why there is unlikely to be any consistent relation between the implications of recalled information and judgments. Suppose subjects are given a series of kind behaviors followed by a series of dishonest ones. Presumably, this will lead to the formation of two trait-behavior clusters, one pertaining to "kind" and the other to "dishonest." Also, in the absence of an a priori trait description of the person, subjects should extract a favorable evaluative person concept (P+) from the implications of the initial (kind) behaviors. Thus, the representations formed should resemble those in Figure 12.4. (For simplicity, only two behaviors of each type are shown.) If subjects are asked to judge the person's honesty and kindness, they should base their

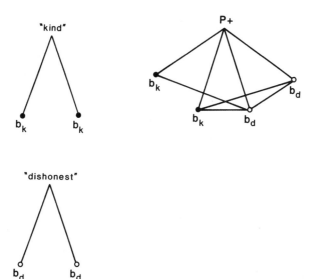

FIGURE 12.4. Cognitive representations formed of a person based on a series of kind behaviors (b_k) followed by a series of dishonest behaviors (b_d). For simplicity, only two behaviors of each type are shown. P+ denotes a favorable evaluative person concept formed on the basis of the first (kind) behaviors presented.

judgments on the concepts defining the trait-behavior clusters that are relevant to these judgments. In addition, they should judge the person's likeableness on the basis of the central concept defining the evaluative person representation (P+). In other words, they should judge the person to be kind, dishonest, and likeable.

But now suppose subjects are asked to recall the behaviors. The behaviors they recall will depend to some extent on which representation they happen to retrieve. If subjects retrieve the evaluative person representation, however, they should recall the last (dishonest) behaviors better than the first (kind) ones, because the last behaviors are inconsistent with the central person concept and therefore have become associated with more other behaviors as a result of inconsistency resolution. This reasoning implies that likeableness judgments will be influenced primarily by the initial behaviors presented, whereas the last behaviors presented will be better recalled. In fact, results of several studies (e.g., Dreben et al., 1979; Riskey, 1979) support this prediction.

To provide a more direct test of the judgment postulates noted above, we have used a procedure that has some interest in its own right. Specifically, we simply tell subjects to disregard different subsets of the behaviors we present under conditions similar to those described above, and determine the effects of this to-be-disregarded information on different types of judgments. To see how this works, suppose for simplicity that subjects are presented the same series of behaviors described above with instructions to form an impression of the person. After the first set of (e.g., kind) behaviors are presented, however, the experimenter interrupts them, tells them that a horrible mistake has been made, that all of the behaviors they have read so far pertain to a totally different person than the one they are supposed to consider, and that they should consequently disregard these behaviors. At the time subjects are given these instructions, the representations they have formed presumably resemble those on the left side of Figure 12.5A. We assume that once representations have been formed, they cannot be erased from memory. However, subjects are presumably able to restart the impression formation process. That is, they form new representations similar to those shown on the right of Figure 12.5A and store them in a new location, thus segregating them from the original, to-be-disregarded representations.

Suppose subjects are now asked to judge the target's traits and general likeableness. They should judge the person to be dishonest and dislikeable, on the basis of the concepts defining the trait-behavior cluster and the evaluative person representation they have retained for consideration. According to Postulate 3, they should also judge the person to be unkind, on the basis of the implications of the evaluative person representation and a partial review of the behaviors contained in it (none of which have descriptive implications for the judgment in this case). In other words, the to-be-disregarded behaviors should have no effect relative to a condition in which these behaviors were never presented in the first place. Nevertheless, suppose subjects are asked to recall the to-be-disregarded behaviors. In doing so, they presumably review the contents of the original memory location containing the representations they had begun to form before being told to ignore the behaviors. Therefore, they should recall the to-be-disregarded behaviors very well, as these behaviors are the only ones in the representations stored at this location.

However, now suppose subjects are presented all of the behaviors without interruption, but then are told to disregard the *last* behaviors in the series (i.e., dishonest ones). In this case, all three representations have already been formed and cannot be erased from memory. However, subjects may segregate the two judgment-relevant representations from the dishonest trait-behavior cluster by copying them into a new location. If this is done, the representations that exist at the original location and the new location should be those indicated in Figure 12.5B. On the basis of the representations stored in this new location, subjects should judge the person to be kind and likeable. However, suppose they are asked to judge the target's honesty. Their judgments should be based in part on the evaluative implications of the central concept defining the evaluative person representation and in part on the descriptive implications of the behaviors contained in it (Postulate 3). Because the to-be-disregarded

A. First Behaviors Disregarded

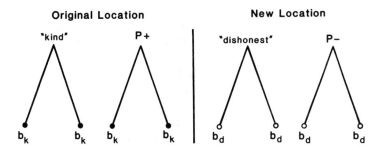

B. Last Behaviors Disregarded

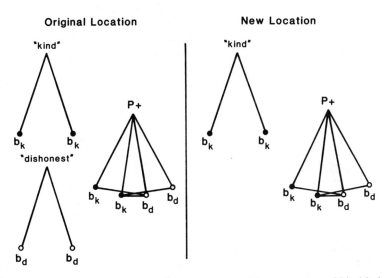

FIGURE 12.5. Cognitive representations constructed from a series of kind behaviors (b_k) followed by a series of dishoenst behaviors (b_d) under conditions in which subjects are (A) told to disregard the first (kind) behaviors presented and (B) told to disregard the last (dishonest) behaviors presented. Representations on the left are those stored at the original memory location (before subjects are told to disregard information) and those on the right are judgment-relevant representations stored at the new location.

behaviors are among the ones contained in this representation, they should in this case influence subjects' judgments.

Finally, suppose subjects are asked to recall the to-be-disregarded behaviors. As before, they should search for these behaviors in the original memory location. In this case, however, not-to-be-disregarded as well as to-be-disregarded behaviors are stored at this location (see Figure 12.5B). Consequently, the to-be-disregarded behaviors should be hard to identify.

In summary, this means that behaviors at the beginning of the series that subjects are to disregard should have little influence on either trait judgments or likeableness judgments, although subjects can recall the behaviors quite well if asked explicitly to do so. In contrast, behaviors at the end of the series that subjects are told to disregard should affect trait judgments but not likeableness judgments, even though subjects cannot recall these behaviors very well when asked to do so. In fact, these predictions were confirmed both by Wyer and Unverzagt (1985) and by Wyer and Budesheim (1987).

Wyer and Budesheim (1987) have also applied the judgment model outlined above to conditions in which subjects are not told to disregard the initial behaviors in the series until the remaining ones have been presented, and to conditions in which the to-be-disregarded and not-to-be-disregarded behaviors pertain to the same trait rather than to different ones. A discussion of the model's predictions under these conditions, which differ in several respects from those outlined above, is beyond the scope of this article. In the course of confirming these predictions, however, a further component of the judgment process was identified. Specifically, when subjects have formed a subjective judgment that they believe may have been influenced by information they have been told to ignore, they appear to adjust their report of this judgment to compensate for the bias. However, the magnitude of this adjustment is less when the to-be-disregarded information is favorable than when it is not. Consequently, behaviors that subjects are told to disregard have greater influence on their judgments when the behaviors are favorable than when they are unfavorable. In fact, unfavorable to-be-disregarded behaviors often have a negative, or *contrast,* effect on subjects' reported judgments, suggesting that subjects sometimes adjust too much.

Although the research outlined above does not provide a complete picture of the model's implications for person memory and judgment, it exemplifies our general research strategy. That is, memory data are used as a tool in understanding the cognitive representations formed from information, and thereby pave the way for research and theoretical analyses of the way these representations are used in judgment and decision making. It is important to note that the model is likely to be applicable under very circumscribed conditions, involving a specific type of stimulus information presented under specific task objective conditions, that is, when subjects receive a list of traits and behaviors with the goal of forming an impression of the person they describe. In fact, *none* of the effects described above occur when subjects receive the same information with instructions to remember it (cf. Hamilton et al., 1980; Srull, 1981; Wyer, Bodenhausen, & Srull, 1984; Wyer & Gordon, 1982).

Moreover, the representations formed from the type of information to which the model is applicable may not resemble those that are formed from the type of information we most often encounter in daily life. This latter information is typically extracted from sequences of temporally and causally related events that occur in a single situation or set of related situations. For this reason, much of our recent work has turned to a consideration of how event sequences are represented in memory and are later used to make judgments. This work is still in its preliminary stages, and the theoretical formulations we have postulated to account for what is going on are not fully developed. It may nevertheless be useful to convey briefly some aspects of our work that make salient the differences that emerge between the processing of event information and the processing of information of the sort to which our person memory model is relevant.

Event Memory and Judgment

Recall

Our conceptualization of the cognitive representation of event sequences has its roots in a more general theory of social information processing proposed by Wyer and Srull (1986). (The person memory and judgment model noted above can also be conceptualized within this broader theoretical context.) According to this theory, the knowledge we acquire is stored in memory in "bins" that pertain to persons and objects to which the knowledge refers. Each unit of knowledge, which may consist of either a single concept or a configuration of several interrelated concepts, is stored in a bin independently of other units. The theory therefore distinguishes between the organization of features and concepts within a knowledge unit and the organization of the knowledge units themselves. Within-unit organization is presumably the result of specific processes that occur at the time information is received that lead different concepts and features to be thought about or otherwise experienced in relation to one another. However, the representations themselves do not have any a priori organization. That is, they are stored in a bin in the order they are formed, and are retrieved independently as the result of a top-down search.

The implications of this for event memory were explored in a study with Galen Bodenhausen (Wyer & Bodenhausen, 1985). Briefly, we constructed a story about a person's experiences at a cocktail party from the time he arrived to the time he went home. Several distinct episodes were described, each consisting of a sequence of events that either occurred at the party or were mentioned in conversations among its participants. Of these, two were target episodes, each consisting of four temporally related events. (One, for example, involved Willa's learning that her father was dying in San Francisco, having too many drinks on the plane, being unable to find the hospital where her father was being cared for, and crying on the streets of San Francisco.) However, the study was constructed so that the events composing target episodes were sometimes described in chronological order and sometimes in the reverse order. Moreover, the events were sometimes described together and in other cases were separated by descriptions of several other unrelated events. Finally, the order of the target episodes was counterbalanced, with one mentioned early in the story and the other mentioned later. Subjects read the story with instructions (a) to form an impression of the party, (b) to empathize with the person from whose perspective the story was written, or (c) to remember what went on. Either 5 minutes or 20 minutes after reading the story, subjects in each condition were asked to recall the events described in it. Then, they were given a list of 25 of these events and were asked to place them in the order they were mentioned.

Impression-formation and empathy-objective subjects were both expected to reconstruct the events pertaining to a given target episode in their order of occurrence in the course of trying to comprehend them. However, empathy-objective subjects, unlike those whose goal was to form an impression of the party as a whole, were expected to treat the episodes as separate units of kowledge,and to store them independently. Data were consistent with these expectations. That is, subjects in both impression-formation and empathy conditions tended to recall the events within a particular target sequence in chronological order regardless of their order of presentation, and to recall the events together rather than apart. However, subjects under empathy conditions, unlike those in other conditions, tended to recall events in the last episode mentioned in the story before events in the first episode mentioned. Perhaps more interesting, these effects were evident under short delay conditions only in subjects' free recall protocols; when asked to order the events in terms of when they were presented, they could do this quite well under all task objective conditions. After a long delay, however, the effects of different processing objectives were evident in subjects' rank orderings as well. This suggests that subjects constructed representations of the event sequence in the course of comprehending it that they used as a basis for free recall, even though they could reconstruct the presentation order of the events on the basis of material still available in working memory. After a delay, however, only the representations they had formed and stored in long-term memory were available, and so these representations were used as a basis for responses to *both* the free recall and the ordering task.

Judgment Processes

Although the above data do not provide a very complete picture of how event sequences are organized in memory, they do suggest that an important factor in this organization is their temporal relatedness (for a similar conclusion, see Barsalou & Sewell, 1985). The question is whether this temporal organization plays a role in judgments, and if so, in what way. The answer may depend on the nature of the judgment. Suppose subjects who have constructed a temporally organized sequence of events are asked to verify the occurrence of some specific event. In this case, it seems reasonable that subjects will engage in a linear search of the representation in order to identify the detail. A similar sequential search may occur if subjects are asked to make a trait judgment; that is, subjects may perform a linear search of the representation until they find sufficient trait-relevant information to make a judgment. In support of these possibilities, Allen and Ebbesen (1981) found that both the time required to verify behavior details and the time required to make trait judgments typically increased with the length of a previously observed videotaped sequence on which judgments were based.[2]

However, other sorts of judgments may invoke quite different processes. For example, suppose subjects are simply given two of the events in a temporally related sequence and asked which one comes first. It is conceivable that subjects in this condition would try to connect the two events in the sequence. If this were so, the time to make the judgment should increase with the distance between them. In fact, however, the opposite is the case. This is true both when the events being compared come from scripted event sequences such as eating at a restaurant (Galambos & Rips, 1982; Nottenburg & Shoben, 1980) and when they are taken from nonscripted, episodic sequences involving a particular person (Wyer, Shoben, Fuhrman, & Bodenhausen, 1985).

In accounting for the data reported in this latter study, we proposed a model that not only specifies the processes involved in making temporal order judgments, but also states in more detail the encoding and organization of the event sequences on which these judgments are based. Suppose subjects read about a sequence of events that occurs to a particular person during the course of a day. We assume that in the course of comprehending this sequence, subjects break it into categories, each of which is defined in terms of a more general concept. They then identify each category with both a descriptive code denoting the name of the concept it exemplifies and a temporal code that indicates its position in

---

[2] In the case of trait judgments, the effect of tape length on response time depended on the type of trait being judged. Specifically, the time to judge traits that (based on normative data) required many behavioral instances to verify increased with tape length. In contrast, judgments of traits that required only one or two instances to verify took the same amount of time regardless of tape length. This suggests that subjects conducted an exhaustive search of the event sequence in the first case, but stopped after identifying the first relevant piece of information in the second case.

relation to other categories. However, subjects do *not* assign temporal codes to the individual events that are contained in each category.

As an example, consider an elaborated version of Willa's experience, consisting of the nine events listed in Figure 12.6. These events may be broken into three categories defined by the concepts "learning her father is dying," "getting drunk on the plane," and "getting lost in San Francisco," and these categories may be assigned temporal codes semantically equivalent to "early," "middle," and "late." However, subjects do not bother to assign distinctive temporal codes to the events contained in each category, as their order can be constructed if necessary on the basis of general world knowledge about the logical and causal relatedness of the type of events involved. Therefore, the representation might resemble that shown at the bottom of the figure. This sequence, as Wyer and Bodenhausen assumed, may then be stored in memory as a single knowledge unit.

Now suppose that some time later, subjects are presented pairs of these events and are asked to decide which one comes sooner, or alternatively, which comes later. A judgment process consisting of three general steps is postulated.

1. *Identification.* The subject first identifies the category in which each event is contained, based on a comparison of the features of the event and those of the concept that the category exemplifies.
2. *Comparison.* The subject then compares the temporal codes assigned

a. The telephone rings
b. Willa gets out of bed
c. Willa learns her father is dying
d. Willa gets on the plane
e. Willa has three drinks
f. Willa feels dizzy
g. The plane lands in San Francisco
h. Willa can't find the hospital
i. Willa breaks into tears

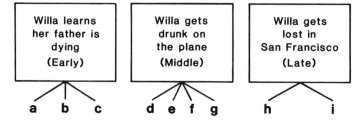

FIGURE 12.6. Example of an episodic event sequence and the cognitive representation formed from it.

to the categories identified on the basis of step 1. If the codes differ (i.e., if the events are in different categories), the temporal order of the events can be determined immediately. If the codes are identical (i.e., if the events are in the same category), further processing is necessary. That is, the subject must compute the temporal order of the actions through a variety of retrieval and reconstructive processes on the basis of general world knowledge.
3. *Response generation.* Finally, the subject generates an overt response to the specific question being asked on the basis of the results of step 2.

Given these assumptions, the response time to judge the order of two events (RT) is simply the sum of the times required to complete these steps, or

$$RT = t_O + t_I + t_{C,1} + t_{C,2} + t_R$$

where t_O is the base time needed to make all judgments and includes factors such as encoding and reading time, t_I is the time required to identify the concepts to which the events to be compared are relevant, $t_{C,1}$ is the time required to compare the temporal codes assigned to these concepts, $t_{C,2}$ is the time required to compute the relative order of the events that exemplify the same concept, and t_R is the time required to transform the results of this subjective comparison into an overt response. Note that when the actions being compared are relevant to different concepts, $t_{C,2} = 0$.

Several predictions can be made on the basis of this conceptualization, based on assumptions about the factors that mediate judgments at each stage of processing.

Influences on Identification

Subjects should take less time to identify the category in which an event is contained if the boundaries of the category are clearly defined than if they are fuzzy. The categories in our example have relatively fuzzy boundaries. For example, "going to the airport" might be relevant to the concept "learning her father is dying" as well as to "getting drunk on the plane." However, suppose the first three events in the overall sequence had been "the alarm rings," "willa gets out of bed," and "Willa eats breakfast," and that the last two were "Willa goes shopping" and "Willa buys a sweater." These categories of events might be encoded in terms of the concepts "gets up in the morning" and "goes shoping," the boundaries of which may be more clearly distinguished from the boundaries of "gets drunk on the plane." Thus, identification time should be less in this case. Consistent with this hypothesis, we found that subjects' judgment times were less when the first and last sets of events pertained to getting up and going shopping, respectively, than when they were thematically related to the middle set.

Similar considerations suggest that it should be easier to identify the category in which an event is contained if the event occurs in the middle of the series of events to which the category refers than it it occurs near the boundaries, or the transition between one category and the next. Consistent with this prediction, judgment times in our study were faster when one of the events compared was in the middle of the center category than when it was near a boundary.

Effects on Comparison Time

A strong implication of the formulation is that it should take less time to compare events if they belong to different categories than if they belong to the same category. This is because in the first case, their order can be determined on the basis of the temporal codes assigned to the categories, whereas in the second case, additional processing is necessary. This was clearly the case in our study.

This latter difference, incidentally, can account for the fact that events are typically discriminated more quickly when they are far apart in the overall sequence than when they are close together. This effect, incidentally, is similar to the "symbolic distance" effect that occurs when comparative judgments are made of other types of stimuli (cf. Banks, 1977; Holyoak & Patterson, 1981). That is, the time to compare two items decreases as the number of items separating them in the series increases. In the present situation, however, note that the likelihood that the events being compared belong to different categories also increases with the distance between them. Therefore, response times on the average should be less at greater distances for this reason alone. According to this interpretation, however, there should not be any effect of symbolic distance on judgment times when comparisons are restricted to either between-category comparisons alone or within-category comparisons alone. This was indeed the case in our study.

Effects on Response Generation Time

In previous research on temporal order judgments, and comparative judgments more generally (Banks, 1977; Galambos & Rips, 1982; Nottenburg & Shoben, 1980), a semantic congruity effect has occurred. That is, events near the beginning of the series are judged more quickly when subjects are asked which comes sooner, whereas those at the end are judged more quickly when subjects are asked which comes later. This difference is presumably a result of factors that come into play during step 3 of the process we postulate. Specifically, if the language in which subjects express the results of their subjective comparisons in step 2 is semantically congruent with the attribute specified in the question being asked, less time is required to translate these results into the language required to make an overt response. If this is so, however, this effect should be most likely to occur when the comparison made in step 2 is based on semantic temporal codes. According to the proposed formulation, the categories used to organize the events being judged are assigned such codes, but the events contained in them are not. Therefore, judgments of events that belong to the same category should not show a congruity effect. The small number of categories into which events were presumably divided in this study prevented us from knowing whether a between-category congruity effect occurred. However, there was clearly no within-category effect. In fact, no congruity effects at all were evident on our study, quite in contrast to results obtained when events composing scripted event sequences are judged on the basis of general world knowledge (Galambos & Rips, 1982; Nottenburg & Shoben, 1980). In combination, data suggest that the individual events composing well-learned sequences of events, such as those involved in eating at a restaurant, may in fact be assigned distinctive temporal codes of the sort assumed to produce congruity effects. However, the events composing episodic sequences of events pertaining to specific persons are not.

Conclusion

The conceptualization we have outlined above is in no way intended to be a complete model of event memory or event judgment. An enormous amount of work must still be done to develop such a model. A critical problem in conceptualizing the representation of events arises when a sequence consists of two conceptually distinct but temporally overlapping experiences. (For example, a couple may begin discussing abortion while eating dinner and finish the discussion in the living room after the dishes have been washed.) Whether such a situation is congnitively represented as a single event sequence, or as two different, overlapping sequences (e.g., "discussing abortion" and "eating dinner") is not at all clear. The representation of events that occur in an interaction between two people, which may also be viewed as either a single event sequence or two separate sequences (one pertaining to each person) is equally unclear. Galen Bodenhausen, Robert Fuhrman, and I are investigating these questions, but as yet we have no answers. Comprehensive models of judgment based on event information may have to await these answers.

Nevertheless, our approach in investigating these problems is philosophically similar to the approach we have taken in investigating person impression formation. That is, we are generally (although not exclusively) relying upon recall data to understand the manner in which event information is organized in memory. Then, given conclusions drawn from this research, we hope to develop judgments models that specify how these representations are used. In both areas we are a long way from attaining a complete understanding of social judgment. However, the approach we have taken holds the promise of ultimately achieving this understanding. In applying this approach, our conceptualizations of social memory are clearly not the end of the story. Indeed, they are just the beginning.

Ackowledgment. The research reported in this paper was supported by grants BNS83-02105 from the National Science Foundation and MH 3-8585, BSR from the National Institute of Mental Health. The author is greatly indebted to Galen Bodenhausen, Lee Budesheim, Bob Fuhrman and Leonard Martin, collaborators in most of the recent research described in this chapter and in the development of the theoretical ideas expressed, and of course to Thom Srull, whose collaboration with the author over the past several years is reflected throughout.

References

Allen, R.B., & Ebbesen, E.B. (1981). Cognitive processes in person perception: Retrieval of personality trait and behavioral information. *Journal of Experimental Social Psychology, 17,* 119–141.

Anderson, N.H., & Hubert, S. (1963). Effects of concomitant verbal recall on order effects in personality impression formation. *Journal of Verbal Learning and Verbal Behavior, 1,* 379–391.

Banks, W.P. (1977). Encoding and processing of symbolic information in comparative judgment. In G.H. Bower (Ed.), *The psychology of learning and motivation* (Vol. 11, pp. 101–159). New York: Academic Press.

Barsalou, L.W., & Sewell, D.R. (1985). Contrasting the representation of scripts and categories. *Journal of Memory and Language, 24,* 646–665.

Cohen, C.E., & Ebbesen, E.B. (1979). Observational goals and schema activation: A theoretical framework for behavior perception. *Journal of Experimental Social Psychology, 15,* 305–329.

Collins, AM., & Loftus, E.F. (1975). A spreading-activation theory of semantic processing. *Psychological Review, 82,* 407–428.

Dreben, E.K., Fiske, S.T., & Hastie, R. (1979). The independence of item and evaluation information: Impression and recall order effects in behavior-based impression formation. *Journal of Personality and Social Psychology, 37,* 1758–1768.

Einhorn, H.J., & Hogarth, R.M. (1981). Behavioral decision theory: Processes of judgment and choice. *Annual Review of Psychology, 32,* 53–88.

Galambos, J.A., & Rips, L.J. (1982). Memory for routines. *Journal of Verbal Learning and Verbal Behavior, 21,* 260–281.

Gick, M.L., & Holyoak, K.J. (1980). Analogical problem solving. *Cognitive Psychology, 12,* 306–355.

Hamilton, D.L., Katz, L.B., & Leirer, V.O. (1980). Organizational processes in impression formation. In R. Hastie, T.M. Ostrom, E.B. Ebbesen, R.S. Wyer, D.L. Hamilton, & D.E. Carlston (Eds.), *Person memory: The cognitive basis of social perception* (pp. 121–153). Hillsdale, NJ: Lawrence Erlbaum Associates.

Hastie, R. (1980). Memory for information which confirms or contradicts a general impression. In R. Hastie, T.M. Ostrom, E.B. Ebbesen, R.S. Wyer, D.L. Hamilton, & D.E. Carlston (Eds.), *Person memory: The cognitive basis of social perception* (pp. 121–153). Hillsdale, NJ: Lawrence Erlbaum Associates.

Hastie, R., & Kumar, P.A. (1979). Person memory: Personality traits as organizing principles in memory for behaviors. *Journal of Personality and Social Psychology, 37,* 25–38.

Hastie, R., & Park, B. (1986). The relationship between memory and judgment depends on whether the judgment task is memory-based or on-line. *Psychological Review, 93,* 258–268.

Holyoak, K.J., & Patterson, K.K. (1981). A positional discriminability model of linear order judgments. *Journal of Experimental Psychology: Human Perception and Performances, 7,* 1281–1302.

Kahneman, D., Slovic, P., & Tversky, A. (1982). *Judgment under uncertainty: Heuristics and biases.* New York: Cambridge University Press.

Lichtenstein, M., & Srull, T.K. (1986). *Processing objectives as a determinant of the relationship between recall and judgment.* Unpublished manuscript, University of Illinois, Champaign.

Loken B.A. (1984). Attitude processing strategies. *Journal of Experimental Social Psychology, 20,* 272–296.

Newtson, D. (1976). Foundations of attribution: The perception of ongoing behavior. In J. Harvey, W. Ickes, & R. Kidd (Eds.), *New directions in attribution research* (Vol. 1, pp. 223–247). Hillsdale, NJ: Lawrence Erlbaum Associates.

Nottenburg, G., & Shoben, E.J. (1980). Scripts as linear orders. *Journal of Experimental Social Psychology, 16,* 329–347.

Riskey, D.R. (1979). Verbal memory processes in impression formation. *Journal of Experimental Psychology: Human Learning and Memory, 5,* 271–281.

Ross, B.H. (1984). Remindings and their effects in learning a cognitive skill. *Cognitive Psychology, 16,* 371–416.

Smith, E.E., Shoben, E.J., & Rips, L.J. (1974). Structure and process in semantic memory: A featural model for semantic decisions. *Psychological Review, 81,* 214–241.

Srull, T.K. (1981). Person memory: Some tests of associative storage and retrieval models. *Journal of Experimental Psychology: Human Learning and Memory, 7,* 440–463.

Srull, T.K., Lichtenstein, M., & Rothbart, M. (1985). Associative storage and retrieval processes in person memory. *Journal of Experimental Psychology: Learning, Memory and Cognition, 11,* 316–345.

Srull, T.K., & Wyer, R.S. (in press). Person memory and judgment. *Psychological Review.*

Srull, T.K., & Wyer, R.S. (1986b). The role of chronic and temporary goals in social information processing. In R.M. Sorrentino & E.T. Higgins (Eds.), *Handbook of motivation and cognition* (pp. 503–549). New York: Guilford Press.

Wyer, R.S., & Bodenhausen, G.V. (1985). Event memory: The effects of processing objectives and time delay on memory for action sequences. *Journal of Personality and Social Psychology, 49,* 301–316.

Wyer, R.S., Bodenhausen, G.V., & Srull, T.K. (1984). The cognitive representation of persons and groups and its effect on recall and recognition memory. *Journal of Experimental Social Psychology, 20,* 445–469.

Wyer, R.S., & Budesheim, T.L. (1987). Person memory and judgments: The impact of information that one is told to disregard. *Journal of Personality and Social Psychology, 53,* 14–29.

Wyer, R.S., Budesheim, T.L. & Martin, L.L. (1986). *Person memory: The priorities that govern the cognitive activities involved in person impression formation.* Unpublished manuscript, University of Illinois, Champaign.

Wyer, R.S., & Gordon, S.E. (1982). The recall of information about persons and groups. *Journal of Experimental Social Psychology, 18,* 128–164.

Wyer, R.S., & Gordon, S.E. (1984). The cognitive representation of social information. In R.S. Wyer & T.K. Srull (Eds.), *Handbook of social cognition* (Vol. 2, pp. 73–150). Hillsdale, NJ: Lawrence Erlbaum Associates.

Wyer, R.S., & Martin, L.L. (1986). Person memory: The role of traits, group stereotypes and specific behaviors in the cognitive representation of persons. *Journal of Personality and Social Psychology, 50,* 661–675.

Wyer, R.S., Shoben, E.J., Fuhrman, R.W., Bodenhausen, G.V. (1985). Event memory: The temporal organization of social action sequences. *Journal of Personality and Social Psychology, 49,* 857–877.

Wyer, R.S., & Srull, T.K. (1986). Human cognition in its social context. *Psychological Review, 93,* 322–359.

Wyer, R.S., Srull, T.K., & Gordon, S.E. (1984). The effects of predicting a person's behavior on subsequent trait judgments. *Journal of Experimental Social Psychology, 20,* 29–46.

Wyer, R.S., & Unverzagt, W. (1985). Effects of instructions to disregard information on its subsequent recall and use in making judgments. *Journal of Personality and Social Psychology, 48,* 533–549.

CHAPTER 13

Thoughts on Interdisciplinary Approaches to Memory

Colleen M. Kelley and Benjamin R. Stephens

The aim of the conference from which this book is drawn is reflected in its optimistic title "Memory: An Interdisciplinary Approach." In pursuit of a complete understanding of memory, we can take advantage of the insights, data, and explanations from diverse areas of psychology: physiological, cognitive, developmental, and social. A number of the participants in the conference were invited not only because they are eminent researchers studying memory, but also because their approach integrates, spans, or straddles two subdisciplines of psychology. The argument ran something along the lines that "if A can talk to B and B can to talk C . . . , then an interdisciplinary approach will follow." We warned all participants that we wanted them to depart from their normal research talk. Instead, we asked them to use their own research to illustrate their areas's approach to memory, to point out what they see as the fundamental questions regarding memory, and to formulate questions they would like to have answered by the other areas of psychology represented at the conference.

The participants ably illustrated their various approaches to memory with examples from their research programs. They also pointed out what they consider to be fundamental questions regarding memory, which ranged from the physiologists' interest in tracing circuits in a model system (Thompson, Chapter 2) to the social psychologists' interest in the supporting role memory plays in impression formation (Hamilton, Chapter 11, and Wyer, Chapter 12). However, it was far more difficult for our participants to find questions that they would like each other to answer. Their interaction could perhaps better be characterized as polite attentiveness than as a meeting of the minds.

One roadblock to interdisciplinary work is the staggering difficulty of mastering several different domains. Most of us have a difficult time keeping up on reading within our subfield, let alone following what's new and interesting in neighboring fields. Two less pragmatic, but no less serious, problems for an interdisciplinary approach emerged from the talks and discussions during the conference. They are the problem of levels of analysis and the problem of defining memory.

The Problem with Levels (of Analysis)

Memory, like any phenomenon in psychology, can be approached at various levels of analysis. Marr (1982) distinguished three levels in his work on vision: computational (e.g., what computation must be performed in vision on incoming stimuli?), algorithmic (what particular algorithm does the visual system use to perform that computation?), and implementational (what hardware implements the algorithm?). Another subdivision delineates another three levels: neural, information processing, and experiential, with perhaps a fourth level that of the larger social and physical environment that people occupy (Massaro, 1986). This volume represents the latter entire spectrum, from the neural basis of behavior to information-processing analyses to collective memory.

These conceptions of the different levels of analysis are not simply descriptive. Marr (1982) used the concept of levels of analysis to reformulate the problem of understanding vision. Pribram (1986) recently used the concept of levels of analysis in an attempt to resolve the mind/body problem. However, the relationships among levels of analysis is not always so felicitous. One unfortunate aspect of taking a particular level of analysis as one's own is that the other levels tend to appear superfluous. For example, those who follow an information-processing approach may feel unconstrained by research on the biological or implementational level, because their information-processing model could be implemented in a variety of ways. Similarly, a model on the biological level can make a cognitive analysis seem redundant and unnecessary (e.g., Thompson's critique in Chapter 2, this volume). What, then, is an appropriate or productive relationship *between* levels of analysis?

Pribram (1986) proposed that the information represented at one level of analysis must be isomorphic to the information represented at another level of analysis. Thus, the order at one level is a transformation of the order at another level. To understand the whole system involves determining the transformation that makes information invariant across levels and, of course, characterizing order or structure on each level. That viewpoint, as in Marr's formulation (1982), stresses the importance of each level for understanding the complete system. No level is redundant. A critical part of understanding a phenomenon is to discover the transformations that link one level to another. With this approach, the psychophysics of vision has yielded an orderly description on the computational level, which is being linked to the algorithmic and implementational levels (Marr, 1982). Memory may be more intransigent to discovery of the links between levels of analysis. Unlike psychophysicists, we haven't yet discovered (or agreed upon) an orderly and complete collection of laws of memory (see Cohen, 1985), and so it is difficult in research on other levels to look to an information-processing analysis for the algorithm that needs to be implemented.

Broadbent (1985) argued for maintaining separation between levels of analysis. He insisted that a model at one level cannot use data from another level for support. For example, a physiological model that proposes distributed rather than specific memory representations cannot rely on data from cross-modality priming studies for support. Instead, such data apply to models at a more abstract level of analysis. Broadbent pointed out that the results from studies at a more abstract level of analysis could be implemented in a variety of ways, and so could not logically be used to confirm any particular implementation. Although the proponents of the model in question convincingly argued that their model was not an implementation model, but a model on the *algorithmic* level (Rumelhart & McClelland, 1985), Broadbent's (1985) argument is echoed by many who work on characterizing information-processing states, rather than neural states.

In contrast, Shallice (1979) made a compelling case for using data from one level of analysis to test models at another level of analysis. He argued that neuropsychological data, in particular evidence of double dissociations, can refute information-processing models. Shallice pointed out that this is not a reductionistic approach; rather the neuropsychological data are interpreted by information-processing models and in turn set limits on the number of feasible models. Baddeley (Chapter 5 in this volume) illustrates the heartening progress that stems from a thoughtful interplay of neuropsychological evidence and experimental analysis.

The Problem of Defining Memory

A second problem for interdisciplinary research in memory is deciding just what it is we are all talking about. The link between conditioning and conscious recollection remains unspecified, although the term *memory* has been applied to both (Hirst & LeDoux, 1986). In this volume, Thompson (Chapter 2), McGaugh (Chapter 3), and Rovee-Collier (Chapter 8) report their studies of memory as measured by conditioned responses. The remaining chapters investigate forms of conscious recollection, as well as semantic memory (Nelson, Chapter 7, and Kail, Chapter 9) and unconscious memory (Mandler, Chapter 5). What are the relationships between these various expressions of past experience?

Memory measured via conditioned responses may differ substantively from memory measured as conscious recollection. For example, Weiskrantz and Warrington (1979) found that amnesic patients express memory for classical conditioning by emitting the conditioned response, all the while denying that they have ever seen the conditioning apparatus. Such data may indicate separable memory systems (e.g., Cohen and Squire, 1980; Tulving, 1983). Multiple memory systems imply that on a neuropsychological level of analysis, dissociations can occur between types of memory. The implication for the cognitive level is that all bets are off. That is, one does not necessarily expect the same functions of encoding, retrieval, or forgetting to apply to both systems. For example, we might ask whether McGaugh's very interesting findings (Chapter 3) regarding the modulation of memory in avoidance conditioning apply also to the process of conscious recollection. Rovee-Collier (Chapter 8 in this volume) notes that infant memory may help bridge the gap between learning and remembering. She applies the terminology, and more importantly, the manipulations of human adult memory studies in her investigations of instrumental conditioned responses in infants. Thus, infants reveal memories by kicking, are reminded by very specific cues, and show forgetting functions over time delays. Her work stresses the commonality between memory measured by learning and memory measured by conscious recollection.

In addition to characterizing the differences and similarities between dichotomies such as conditioning and remembering, or between unconscious and conscious forms of memory, one can ask what, if any, is the relationship between the two. For example, Warrington and Weiskrantz (1982) suggested that amnesia represents a disconnection syndrome. The temporal lobe may be responsible for unconscious memory effects, whereas awareness of the past in conscious remembering may depend upon a "mediational memory system" in the frontal lobe. They proposed that in some amnesics, the connections between temporal lobe and frontal lobe functioning are severed. Although the amnesics can continue to show the effects of the past in their performance, they cannot consciously recollect. Mandler's model (Chapter 4 in volume) points to similar distinctions, but on a cognitive rather than a neuropsychological level of analysis. He proposes that conscious memories depend on elaboration between units in memory, whereas unconscious memories reflect the activation and integration of preexisting units.

One speculative account of the relationship between unconscious memory and conscious memory posits a functional relationship between the two (Jacoby, Kelley & Dywan, in press). Conscious recollection may be an attribution of the effects of the past to a particular source in the past. By this account, the past is expressed in very specific ways in behavior, perception, and thinking. Essentially, people respond more fluently when they repeat an experience (Jacoby & Dallas, 1981). Such fluency of perception and thinking is detectable and may be correctly attributed to the past, and so experienced as remembering. However, if the current situation biases people's attributions toward a source other than the past (c.f., Witherspoon & Allan, 1985; Jacoby, Allan, Collins, & Larwill 1988), they may instead misattribute their fluent performance to a quality of the current stimulus. Such a theory of conscious remembering as an attribution of changes in performances stemming from past experience is modeled on a social psychological theory of emotion as an attribution (Schachter & Singer, 1962). In that theory, a particular emotion such as anger or euphoria is experienced when people attribute their physiological arousal to a particular situational cause. The memory as attribution hypothesis predicts some common parameters for conscious and unconscious forms of memory, since a conscious memory is a particular interpetation of effects of the past that otherwise would be experienced as an unconscious memory. However, the two forms of memory would behave differently because the attribution process is unique to the generation of conscious memories. Although such an interpretation of the link between remembering and other effects of the past on performance remains speculative, we expect explorations of the relationship between memory in the strict sense and memory in the broad sense will be an important area for interdisciplinary research.

Integration Across Domains: Shared Models as Research Tools

One important exchange across areas of psychology involves the application of models of memory to domains that find them useful for investigating very different questions. This exchange is exemplified in this volume by Hamilton (Chapter 11), Kail (Chapter 9), Ostrom (Chapter 10), and Wyer (Chapter 12) (although Wyer and his colleagues have also developed their own models of memory). These chapters illustrate how researchers in social and developmental psychology use cognitive models and concepts, such as network structures and spreading activation, as tools to probe issues such as impression formation, social judgments, and language disorders. Clearly the goal of this research is not to evaluate the validity of the models per se, but rather to use the models to design tasks and guide thinking in the particular area of interest. In a sense, then, the model-building process undertaken by researchers in cognitive psychology serves as the basis of work in other domains, which borrow the work and apply it to other problems. This type of exchange across domains is the primary type of integration observed in symposia that focus on interdisciplinary research.

One attribute of such integration between the cognitive and other areas is that the exchange often is a "one-way street." The transfer of ideas and observations is mainly from the cognitive area to the other areas. There is little if any feedback from the efforts of the social and developmental psychologists to the cognitive psychologists. There are many possible reasons for this one-way interaction. One is that the current work of the cognitive psychologists seems to be a few steps beyond the particular models that the other psychologists use in their research. Researchers in other domains may be cautious and unwilling to embrace new concepts and ideas in their quest for useful research tools. Alternatively, the older models may be sufficient for many of the questions that researchers are addressing. Kail provides a good example of this second alternative. His work, aimed at identifying the locus of language disorders involved in word-finding problems, seems well-served by concepts such as distinctions between controlled and automatic processes, which help him delimit the processes likely to be involved in developmental language disorders.

The time lag between new models and applications to other questions is eliminated when people work collaboratively or cross domains. For example, Baddeley's model of working memory with separate visuospatial and articulatory loops seems promising in his laboratory work with normal subjects, and he is quickly testing it in clinical populations. Similarly, Mandler has applied his distinction between conscious and unconscious memory processes to clinical neuropsychological populations. Such integrative and collaborative work across domains allows the line between model building and application to blur, as insights from applications shape the models.

One attractive aspect of a symposia such as the G. Stanley Hall meeting is that there is an exchange of information concerning current models of memory. Thus, researchers in other domains have information needed to develop tests in their areas that might evaluate the more current models.

Testing Memory Models in New Domains

Several chapters in this book represent attempts to examine directly the structure and function of memory in different domains. Chapter 7 by Nelson, for example, looks at the concept of distinctions between types of memory (autobiographical and semantic memory) through development. Nelson's research meshes nicely with Neisser's (Chapter 4). Neisser argues that such memoria are fundamental to an understanding of mature memory. The implication that autobiographical memory may follow a separate developmental course than semantic memory offers some support for Neisser's claim that it may involve a separate memory system.

Rovee-Collier (Chapter 8) also provides developmental evidence concerning traditional thinking about memory processes. Her evidence concerning the presence of context effects in infant memory may challenge some currently held beliefs that infantile amnesia results from the development of qualitatively different memory structure and function. Indeed, Nelson and Neisser present thinking that is in part inconsistent with some of the data reported by Rovee-Collier. This seems to be a fruitful exchange and offers some glimmer of real integration. Both domains are providing evidence concerning the utility of distinctions between forms of memory.

The neuropsychological contributions also provide rich evidence of the potential exchange between cognitive models and the possible neurological underpinnings of such models. The main problem with this integration concerns the issue of definition of memory, as we have previously noted.

The implications of this difference in the definition of memory are important if there is to be some integration of the two areas. Much neurophysiological work assesses the utility of concepts and processes most closely associated with learning theory. Perhaps this is due to the specificity of those models that involve classical conditioning. In other words, those models tend to be quantitative enough to allow them to be translated to a physiological domain. Other phenomenon such as conscious remembering may be more complex, and may even lack an appropriate animal model. Thus the difference in phenomenon studied in these two areas may mitigate against interaction.

Points of Connection: Using Memory

One theme that recurs in this volume is emphasis on the study of memory as it is used, rather than as an isolated process. For example, the social psychologists study memory as it is used in impression formation and social judgment. Kail illustrates the use of memory in his studies of word accessibility in language-impaired children. Neisser notes a new emphasis on the everyday uses of memory and the memory demands of the environment. Baddeley focuses on the question, "What is STM used for?," in his investigation of the role of working memory in interpreting speech. This theme of the uses of memory directs investigators to tasks that are likely to capture the truly important and enduring aspects of memory. As Neisser notes, such an approach broadens the phenomenon under investigation to include what he terms new *memoria*.

Nelson (Chapter 7 in this volume) also exemplifies a functionalist approach to memory and explicitly asks: What purposes does memory serve? She answers that one critical function is to provide people with a self-history that is worked out in social interaction. Parents and other important people direct the child's encoding of events, helping to determine what will be a part of the child's history. The important role of other people for one's own memory does not end with early memory development. Ostrom (Chapter 10) also expands the "memory system" beyond the individual to include the important people who corroborate, invalidate, or even substitute for one's memory, in a form of collective memory. Thus, the social context highlights previously unconsidered uses of memory, which may provide new insights into the functioning of memory in general.

Summary

Interdisciplinary work is not an easy enterprise. It is far more straightforward to specialize narrowly and ignore research beyond one's subspecialty. G. Stanley Hall (1923) wrote admiringly of attempts by a president of Johns Hopkins to avoid "excessive specialization" among students and faculty, and noted that:

This work, although welcomed by broader minds, always encountered some opposition and more inertia. . . . Some of the professors found it irksome to summarize their technical studies in a way intelligible to cultured minds in other fields. (p. 250)

Our participants were of broader minds, rather than irksome characters, but nonetheless the task of interdisciplinary communication was not an easy one. It becomes clear that the best impetus to interdisciplinary research in memory is not the good intentions of conference organizers. Instead, the most powerful motivator appears to be a research question that yields to no other approach, and pulls the research toward interdisciplinary considerations.

References

Broadbent, D. (1985). A question of levels: Comment on McClelland and Rundhart. *Journal of Experimental Psychology: General, 114,* 189–192.
Cohen, R.L. (1985). On the generality of the laws of memory. In L.G. Nilsson & T. Archer (Eds.), *Perspectives on learning and memory.* Hillsdale, NJ: Lawrence Erlbaum Associates.
Cohen, N.J., & Squire, L.R. (1980). Preserved learning and retention of pattern-analyzing skill in amnesia: Dissociation of knowing how and knowing that. *Science, 210,* 207–210.
Hall, G.S. (1923). *Life and confessions of a psychologist.* New York: Appleton.
Hirst, W., & LeDoux, J.E. (1986). Cognitive neuroscience: Final considerations. In J.E. LeDoux & W. Hirst (Eds.), *Mind and brain: Dialogues in cognitive neuroscience.* New York: Cmabridge University Press.
Jacoby, L.L., Allan, L.G., Collins, J.C., & Larwill, L.K. (1988). Memory influences subjective experience: Noise judgments. *Journal of Experimental Psychology: Learning, Memory and Cognition, 14,* 240–247.
Jacoby, L.L., & Dallas, M. (1981). On the relationship between autobiographical memory and perceptual learning. *Journal of Experimental Psychology: General, 3,* 306–340.
Jacoby, L.L., Kelley, C.M., & Dywan, J. (in press). Memory attributions. In H.L. Roediger III & F.I.M. Craik (Eds.), *Varieties of memory and consciousness: Essays in honor of Endel Tulving.* Hillsdale, NJ: Lawrence Erlbaum Associates.
Marr, D. (1982). *Vision.* San Francisco, CA: W.H. Freeman.
Massaro, D.W. (1986). The computer as a metaphor for psychological inquiry: Considerations and recommendations. *Behavior Research, Methods, Instruments and Computers, 18,* 73–92.
Pribram, K.H. (1986). The cognitive revolution and mind/brain issues. *American Psychologist, 41,* 507–520.
Rumelhart, D.E., & McClelland, J.L. (1985). Levels indeed! A response to Broadbent. *Journal of Experimental Psychology: General, 114,* 193–197.
Schachter, S., & Singer, J. (1962). Cognitive, social, and physiological determinants of emotional state. *Psychological Review, 69,* 379–399.
Shallice, T. (1979). Neuropsychological research and the fractionation of memory

systems. In L.G. Nilsson (Ed.), *Perspectives on memory research*. Hillsdale, NJ: Lawrence Erlbaum Associates.

Tulving, E. (1983). *Elements of episodic memory*. New York: Oxford University Press.

Warrington, E.K., & Weiskrantz, L. (1982). Amnesia: A disconnection syndrome? *Neuropsychologia, 20*, 233–248.

Weiskrantz, L., & Warrington, E.K. (1979). Conditioning in amnesic patients. *Neuropsychologia, 17*, 187–194.

Witherspoon, D., & Allan, L.G. (1985). The effects of a prior presentation on temporal judgments in a perceptual identificationt task. *Memory and Cognition, 13*, 101–111.

Author Index

Subject Index